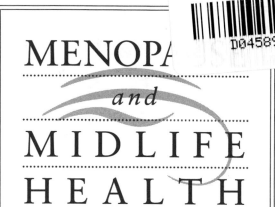

MENOPA
and
MIDLIFE
HEALTH

Also by Morris Notelovitz, M.D., Ph.D. (with Marsha Ware)

Stand Tall! The Informed Woman's Guide to Preventing Osteoporosis

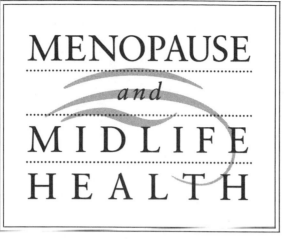

MENOPAUSE *and* MIDLIFE HEALTH

Morris Notelovitz, M.D., Ph.D.

Diana Tonnessen

Illustrations by
Aher/Donnell Studios

Chart graphics by
Douglas Reinke

St. Martin's Press
New York

Design by Robin Hessel Hoffman

Library of Congress Cataloging-in-Publication Data

Notelovitz, Morris.
   Menopause and midlife health / Morris Notelovitz and Diana
Tonnessen.
      p. cm.
  ISBN 0-312-09337-3
  1. Menopause—Popular works. 2. Middle aged women—Health and
hygiene. I. Tonnessen, Diana. II. Title.
RG186.N68 1993
618.1′75—dc20   93-679
                                           CIP

10 9 8 7 6 5 4 3 2

To climacteric medicine and the patients who
helped formulate the concept.—M.N.

To the women in my family and in my
extended family of friends.—D.T.

And to the well-being of all women
in their prime years.—M.N. and D.T.

Contents

....

Acknowledgments

·······································

A work of this size and scope is a culmination of a lifetime of research and clinical experience on the part of the physician, and of years of writing and editing on the part of the writer. We are deeply indebted to our families, educators, professional colleagues, patients, and personal friends who helped shape our lives and our careers over the years.

We wish to extend a special thanks to Farouk Khan, M.D., for his willing assistance; to registered dietitian Kathryn Parker for contributing some of her painstakingly assembled low-fat menus and for sharing her "slim-trim" weight-loss program; to physical therapist Vibeke Vala for sharing her expertise on exercises and good body mechanics for women with osteoporosis; to Alex Macgregor, M.D., for reviewing the surgery section of the chapter on obesity; to Michael Pollock, Ph.D., and Jay Graves, Ph.D., for their many contributions to the sections on measuring body composition and the chapter on exercise; to Ann Voda, Ph.D., for generously offering suggestions on how to cope with hot flashes; to Ruth Mooney, M.D., for explaining how to assess the strength of the pelvic-floor muscles; to Betsey Neis for making countless trips to the library and for the tedious job of compiling the data for many of the tables and charts in the book; to the staff of the Women's Medical and Diagnostic Center and the Climacteric Clinic; and, finally, to the patients who allowed us use of their records and who graciously shared with us and with you their feelings and experiences.

We would also like to thank the following important people in our lives.

From Morris Notelovitz: To my wife, Beryl, whose selfless dedication freed me to pursue my interest in climacteric medicine and menopause-related research; to my children Selwyn, Sandra, and Gillian, who sacrificed decades of "togetherness time"; and to my scientific colleagues and coworkers, who shared their time, ideas, and clinical experience with me.

From Diana Tonnessen: Many thanks to my agent, Barbara Lowenstein, for getting us together and for knowing whom to have lunch with; to Ted Burt,

Barbara Cox, Bonnie Prescott, Diana Reese, and especially to Josleen Wilson for their guidance and professional hand-holding; to Pauline Cowart, Evelyn Tanner, and especially to Norma Morales for providing hours of worry-free child care while I worked; to Darcy Meeker for giving me a leg up as a fledgling science writer; to my parents, who taught me the self-discipline I needed to complete such a project; to my children, Casey and Vijay, for putting up with a part-time mom; and to my husband, Pradeep Kumar, for the untold ways in which he has lent his support.

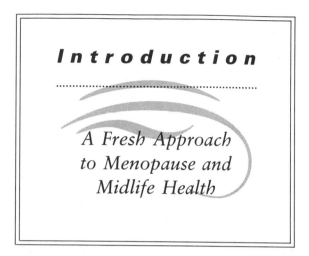

Introduction

A Fresh Approach to Menopause and Midlife Health

Perhaps you've already felt the subtle stirrings of change within you. Indeed, by the time you turn thirty, your body has already begun preparing for one of the most monumental physical changes of your life: menopause.

Few other biological milestones will have as great an impact on your health as your final menstrual period. Levels of the reproductive hormones estrogen and progesterone start to decline some fifteen years before you feel your first hot flash, and they influence numerous tissues in your body. As a result, everything from your hair and skin to your heart and bones will be affected by your menopause.

The health consequences of these hormonal changes range from the annoying symptoms of premenstrual syndrome (PMS) in your thirties and forties to such life-threatening illnesses as heart disease and osteoporosis in your later years. What's more, these menopause-related changes occur at a time when aging naturally increases your risk of other chronic and potentially terminal illnesses such as diabetes and cancer.

If you're beginning to think that, as far as your physical health is concerned, your menopause is a major midlife crisis, relax. New research shows that most of these disease risks can be easily managed—many of them simply by taking preventive measures in your middle years. Ideally, you should start preparing for menopause in your late twenties and early thirties. But it's never too late to begin. Whether you're thirtysomething, fortyish, fifty-plus, or over sixty, there's a tremendous amount you can do—right now—to make your middle years more comfortable and to increase the length and, perhaps more important, the *quality* of your later years.

Few women realize how far-reaching their menopause is or that they can exercise any control over it. Indeed, the real crisis for the 53 million American women over thirty today may not be menopause so much as a shortage of information about how to manage its long-term effects on their health. When in 1980 we opened the Center for Climacteric Studies at the University of Florida—the nation's first research center devoted entirely to women in mid-life—we were astounded by the lack of medical research that had been conducted on women ages thirty to sixty-five. Hundreds of thousands of studies had been done on women of childbearing age. A growing body of research dealt with the debilitating illnesses of women over age sixty-five. But we found only a handful of studies on midlife health. In effect, we knew virtually nothing about women's health needs during one of the most critical times of their lives—the middle years.

This shortage of information was rivaled only by an abundance of misinformation perpetuated by generations of mothers, the media, and sometimes by physicians. One woman who participated in a study at our center, for instance, thought menopause was a disease caused by a shortage of hormones. Another related that her mother, who had suffered a miserable menopause, told her to prepare for the worst. "I kept bracing myself for the beginning of the end," she said. "But the end never came. After my menopause, I felt better than ever."

In addition, we found many of these women voicing legitimate concerns that, until recently, had been brushed off as "all in your head." One thirty-six-year-old nursing student who was suffering from a severe estrogen deficiency after having her ovaries removed recalls, "I felt like a jigsaw puzzle with several major pieces missing. I kept looking for other reasons for why I felt this way, like pressures at school."

Clearly, we had our work cut out for us. Our objective at the center was to find out as much as we could about menopause and its long-term effects on a woman's health and to find ways to meet the health needs of women in the middle years. This involved, first of all, recognizing that menopause is not a disease but a natural part of aging—a fact of life, much like the onset of menstruation at puberty. And while menopause is a single event (the final menstrual period) that occurs around age fifty, the process leading up to it begins some fifteen years earlier—usually in your early thirties. Physical changes continue for at least another fifteen years after menopause, until about age sixty-five. The entire spectrum of changes can be broken down into three stages: the *premenopausal* (ages thirty to forty-five), *perimenopausal* (ages forty-five to fifty-five), and *postmenopausal* (ages fifty-five and over) years. The medical term for this time in a woman's life—what most of us refer to as midlife—is called the *climacteric*. When we talk about menopause, we usually mean the myriad changes that take place during the thirty to thirty-five years of the climacteric and the health needs that arise as a result.

We also realized early on that menopause was much more than a hormone deficiency to be treated with hormone therapy. Our research revealed that nutrition and exercise can have a tremendous influence on your health and well-being throughout the second half of your life. For instance, studies have shown that lacto-ovo vegetarian women, who consume dairy products and eggs but no meat, have more bone mass—and therefore are at a lower risk of developing the bone-thinning disorder osteoporosis after menopause—than meat eaters.

In the course of our research, we also discovered that we could no longer ignore the emotional needs of women in the middle years. The physical changes associated with menopause, such as premenstrual syndrome and hot flashes, can have a tremendous influence on a woman's emotional health. What's more, menopause often occurs at the same time a woman experiences changes at work (a promotion or retirement from her job, for example) and at home (loss of her spouse through divorce or death). Of course, few researchers recognized until recently that menopause can also have a *positive* effect on a woman's emotional well-being. For instance, many postmenopausal women are relieved that they don't have to worry about birth control anymore.

After five years of research involving thousands of women at the center, one fact became painfully clear to us: The health needs of women in midlife extend far beyond the standard pelvic exam and Pap smear. For this reason, we decided to put our medical findings to work in a clinical setting. In 1986, we opened the Women's Medical and Diagnostic Center and Climacteric Clinic in Gainesville, Florida, where we began practicing a new kind of medical care: *climacteric medicine*. The concept is based on our research and clinical experience involving nearly 11,000 women. Although the name sounds complicated, the principles are simple: Climacteric medicine takes an integrated approach to health care, considering the woman as a whole (including her lifestyle and environment) and not just her reproductive parts.

There are only a handful of other centers like ours in the country, so, until recently, climacteric medicine has been available only to the women who lived closest to us. Our goal in writing this book has been to make the knowledge gained at our research center and clinic available to all women, no matter where they live. In the following pages, you'll find the most up-to-date, medically sound information you need to prepare for a comfortable menopause and healthy postmenopausal years. Part I gives you a thorough understanding of aging and menopause and the impact they have on your health. In Part II, you'll learn the principles of climacteric medicine and will find practical advice on how to apply the concepts to your everyday life.

You'll also find troubleshooting sections in Parts III and IV that deal with specific problems you may face as you journey through midlife: contraception, midlife pregnancy, premenstrual syndrome, menopause, heart disease, osteoporosis, and cancer, to name a few. Finally, in Part V you'll find the latest scientific data on hormone therapy's benefits and risks to help you make an informed decision about whether to take postmenopausal hormones.

This book was written for you. But the best health care comes when you and your doctor work together as a team. Read the book, discuss the concepts described here with your doctor, and start now to make your middle and later years the best years of your life.

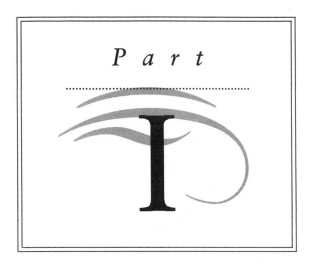

Part

I

Reaching
Your Prime

```
┌─────────────────────────────────────┐
│                                     │
│     C h a p t e r   1               │
│     ..............................  │
│                                     │
│     The Misunderstood               │
│       Middle Years:                 │
│      No More Myths                  │
│                                     │
└─────────────────────────────────────┘
```

Congratulations! You've made it to the middle years—your prime years. By now, you've probably managed to resolve many of the uncertainties of young adulthood. You've most likely established yourself in your job or career. You've probably achieved some measure of financial security. And if your children aren't already almost full-grown, you have likely started your family. In many ways, the middle years have earned the name "prime of life." So why do so many women still worry about those birthdays ending in zero?

Old myths die hard, and the middle years have more than their share of misunderstandings: the so-called midlife crisis; the ticking of your biological clock; the "empty nest" syndrome, and, perhaps the biggest of all for women to contend with, menopause. In terms of scientific research, the middle years are largely uncharted territory. While the scientific community has conducted a tremendous amount of research on other stages in the human life cycle—infancy, childhood, adolescence, and old age—it has not focused on the physical and mental health issues of the middle years—until now.

As the first of the 72 million baby boomers enter midlife, more and more experts are turning their attention to the middle years. And they're finding that many of our long-held grudges against middle age are largely the result of myth. Indeed, these may well be some of the best years of your life. Let's take a look at a few of the myths behind some of your most common midlife concerns.

"I haven't gone through a midlife crisis—yet. But I've often stepped back and tried to reassess what I'm doing and where it's leading. I'm probably more than halfway through my life . . . have I accomplished what I thought I would?"

It's not unusual to step back periodically and reflect on where you've been and where you're going with your life. And the middle years seem to be a prime time for this kind of introspection. However, the major identity crisis that most

3

of us have come to expect—the so-called midlife crisis—may never be a part of your middle years. Mounting evidence now suggests that, for most people, the transition into middle age is not nearly so traumatic as it has been made out to be.

Susan Krauss Whitbourne, Ph.D., a psychologist at the University of Massachusetts in Amherst, recently interviewed ninety-four men and women over age twenty-four and found that none in their forties had experienced anything that qualified as a real midlife crisis. Rather, she found that identity crises can happen to anyone at any age.

And a fifteen-year study of seven hundred men and women by University of Chicago psychologist Bernice Neugarten, Ph.D., also turned up little evidence of a predictable midlife crisis. She found that as adults enter middle age, they become more introspective and think more about issues having to do with family roles, work, and "generativity" (the idea of "making your mark," or "leaving something behind for posterity"). But this kind of introspection does not generally lead to a major life crisis.

Dr. Neugarten points out that expected life events—leaving home, marriage, parenthood, career achievements, having your own children leave home, the menopause—are "normal turning points, punctuation marks along the life line." These anticipated events aren't life crises for most men and women. Rather, it's the unexpected turn of events—the early death of a parent or a car accident, for example—that is more likely to trigger a psychological crisis.

A growing number of researchers now feel that most people *don't* have a midlife crisis. They point out that a crisis can occur at any age, and that, typically, the people who have a life crisis during the middle years have experienced crises all their lives. They simply label the one in their forties a "midlife crisis."

"I've heard so many horror stories about women who lost all interest in sex after menopause. Is it true that after age fifty your sex life is basically over?"

Nothing could be further from the truth. Although both men and women experience a decline in sexual responsiveness as they grow older, there's no physiological reason why you can't continue to enjoy sex throughout the middle years and well into your later years.

On the other hand, sexual problems can arise at any time during your life (remember the first time you had sex?). And some problems crop up more frequently in the middle and later years. But most are minor and can be fairly easily resolved. A key is to keep the lines of communication open with your partner *and* your physician. It's essential, too, that you speak up *before* minor problems turn into major headaches.

For many couples, a frank discussion with your physician may reveal a physical problem that's as easy to resolve as writing a prescription. Others may find a few sessions with a sex counselor enormously helpful. (We'll review some of the more common sexual problems—and their solutions—in Chapter 14.)

"I'm forty-two and have finally decided I'd like to start a family. But I'm worried that my biological clock is about to run out. And isn't pregnancy this late in the game a little risky?"

If you've postponed starting your family until after age thirty-five, you're in good company. Between 1978 and 1988, the number of women ages thirty to forty-four giving birth to their first child rose by 50 percent.

You should be aware that as you grow older, your fertility *does* decline somewhat and it may take you a little longer to conceive. So don't expect to get pregnant on your first try. If infertility is a problem, keep in mind that in the last ten years, the process of conceiving a child has gone high-tech; often with a little patience and perseverance, even complicated cases of infertility can be overcome.

Yes, pregnancy in midlife *is* more risky to mother and baby. Fortunately, early prenatal tests, such as ultrasound, amniocentesis, and chorionic villus sampling, are helping take some of the worry out of pregnancy for those over thirty-five by allowing doctors to screen for potential birth defects early in pregnancy. Plus, we have a better understanding of the importance of nutrition, exercise, and regular medical checkups, which will help you manage safely through pregnancy and deliver a healthy baby. (For details on midlife pregnancy, see Chapter 10.)

"I haven't had a period in several months. Does this mean I've experienced menopause and don't have to worry about contraception anymore?"

Don't be lulled into a false sense of security by irregular menstrual patterns. Your periods will become more irregular as you approach menopause. But as long as you're menstruating—even sporadically—you can *still* get pregnant.

Technically, you're not considered past menopause until you haven't had a period for at least one year. (However, your physician can administer a simple blood test that can also tell you whether you are menopausal. See page 36.) Until this time, it is essential that you use some type of contraception to protect against pregnancy.

Fortunately, your contraceptive choices have broadened—even the newer, low-dose birth-control pills are considered safe for women over forty. (We'll discuss the pros and cons of various contraceptive methods in Chapter 9.)

"When I started having hot flashes, I kept bracing myself for the beginning of the end. But the end never came. After my menopause, I felt great!"

Even a generation or two ago, the end of your reproductive years had come to symbolize the end of the most productive years of your life. However, most women today recognize that menopause isn't the beginning of the end. For many women, it's the beginning of some of the best years of their lives.

New research is finally dispelling some of the most common and stubborn myths about menopause. Our research clinic was among the first to show that women don't simply "fall apart at the seams" after menopause. With funding from the National Institute on Aging, we recruited 145 women ages thirty-six to seventy-five to investigate the emotional *and* physical effects of menopause and aging on women in midlife. To see whether there might be a correlation between any psychological changes and biological ones, we checked the womens' blood levels of various reproductive hormones, including estrogen, progesterone, and the "male" hormone testosterone. We then asked the women to judge themselves on their levels of stress, depression, life satisfaction, and self-esteem. In addition, we administered a standardized test for a more objective measure of how psychologically well adjusted the women were. Finally, to get a general idea of social and personal issues that may affect women at the time of menopause, we asked study participants to name the happiest, saddest, and most important occurrences during the previous year.

Contrary to the belief that menopause causes depression, we found no increased incidence of depression among the older women in our study. What's more, only a minority of women experienced a drop in their overall sense of well-being that could be correlated to a menopause-related drop in hormones. Surprisingly, the hormone responsible was not estrogen or progesterone, but testosterone. This finding supports clinical observations and a few preliminary studies showing that postmenopausal women who take testosterone experience a definite feeling of well-being.

As for handling stress, while the source of stress changed over time, we found no age- or menopause-related differences in the women's ability to cope with stress.

And contrary to the belief that menopausal women regret losing their ability to bear children, none of the postmenopausal women in our study mentioned menopause or the end of their childbearing years as a significant change in their lives. What's more, the frequent comments these women made relating to their children rarely had to do with children leaving home. So much for the "empty nest" syndrome!

Other studies now support our preliminary findings. An ongoing survey of 2,300 healthy middle-aged women by Sonja McKinlay, Ph.D., and John McKinlay, M.D., at the New England Research Institute in Watertown, Massachusetts, also found that menopause has no significant effect on depression. About 10 percent of the women said they experience occasional depression—a similar rate of depression found in the general population.

The McKinlays' study also supports our findings that not all changes resulting from menopause are perceived as negative. Seventy percent of the women reported they felt relief or neutral feelings about the cessation of menstruation. And the biggest source of frustration for menopausal women was *not* having their children leave home but *having their grown children return to the roost.*

Other researchers point out that there are numerous positive counterbalances at this time in a woman's life: the arrival of grandchildren, freedom from unwanted pregnancy, and the chance to pursue other activities, such as finishing an education or reentering the work force.

For a majority of women, menopause will mark the beginning of the best years of their lives. Nevertheless, the middle years *are* a time of transition. And menopause is just one of many life changes you may contend with in the middle years. To cope with the stress that often accompanies change, it's wise to learn all you can about some of the physical changes your body is going through. (Some studies have shown that better-educated women experience less severe menopausal symptoms.) Let's take a look now at exactly what happens when you experience menopause, and at its long-term implications for your health.

Chapter 2

The Facts
About Menopause
and Aging

There's really nothing mythical about menopause. It's simply a biological milestone marking the end of your reproductive years—just as your *menarche* (start of menstruation) marked the beginning.

Technically, menopause lasts about a week—the week of your final menstrual period. But menopause is actually a culmination of changes in your ovaries that begin as early as your mid- to late thirties. Changes continue for up to fifteen years after menopause. To understand what happens during menopause, it helps to know something about your reproductive system and menstrual cycle.

Your Reproductive System

Your reproductive system—ovaries, Fallopian tubes, uterus, and vagina (see Figure 2.1)—begins to form just seven or eight weeks after conception. By the time you are a seven-month-old fetus, your developing ovaries contain some 6 to 7 million eggs—a lifetime supply.

Throughout your life, the number of eggs diminishes as they fail to develop and are reabsorbed back into the ovaries. By the time you are born, the number of eggs in your ovaries has already been reduced to about 2 million. At puberty, your ovaries contain just 300,000 eggs, each surrounded by a casing of cells called a *follicle*.

During your childbearing years, only about 450 eggs will reach maturity and travel through the Fallopian tubes, where they can be fertilized by sperm. The rest slowly disintegrate. By the time you reach menopause, only about three thousand ova remain.

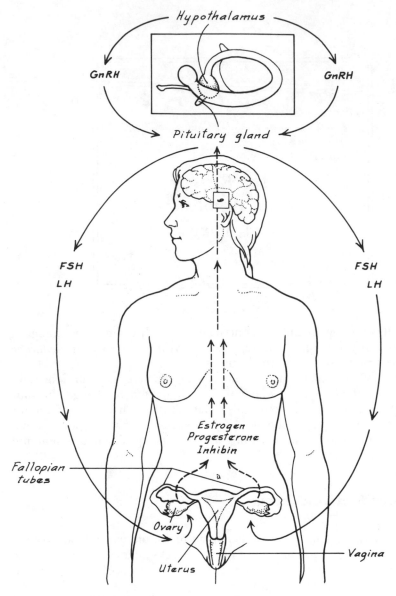

Figure 2.1   Female Reproductive System

How Your Menstrual Cycle Works:
The Interplay of Hormones

Your menstrual cycles are governed by hormones, chemical messengers that circulate throughout your bloodstream. Menstruation is initially triggered by hormones released from the *hypothalamus* years before you begin menstruating. The hypothalamus is the part of the brain that controls the endocrine (glandular) system and other bodily functions. Around the time of puberty, the hypothalamus begins releasing *gonadotropin-releasing hormone* (GnRH). Eventually, the hypothalamus produces enough GnRH to signal the pituitary gland to churn out *follicle-stimulating hormone* (FSH) and *luteinizing hormone* (LH). These two hormones communicate with your ovaries and help orchestrate your menstrual cycles.

In the first phase of your menstrual cycle, the *proliferative phase,* your pituitary releases more FSH than LH. When FSH reaches your ovaries, it stimulates several eggs in the ovaries to grow and mature. The follicles surrounding the eggs absorb fluid and swell as they work their way to the surface of the ovary. Only one egg will grow sufficiently to ripen and be released from one of your ovaries. The others will slowly disintegrate.

As the follicles mature, they begin producing two types of *estrogen: estradiol,* the more potent of the two, and *estrone.* These are very powerful hormones that stimulate the growth of specific cells in your body. Rising estrogen levels around the time of menarche are responsible for the growth and maturation of your reproductive organs and your breasts. Estrogen also causes you to start storing fat in your buttocks and thighs. Estrogen stimulates bone growth and is largely responsible for the growth spurt associated with puberty. During each menstrual cycle, estrogen stimulates the cells lining your uterus (the *endometrium*) to grow and thicken, helping to prepare the uterus for pregnancy.

In the middle of your menstrual cycle, a surge of luteinizing hormone is released from the pituitary gland. It's not certain what signals the pituitary suddenly to secrete large amounts of LH, although it is suspected that rising levels of estrogen in the first phase of the cycle play a role. At any rate, the surge of LH causes rapid swelling of the follicle. It also causes the wall of the follicle to weaken. Eventually, the follicle ruptures and the ovum is released into your abdominal cavity—this is what is known as *ovulation.* The tiny hairs (or *cilia*) at the opening of the Fallopian tubes almost always draw the egg into the tube, where it can be fertilized.

In the second, or *luteal* phase of the menstrual cycle, the cells lining the space once occupied by the egg form the *corpus luteum.* Beginning just a few hours after ovulation, this mass of yellow cells secretes small amounts of estrogen and large amounts of progesterone, which further help thicken the uterine lining. The corpus luteum also produces *inhibin.* This hormone, along with estrogen and progesterone, signals the pituitary to stop secreting FSH and LH. As a result, both FSH and LH in the blood fall to very low levels.

The corpus luteum depends on FSH and LH to sustain it, and the low levels of FSH and LH cause the corpus luteum to degenerate. When this happens—about two days before menstruation—estrogen, progesterone, and inhibin levels fall. The sudden drop in estrogen and progesterone, in turn, causes the endometrial lining to degenerate. A day or two later, the uterine lining is shed from the walls of the uterus and you begin menstruating.

In the meantime, the pituitary gland, without estrogen, progesterone, and inhibin to suppress it, once again starts to secrete FSH and LH, stimulating more follicles and beginning the cycle all over again. The whole process takes about twenty-eight days. But a "normal" cycle can range from twenty-one to thirty-five days.

The Effect of Aging on Your Menstrual Cycle

By your mid- to late thirties, the number of follicles in your ovaries has gradually declined. At about the same time, the remaining follicles become less responsive to FSH and LH. As a result of these changes, your ovaries produce less and less of the reproductive hormones estrogen and progesterone. A typical pattern: Levels of estradiol begin to fall first, resulting in a gradual shortening of the luteal (second) phase of the menstrual cycle. This is followed by a drop in progesterone, which increases the overall length of the cycle and often results in heavier periods. In response to these changes, the pituitary secretes higher levels of FSH and LH to stimulate the ovaries.

You may not notice any difference in your menstrual cycles at first. But anywhere from two to eight years before menopause, your menstrual flow may change, becoming heavier one month and lighter the next. Your menstrual cycles themselves may become more erratic. You may even skip periods altogether.

Eventually (around age fifty-one for the average American woman), the levels of estrogen and progesterone produced by the ovaries drop so low that you stop menstruating altogether. You (and your physician) will know you've experienced menopause when you start having menopausal symptoms, such as hot flashes, or when you haven't had a period for twelve or more consecutive months. A blood test showing elevated FSH levels can also help your physician determine whether you are menopausal.

Postmenopausal Hormone Levels

Although it may seem that your ovaries have completely shut down after menopause, they still produce small amounts of estrogen (see Table 2.1, especially the columns for estrone and estradiol). What's more, your ovaries continue to produce substantial amounts of the "male" androgens (testosterone and androstenedione) after menopause, some of which are converted to estrogen by body fat. Most of the estrogen circulating in your bloodstream after menopause comes from these androgens. Your adrenal glands also produce minute amounts of estrogen.

The predominant type of estrogen changes after menopause, too. Premenopausal women have higher levels of estradiol, produced by the ovaries. After menopause, estrone is the principal type of estrogen circulating in your bloodstream.

On the other hand, since you've stopped ovulating and no corpus luteum is formed, your ovaries produce virtually no progesterone or inhibin.

Menopause and Aging: What's The Connection?

The chief role of estrogen and progesterone is to help regulate your menstrual cycle and prepare your uterus for pregnancy. But like all hormones, these chemical messengers circulate throughout your body, interacting with other

TABLE 2.1 *Pre- and Postmenopausal Hormone Levels*

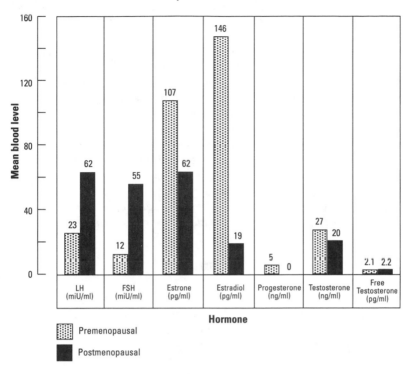

hormones and with your body's metabolism. Estrogen *receptors*—specialized parts of cells that allow various hormones to lock into the cell and influence its activity—have been found in many tissues throughout the body, including the mucous membranes, the urethra, breasts, bones, skin, and even the lung and coronary arteries (which supply the heart muscle with nutrients and oxygen). So you can see how your menopause can have a major impact on your health, your looks, and your sense of well-being.

Menopause also occurs at a time when your body is already undergoing various other changes related to normal aging, a process that has been ongoing from the moment you were born. Of course, as you've already seen, menopause *is* one of the changes of aging—the aging of your reproductive organs. Still, it's important to make a distinction between normal aging and menopause, because menopause can *accelerate* the natural aging process of certain organs (notably your cardiovascular system and bones).

What do we mean by "normal" aging? Surprisingly, the science of aging is still fairly young, and researchers are still puzzling over exactly how the aging process unfolds. However, we do have a pretty good handle on what happens to your body as you age. Generally, your body's organ systems (including your bones, heart, brain, and other vital organs) grow and mature from birth until they reach a peak around age thirty. After that time, bodily functions begin to decline, and the biological changes we associate with aging, such as skin wrinkling, middle-age spread, stiff joints, and "brittle" bones, become more problematic. Most of these changes occur gradually over time and are

11

barely noticeable from day to day or even from year to year. In fact, it often takes ten years or more before you'll see a measurable difference in many of the physical changes associated with aging. (Perhaps this is why we dread those birthdays ending in zero!)

How "well" you age is also influenced by your environment and just about everything that happens to you from the moment you're born. Heredity, diet, hormones, physical activity, stress, injury, disease, and drugs—all have some effect on the aging process. In fact, we're now discovering that many of the changes we chalked up to "normal" aging are more often a result of environmental assaults and poor lifestyle habits. For instance, up to 90 percent of skin wrinkling, one of the most visible signs of aging, is now known to be a result of excessive sun exposure and cigarette smoking, *not* normal aging.

Other so-called changes of aging, such as joint stiffness, muscle weakness, and even middle-age spread, also appear to be related more to behavior than biology. So in effect, *by taking good care of yourself, particularly in the middle years, you can slow—and sometimes even reverse—many of the most common changes of aging.*

The Aging Process: What's Normal, What's Not

Much of what we know about how the body ages is based on studies of large numbers of healthy adults, from which scientists describe the "normal" aging patterns of "average" adults. But how normal is normal?

The studies themselves are conducted either by tracking changes in a single group of volunteers as they age (*longitudinal* studies) or by comparing groups of people of different ages (*cross-sectional* studies). Cross-sectional studies are much cheaper and easier to perform, since they don't involve keeping tabs on a large number of people over the course of several decades or more. One shortcoming of cross-sectional studies, however, is that they don't account for differences in lifestyle habits over the generations. For example, a seventy-year-old woman, born a full half century earlier than a twenty-year-old, probably had quite a different diet from the younger woman, and the nutritional status of both women affects the way they age.

Comparing various age-related changes between cultures can also be an eye-opener. For example, normal blood-cholesterol levels in the United States, where heart disease is the leading cause of death, are 205 milligrams per deciliter (mg/dl) of blood. In Japan, however, where heart disease rarely develops, average blood-cholesterol levels are between 125 and 165 mg/dl. Which is more normal?

Likewise, charts that describe "average" bone mass for women in the United States are based on studies that include women who have lived sedentary lives. Yet exercise increases bone mass; if the studies were based on groups of women who have been active all their lives, "normal" values would undoubtedly be much higher than what they are now.

The good news is that most women today are healthier than ever before. On the whole, they're more physically active and better nourished than their mothers and grandmothers, and this is bound have a positive effect on the way they age.

TABLE 2.2 *How Menopause Affects Blood-Cholesterol Levels*

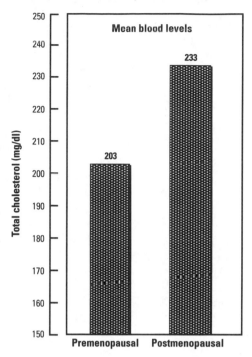

Because menopause occurs around the same time that gray hairs and wrinkles begin to appear, it has often been implicated in causing these and other aging changes. With a few notable exceptions, however, menopause has no perceptible effect on aging. In our study, supported by a grant from the National Institute on Aging, we documented that menopause per se has no significant effect on blood pressure. Rather, the gradual rise in blood pressure as you grow older appears to be a part of the normal aging process. We also found that menopause has no effect on your ability to become (or stay) physically fit.

On the other hand, estrogen does have a potent effect on blood cholesterol and bone. Lower estrogen levels after menopause often raise blood-cholesterol levels, which appears to be one reason why the risk of developing heart disease rises after menopause (see Table 2.2). (Estrogen may protect your heart in other ways, too. See Chapter 16.) Estrogen also has a protective effect on bone, and the drop in estrogen after menopause accelerates bone loss, which increases your risk of developing the bone-thinning disorder osteoporosis (See Table 2.3). As you'll see in the chapters to come, however, even these menopause-related changes can be offset by making healthy changes in your lifestyle now and, if necessary, by taking postmenopausal hormones.

We still don't know what effect, if any, the drop in estrogen associated with menopause has on your risk of developing breast cancer. The breasts themselves do shrink in size when estrogen levels fall after menopause. The *alveoli*, the tiny sacs where breast milk is made and stored, begin to disappear, and the milk ducts leading out of the breast decrease in number, as well. But

	What to expect	What you can do
Brain and Central Nervous System	Slower reflexes and reaction time. (Note: Senility, or gross memory loss, is a disease and *not* a part of normal aging.)	Exercise, during which your central nervous system coordinates the movement of your muscles and improves reflexes and reaction time. Exercise also increases blood flow to the brain. Certain nutrients may also affect mood and behavior (see page 67).
Skin	Connective tissues *collagen* and *elastin*, which maintain skin tone, become less elastic; collagen production declines, resulting in wrinkles.	Avoid excessive sun exposure and cigarette smoking, both of which accelerate these changes.
Cardiovascular System	Gradual narrowing of arteries, decreased pumping efficiency of heart; less blood flow to major organs; gradual rise in blood pressure, blood cholesterol, and other fats (*lipids*) in the blood.	Exercise lowers blood pressure, increases efficiency of heart. A diet low in fat, cholesterol, and sodium and high in antioxidants can help offset age-related rises in blood pressure and blood cholesterol. Avoid cigarette smoking, which raises heart-disease risks in several ways.
Immune System	Produces fewer antibodies, more autoantibodies. May increase the risk of infections, cancer, and autoimmune diseases.	Muscle-strengthening exercises may boost immunity (see page 102). Avoid chronic stress, which may depress immunity.
Digestive System	Calcium absorption declines, possibly contributing to bone loss; colon wall weakens, increasing the likelihood of constipation.	Increase calcium intake; increase intake of high-fiber foods; drink plenty of fluids; exercise.

Metabolism	Basal metabolic rate (amount of calories you burn at rest) declines, possibly contributing to weight gain as you grow older.	Exercise raises metabolism by increasing (or maintaining) muscle mass, decreasing body fat.
Reproductive System	Ovaries' production of estrogen and progesterone declines, leading to hot flashes, vaginal dryness, and other symptoms. Lower levels of reproductive hormones also change cholesterol levels and accelerate bone loss.	Menopausal symptoms can be managed with various nondrug and drug treatments (see page 244), including postmenopausal hormone therapy. Rise in risk of heart disease and osteoporosis can be reduced with proper diet, exercise, and other lifestyle changes; postmenopausal hormone therapy may provide added protection for women who need it.
Bones, Muscles, Joints	Breakdown of old bone begins to out-pace formation of new bone, resulting in a loss of bone mass and gradual weakening of bones. Muscle mass declines, resulting in a loss of muscle strength and tone. Lost muscle is replaced by less-metabolically active fat. Connective tissues in joints become less elastic, leading to stiffer joints, decreased flexibility.	Exercise builds bone and can slow or reverse age-related decline in bone mass. Muscle-strengthening exercises can offset loss of muscle mass and strength associated with aging. Flexibility exercises can relieve joint stiffness, increasing range of motion of joints. A sensible, calorie-restricted diet along with exercise can help control increases in body fat.
Senses (hearing, vision)	Changes in the lens of the eye make it less flexible, less able to shift focus quickly from near to far, resulting in *presbyopia*, or far-sightedness. Changes in the ear cause a gradual decline in hearing, particularly in the ability to distinguish high-pitched sounds.	Have vision and hearing tested annually. Corrective eyewear and hearing aids are readily available for these nuisance changes.

TABLE 2.3 *How Menopause Affects Bone Density*

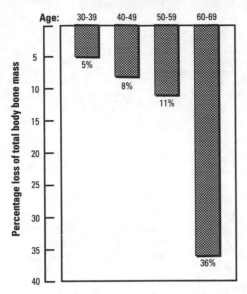

since hormones *and* aging play a role in the development of many kinds of breast cancer, it's hard to tell what impact these menopause-related changes have on your risk for developing this disease. It would seem that your risk of developing estrogen-dependent cancers of the breast would be reduced after menopause. But statistics show that the number of estrogen-dependent cancers increases steadily until ages sixty to seventy-four—some ten to fifteen years after estrogen levels fall. And for reasons that aren't clear yet, breast cancer is far more prevalent in women over fifty. There's still a lot you can do to protect yourself from breast cancer, however. (See Chapter 18.)

Climacteric Medicine: The Promise of Prevention

Few of us relish the prospect of growing older. But it's a fact of life. Indeed, thanks to better health care and medical advances, women today can expect to live longer than women of any previous generation. The average life expectancy in the United States has reached seventy-five years. And for reasons not yet known, women can expect to live an average of seven years longer than men. *Women who reach age sixty-five today can expect to live another 18.6 years.*

It would be wonderful—but not probable—for all of us to live *beyond* the human life span—the biological limit to human life (roughly ninety to one hundred years). You can increase your chances of reaching this milestone by starting *now* to take the precautions that research scientists tell us will improve the quality of our later years. Doing so is particularly important when you consider the fact that for many women today, the later years are an age of disability and dependence. Older women are prone to suffer from chronic, often life-threatening illnesses—such as heart disease, cancer, arthritis, and osteoporosis—that are more likely to be debilitating and to require long-term care. Women are also the primary users of long-term care, including in-home services, adult day care, care in resident facilities, convalescent homes, and nursing homes. While just 5 percent of the elderly are institutionalized in a nursing home at any given time, nearly 75 percent of them are women.

Many baby boomers who joined the health and fitness craze of the last twenty years are ahead of the game already. These women will probably be healthier, more energetic, and more independent as seniors than any prior generation. In fact, as this generation of women grows older, they may redefine many of our ideas about what constitutes "normal" aging—for the better.

If you haven't already become more health-conscious, it's not too late to begin. If you begin exercising and eating a low-fat, low-cholesterol diet right now, in two years you can have stronger bones and cleaner arteries. If you quit smoking now, your cancer risks will return to normal within eight to ten years.

In Part II, you'll find a complete program of prevention that we developed specifically for women in their middle years, based on our own studies and the research of other experts around the country. The section begins where you should begin—with a complete physical exam designed to evaluate your special midlife health needs. In subsequent chapters, you'll learn how to reduce your risk of chronic and life-threatening diseases and keep healthy and active through diet, exercise, stress management, and more.

By following our program, we can't promise that you'll live forever. But you will dramatically increase your odds of living a fuller, healthier life well into your later years. *The worst you can do is nothing at all.*

··
Resources and Support
··

American Association of Retired Persons (AARP), 601 E Street, NW, Washington, D.C. 20049. Phone: (202) 434-2277. Provides a wide range of information on and services for issues concerning older and retired people. The AARP publishes *Modern Maturity,* a bimonthly magazine; the *AARP News Bulletin,* a monthly newspaper; and a number of books and pamphlets. Check the phone directory for a local chapter or write the national office.

American College of Obstetricians and Gynecologists, Resource Center, 409 12th St., SW, Washington, D.C. 20024. Provides free brochures on a wide range of women's health topics, including menopause and pregnancy after age thirty-five. Send a stamped self-addressed business envelope along with your request for information.

....
Suggested Reading
....

The Boston Women's Health Collective. *The New Our Bodies, Ourselves.* New York: Simon & Schuster, 1992.

Dordis, Paula Brown, Diana Laskin Siegal, and the Midlife and Older Women Book Project, in cooperation with the Boston Women's Health Collective. *Ourselves, Growing Older.* New York: Simon & Schuster, 1987.

Henig, Robin Marantz. *How a Woman Ages.* New York: Ballantine Books, 1985.

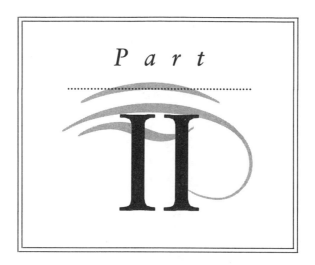

Part

II

*Staying Healthy:
An Easy-to-Follow
Program for
Your Prime Years*

Chapter 3

....

*Your Annual
Physical:
Beyond the Pelvic
and Pap*

Your prime years good health program begins with a complete physical examination. This typically includes such routine tests as blood counts, urinalysis, hearing, vision, blood pressure, a breast exam by your physician, and a pelvic exam and Pap smear. In addition to these procedures, certain other screening and diagnostic tests are essential for your pre-, peri-, and postmenopausal years, for, as you've already seen, the health needs of women in the middle years extend far beyond what a pelvic exam and Pap smear can tell you.

In the pages that follow, we'll highlight the procedures and tests above and beyond those routinely offered during an annual physical that would be most helpful to premenopausal, postmenopausal, and older women (see Recommended Screening Tests for Women in Midlife on pages 24–26). We'll explain why these tests are important to you now, how they're conducted, and how reliable the test results are.

As you'll see, some of the tests described here are quite simple and can be performed in virtually any physician's office. (A few you can even do yourself!) Others are more sophisticated and may not yet be widely available. Ask your doctor about which tests may be available to you. (We'll alert you to any medical organizations that provide referrals to centers that perform some of the more advanced tests described here.)

First Things First: Finding the Right Physician

The best medical care comes when you and your physician work together as a team. Obviously, it's important that you trust your physician and have a sense that he or she cares about you. You should also look for reputable credentials. Part of your trust in your physician will come from the knowledge that he or she has a sound medical background and experience. Here are the steps you'll need to take in choosing your health-care team.

1. Decide which specialists are best for your needs. Virtually all physicians today are specialists, which means that in addition to their regular medical training they have had three or four years of specialized training in a specific field, such as obstetrics and gynecology, family medicine, internal medicine and so on.

Many women today rely on their gynecologist as their primary-care physician. This is fine as long as your gynecologist refers you to an outside specialist should you develop a health problem beyond his or her area of expertise.

Because your health needs now are becoming broader, you may want to consider adding an internist (a specialist in adult medicine) or a family physician to your health team. However, if you do decide to see an internist or family physician rather than a gynecologist, make sure these specialists also perform an annual pelvic exam and Pap smear. If they don't, you should continue to see your gynecologist on a yearly basis, as well.

2. Begin your search by compiling a list of names. To find a doctor with whom you are comfortable and whom you can trust, ask friends or coworkers for recommendations. If you have moved, your former physician might be able to recommend a doctor in your new area. You might also call a local hospital to get the names of doctors who are affiliated with it. Other good sources can be found at your local library. Look for the *Directory of Medical Specialists* and the *Compendium of Certified Medical Specialists*, which list physicians' credentials and whether they are board-certified. (Board-certified physicians have undergone additional training in their specialty field and have taken written and oral exams before specialty boards composed of their professional peers.)

3. Make a list of your personal preferences. Once you have the names of several doctors, make a list of qualities that you are looking for in both the doctor and in his or her practice. Some questions and issues to consider might include:

- Do you prefer a male or female? Does age make a difference?
- Is the physician in a group or solo practice? (With a group practice, you can usually see another doctor if your own is unavailable.)
- Does the physician have admitting privileges to a good hospital?
- Are the fees reasonable? Will the doctor accept your medical insurance?
- Is the doctor easy to talk to? Are you comfortable asking questions? Does the doctor answer them in terms you can understand?
- Is the doctor up-to-date on the special health needs of a woman your age?
- Does the doctor provide follow-up reports in the form of a letter, an office visit, or a phone call?
- If the doctor is unavailable to speak with you when you call with questions, is there someone else (a trained nurse, for example) who can field your questions?

4. Schedule an office visit. You first may want to have telephone or office consultations with several of the physicians on your list. You may not know which physician is best for you, however, until you actually schedule an office visit and see how the doctor deals with you as a patient. If, for instance, you are over age fifty and he or she doesn't recommend mammograms, the physician may not have a full understanding of the particular health needs of women in midlife.

5. Consider a menopause clinic or women's health center. Many institutions and physicians are now setting up clinics that provide a wide array of health-care services under one roof. When deciding whether one of these specialty clinics is best for you, you should apply the same criteria that you would for a doctor in private practice.

How to Prepare for Your Checkup

To get the most out of your visit, make a list of questions and concerns you have before you walk into your doctor's office. Plan to share the list with your physician during your visit. By doing so, you'll feel less anxious about your visit and will be more satisfied with the care you receive.

Let your doctor know whether you're there for a checkup or if you have a specific problem. If you have a problem, ask about it directly rather than allude to it. Although it's not always easy to talk about subjects such as sex or loss of bladder control—especially to someone you may not know very well—help is readily available for these problems. Remember that not all problems are readily apparent to your doctor—even after a complete physical. You need to tell him or her about any unusual symptoms or patterns.

If this is your first visit with a new physician, be prepared to spend some time talking about your past medical and family history. Better yet, arrange to have your medical records transferred to the new office ahead of time. Whenever possible, try to ferret out the relevant information, since some medical records can be quite lengthy.

Since you'll need to undress completely for your annual physical, wear comfortable clothes that you can easily slip off and on.

Preliminary Tests for All Women in Midlife

In addition to the routine blood-pressure check, urinalysis, and blood tests that are usually performed by a nurse or assistant before you see your physician, you should also consider undergoing the following procedures.

Height

Your total height (measured *without* shoes) is important in determining your ideal weight—the body weight associated with the lowest health risks and the highest life expectancy. You should also have the following measurements taken in addition to your total height:

23

RECOMMENDED SCREENING TESTS FOR WOMEN IN MIDLIFE*

Type of test	Covered by insurance?†	In your premenopausal years (35–45)	In your perimenopausal years (45–55)	In your postmenopausal years (55–65)	In your later years (65 and older)
Crown-to-rump height	Yes, if office visit is covered	Every 5 years	Every 5 years	Every year	Every year
Weight and body composition (skin-fold test; girth measurements; BIA; DEXA)	No	Every 5 years; more often if you have a weight problem (DEXA only if there is a significant change in your weight)	Every 5 years; more often if you have a weight problem (DEXA only if there is a significant change in your weight)	Every 5 years; more often if you have a weight problem (DEXA only if there is a significant change in your weight)	Every 5 years; more often if you have a weight problem (DEXA only if there is a significant change in your weight)
Blood pressure	Yes, if office visit is covered	With every exam (or once a year)	With every exam (or once a year)	With every exam (or once a year)	With every exam (or once a year)
Pelvic exam	Yes	Every year	Every year	Every year	Every year
Pelvic-floor muscle strength	Yes	Every 3–5 years	Every 3–5 years	Every year	Every year
Pap smear	Check with your insurance carrier	Every year	Every year	Every year	Every year
Vaginal pH/Maturation index	No			With every exam (or once a year)	With every exam (or once a year)
FSH blood test	Yes	If you have menopausal symptoms	If you have menopausal symptoms	If you take postmenopausal hormones, to determine biological efficacy	

Type of test	Covered by insurance?†	In your premenopausal years (35–45)	In your perimenopausal years (45–55)	In your postmenopausal years (55–65)	In your later years (65 and older)
Progestogen challenge	Yes			Once a year (if you have not had a hysterectomy) until the test is no longer positive	
Breast exam by physician	Yes	Every year	Every year	Every year	Every year
Mammogram	Yes, in most states; check with your insurance carrier	Baseline test between ages 35 and 39; then every 3 years	Every 2 years until age 50; then every year	Every year	Every year
Lipid profile (cholesterol screen)	Check with your insurance carrier	Baseline test at age 35; then every five years	Every 3 years until menopause, then every other year	Every other year	Every other year
Digital rectal exam	Yes	Every year	Every year	Every year	Every year
Stool test (occult blood)	Check with your insurance carrier	Every year after age 40	Every year	Every year	Every year
Sigmoidoscopy	Check with your insurance carrier		Each year for 2 years in a row, then every 3 to 5 years if the first two exams are negative	Every 3 to 5 years	Every 3 to 5 years

RECOMMENDED SCREENING TESTS FOR WOMEN IN MIDLIFE* *(cont.)*

Type of test	Covered by insurance?†	In your premenopausal years (35–45)	In your perimenopausal years (45–55)	In your postmenopausal years (55–65)	In your later years (65 and older)
Iron status (hemoglobin/ hematocrit; CBC; ferritin)	Check with your insurance carrier	Every 5 years	Every 5 years	Only if you have symptoms of an iron deficiency	Only if you have symptoms of an iron deficiency
Bone-density screening (SPA, radiographic densitometry, DEXA)	No	Baseline test around age 35; then every 5 years	Every 3 years until menopause; then every year. Also baseline DEXA at age 50.	Every year	Every year

* The recommendations here are for healthy women. If you have a family history or other risk factors for heart disease, cancer, osteoporosis, or other illnesses, your physician may recommend that you undergo certain screening tests more often or that you undergo additional diagnostic tests.

†The costs of medical tests vary widely and depend on the type of insurance you have. Until recently, most insurance carriers did not cover screening tests for preventive care. In 1991, however, Blue Cross and Blue Shield, one of the nation's leading insurance carriers, issued guidelines for a lifetime schedule of medical tests to detect such diseases as cancer and heart disease and said it would offer coverage of these services. (The 73 independent nonprofit Blue Cross and Blue Shield plans will be strongly encouraged to offer the additional coverage but are not required to do so.) Medicare, the federal health-insurance program for the elderly, has also added coverage for a few selected screening tests, such as mammography. If you are in doubt about whether a screening test is covered by Medicare or your insurance policy, check with your local Medicare office or your individual insurance carrier. You may be in for a pleasant surprise.

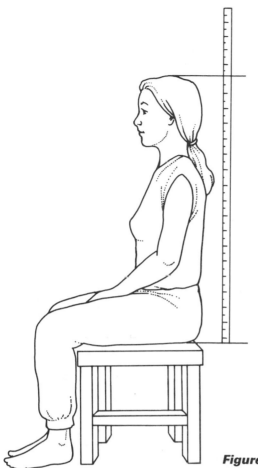

Figure 3.1   Crown-to-Rump Height

• **Crown-to-rump height:** This measure is taken from the top of your head to the bottom of your spine while you're seated on a stool (see Figure 3.1). When crown-to-rump measurements are compared over a number of years, they can help assess whether you're experiencing more than the average loss of stature that occurs with normal aging—a possible sign of vertebral fractures and osteoporosis.

• **Skeletal-frame size:** The overall size of your bones gives a clue as to whether you may be at increased risk of developing osteoporosis. Small-boned women are typically at greater risk because they have less bone to lose than women with medium or large bones. The size of your skeletal frame also helps determine your ideal weight in standardized height and weight tables (see page 472). Women with large frames naturally weigh more because they're "big-boned."

To find your skeletal-frame size, extend your arm and bend the forearm upward at a 90-degree angle. Keep your fingers straight and turn the inside of

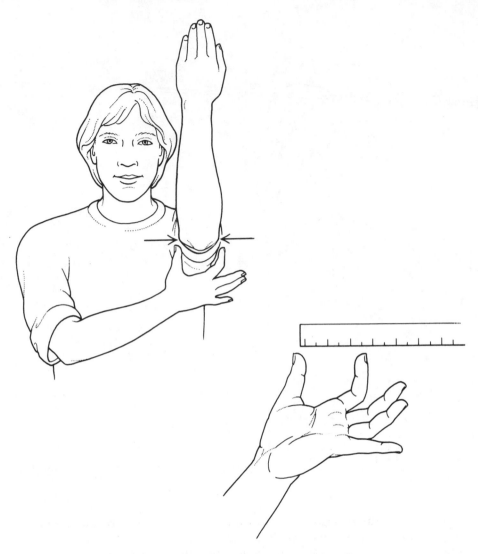

Figure 3.2   Determining Your Skeletal Frame Size

your wrist toward your body. Place the thumb and index finger of your other hand on the two prominent bones on either side of your elbow (see Figure 3.2). Measure the space between your fingers against a ruler or tape measure. (For the most accurate measurement, have your physician measure your elbow breadth with calipers.) Compare this measurement with those in the table on page 472.

•   **Leg length:** The length of both your legs should be measured, from the top of the hipbone to the top of the inner ankle (see Figure 3.3)—especially if you've been experiencing low back pain. Disparities in leg length are a simple and often overlooked cause of low back pain, which can easily be remedied by inserting a lift in the shoe of the shorter leg.

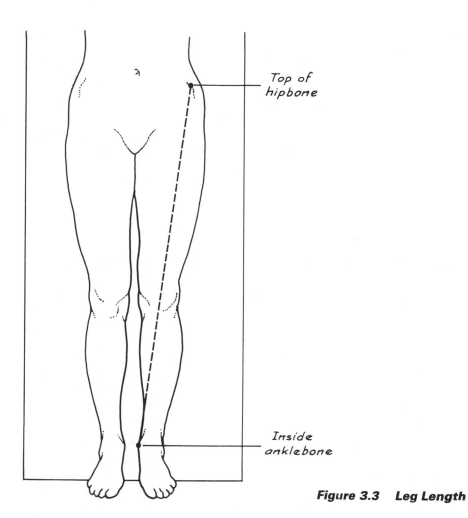

Top of
hipbone

Inside
anklebone

Figure 3.3   Leg Length

Weight and Body Composition

Conventional scales tell your overall weight and give you an idea as to whether you're overweight. (You'll find standardized height and weight tables on page 472.) But there's a lot the scales *don't* tell you. For example, you can be overfat without being overweight; that is, you can have a high percentage of body fat and still register normal weight on the scales. Yet body fat, not overall weight, is a more telling indicator of potential disease risks.

In addition to weighing in on conventional scales, the following tests of body composition may also be helpful to women in midlife. The results can be used to help determine whether you're eating right, how physically fit you are, and whether you need to lose weight.

•   **Body-mass index:** The easiest way to estimate your percentage of body fat is by calculating your *body-mass index* (BMI). To determine your body-mass index, find your present weight in the left-hand column of the table on page 473. Then read across to the column with your height.

A body-mass index over 27.3 means that you're moderately obese. A BMI over 32.3 indicates severe obesity. Remember, however, that BMI is based on charts of average women and is only an estimate of your percentage of body fat. But it's a start.

• **Skin-fold test:** Another estimate of your fat content can be obtained by measuring your *skin-fold thickness*, or "pinching an inch" with skin-fold calipers. Since about half of your total body fat is in the tissues just under your skin, the calipers are used to pull the skin and fat away from the muscle and measure its thickness. Measurements are taken from the upper arm, the abdomen just above the hipbone, and the thigh, then averaged. The accuracy, however, depends on how experienced the health professional is at taking measurements. And in a study we participated in with Michael Pollock, Ph.D., director of the Center for Exercise Science at the University of Florida, skin-fold measurements became increasingly inaccurate among more obese and older women. (See Body-Fat Measurements: How Do the Methods Measure Up? on page 33.)

• **Girth measurements:** This is a quick and surprisingly accurate way to measure your total body fat. A health professional will measure the circumference of your abdomen, right thigh, and right calf with a cloth measuring tape. These numbers are then used in a formula and with special conversion tables to calculate your percentage of body fat. Since girth measurements are easy to take, there's less room for error, too. Instructions for taking your own girth measurements, as well as the conversion tables needed to interpret the results, can be found in *Nutrition, Weight Control and Exercise*, Frank I. Katch and William D. McArdle (Philadelphia: Lea and Febiger, 1988).

• **Waist-to-hip ratio:** This measurement won't tell you how much body fat you have, but it can give you an idea of *where* fat is accumulating on your body, which has become an important barometer of certain disease risks. Fat that accumulates around your waist and lower abdomen appears to be metabolically more active and is frequently associated with an increased risk of high blood cholesterol, coronary heart disease, diabetes, hypertension, and possibly breast cancer. You can *reduce* your risk of developing many of these illnesses by losing weight and reducing your waist-to-hip ratio.

To determine your waist-to-hip ratio, use a cloth measuring tape to measure your waist about an inch above your navel (see Figure 3.4). Measure your hips at the widest point between your hips and buttocks. Now divide your waist measurement by your hip measurement. (For example, if your waist measurement is 32 and your hip measurement is 36, your waist-to-hip ratio would be calculated in this way: $32 \div 36 = 0.88$). A waist-to-hip ratio greater than 0.80 may signal greater health risks.

• **Muscle (lean-tissue mass):** Our concern about having too much body fat often overshadows another, equally important component of body composition: muscle mass. The more muscle you have, the more efficiently you will burn calories, which may help provide built-in protection against weight gain in the middle and later years. Our preliminary research suggests that increasing muscle mass may also help strengthen the immune system (see page 102), possibly giving you better protection against illness. Muscle is particularly

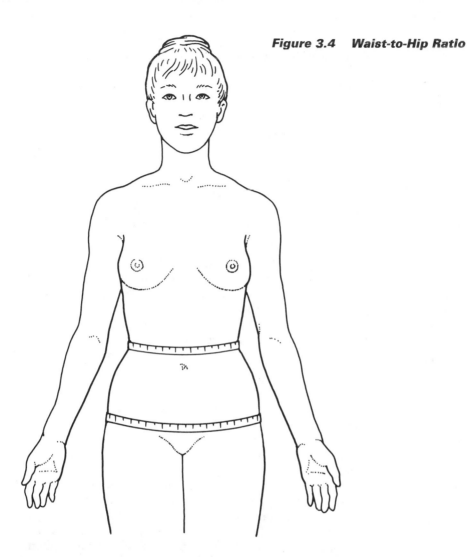

Figure 3.4   Waist-to-Hip Ratio

important as you grow older: Maintaining your muscle mass may help improve balance and so protect you from falls, a major cause of debilitating bone fractures in later life. You tend to lose muscle mass as you grow older, an age-related change that can be *reversed* with muscle-strengthening exercises (see page 99).

To determine your percentage of muscle mass, a health professional uses skin-fold calipers and a cloth tape measure to determine the fat content and circumference, respectively, of your upper arm. The numbers are then used in a formula along with your total weight to calculate your percentage of lean body weight. This measurement, when used along with measures of body fat, is an excellent way to monitor weight-loss efforts geared toward losing body fat and retaining muscle.

The most accurate measure of body composition is *underwater weighing,* which has become the "gold standard" with which all other methods are compared. However, this is also the most cumbersome and inconvenient method and is usually available only in sophisticated laboratories. You are first weighed on a conventional scale (dry weight). You are then weighed while totally submerged in a tank of water. Since fat weighs less than water, your percentage of body fat can be calculated by using a formula that compares your underwater weight with your dry weight.

Newer, more advanced methods of measuring body composition are now becoming available. These include the following:

- **Bioelectrical-impedance analysis (BIA):** Low-level electrical currents are sent through electrodes attached to your foot and hand. The greater the resistance to electricity, the more body fat you have. Although BIA is now being used in some health spas and fitness centers to determine body composition, its accuracy has been called into question. (See Body-Fat Measurements: How Do the Methods Measure Up? on page 33.)

- **Ultrasound:** A lightweight, portable ultrasound meter that emits high-frequency sound waves can be used to measure your percentage of body fat. The sound waves pass through the skin and fat tissue until they reach the muscle layer, where the sound impulses bounce back, creating an "echo" that returns to the ultrasound unit. The time it takes the sound waves to pass through the tissues and back is displayed on the ultrasound meter and is used to determine your percentage of body fat. This method of measuring body composition is not widely available.

- **Dual-energy X-ray absorptiometry (DEXA):** Low-dose X rays can now be used to determine your percentage of body fat, muscle, and bone mass. During the twenty-minute test, you simply lie quietly on an examining table as a scanner positioned about twelve inches overhead moves back and forth, gradually working its way from the top of your head to your toes. The scanner gives you a complete analysis of your body composition, including the amount of fat, muscle, and bone mineral in various regions of your body (arms, legs, and trunk) and in your total body (see Figure 17.4 on page 348). Again, the technology is fairly new and the machinery expensive, so this method of measuring body composition may not be available everywhere. For a referral to a clinic, hospital, or physician near you who has a DEXA scanner, write to either Lunar Radiation Corporation (313 West Beltline Highway, Madison, WI 53713), or Hologic, Inc (590 Lincoln Street, Waltham, MA 02154).

Once you know your percentage of body fat, compare it with Table A.1 on page 474 to determine whether you are overfat and need to lose weight.

The Premenopausal Checkup

The objective of a premenopausal checkup is simple: It lets you know how healthy you are *before* menopause and alerts you to potential health problems that may worsen after menopause—many of which can be prevented by acting *now*. Many of the following tests can be used as a baseline from which to compare the impact of menopause on your health and to develop preventive

Body-Fat Measurements: How Do the Methods Measure Up?

What's the best way to determine your body composition? It depends partly on your weight and your age, according to a study we participated in comparing the effectiveness of various methods of measuring body composition. In this study, directed by Michael Pollock, Ph.D., skin-fold thickness, BIA, and DEXA were compared with the "gold standard," underwater weighing.

As you can see from the graphs in Table 3.1, parts A and B, skin-fold thickness and BIA became increasingly inaccurate among the more obese women in the study. Indeed, BIA was far too inaccurate to be a useful screening tool among women with more than 35 percent body fat. These two procedures became more inaccurate among older women, as well. For these women, girth measurements or DEXA may be more reliable methods of determining body composition. DEXA may be most useful in measuring and monitoring muscle mass.

TABLE 3.1A *Accuracy of Various Methods of Measuring Body Composition Among Normal Weight and Overweight Women*

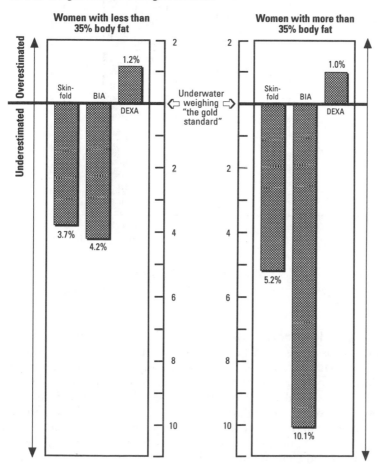

33

TABLE 3.1B *Accuracy of Various Methods of Measuring Body Composition Among Younger and Older Women*

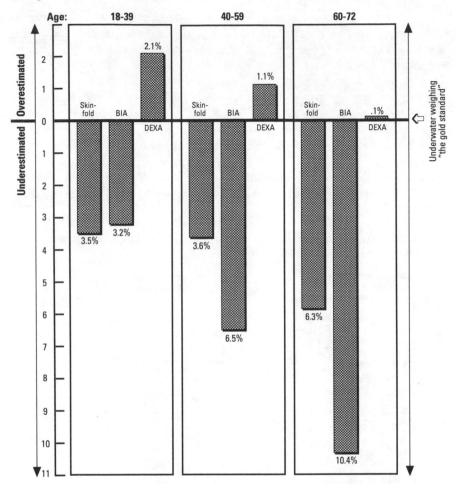

and treatment strategies. Most of the following tests should be performed at least once between ages thirty-five and forty-five; they can be handled by your gynecologist.

• **Check for iron deficiency:** Those old Geritol advertisements suggesting that women over age fifty should take a supplement to ward off "iron-poor blood" were somewhat off the mark. Actually, premenopausal women are much more likely to need iron than postmenopausal women (see Table 3.2). For this reason, you should undergo a periodic check for iron deficiency in your premenopausal years, particularly if you have heavy menstrual periods.

An iron deficiency may result from eating a diet low in iron; chronic blood loss due to a peptic ulcer; hemorrhoids, cancer, or from pregnancy (in which the developing fetus and changing metabolic requirements increase your need

TABLE 3.2 *Pre- and Postmenopausal Iron Levels*

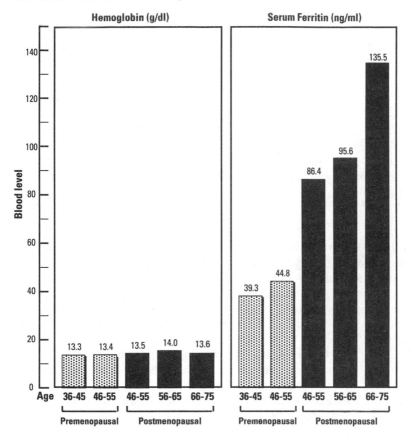

for iron). However, the most common cause of iron deficiency among women in midlife is heavy menstrual bleeding that often occurs in the years just preceding menopause.

The condition usually develops slowly over months or even years. The earliest phase, *storage depletion,* occurs when the body's iron stores in muscles and tissues become exhausted. Once iron stores are fully exhausted, any further decline in body iron results in a curtailment of the iron supply to developing red blood cells, known as *iron-deficient erythropoiesis.* In the final stage, *iron-deficiency anemia,* hemoglobin circulating in the bloodstream falls. It is not until this stage that symptoms—fatigue, dizziness, breathlessness, and sometimes heart palpitations—appear.

To check for an iron deficiency, your physician may test either your *hemoglobin* or *hematocrit.* Hemoglobin, the main component of red blood cells, is the essential protein that combines with and transports oxygen to the body cells for nourishment. Normal values are 12 to 16 grams per deciliter of blood (g/dl). *Hematocrit* is the percentage of red blood cells in whole blood. Normal values for women are 37 to 47 percent.

If levels of serum ferritin	and hemoglobin are . . .	Then you have . . .
Normal	Normal	No iron deficiency
Low	Normal	Depleted iron stores
Low	Low	Iron-deficiency anemia
Normal or high	Low	Other causes of anemia

If you *are* found to have an iron deficiency, you'll be advised to eat plenty of foods rich in iron (see page 83) and take an iron supplement (see page 82) for at least six months.

Your level of hemoglobin or hematocrit can be determined from either a drop of blood taken through a finger prick or from blood drawn through a vein. If your doctor plans to do a *complete blood count* (a routine part of many physical examinations), the blood will be taken from a vein in your arm.

The main drawback to these tests is that they detect only the final stage of iron deficiency: full-blown anemia. For a more accurate—and early—assessment of iron deficiency, your physician may test the level of *ferritin* in your blood. This is a highly specialized protein that reflects the amount of iron stored in body tissues. A low blood-ferritin level (below 12 nanograms per milliliter) means you have depleted your iron stores. A low serum-ferritin level in addition to a low hematocrit or hemoglobin level indicates that you have iron-deficiency anemia (see Screening for Iron Deficiency, above).

• **Check for menopausal status:** Menopause is a gradual transition that occurs over many years, so obviously you won't simply wake up one morning and discover that you've experienced it. Symptoms of menopause, including hot flashes, may begin several years before your final menstrual period. Moreover, many premenopausal women may develop symptoms suggestive of either premenstrual syndrome *or* menopause, such as mood swings and insomnia. Women over forty who take birth-control pills may not experience *any* telltale signs of menopause, for the hormones in birth-control pills tend to mask many of the symptoms associated with declining levels of estrogen and progesterone, such as irregular menstrual patterns. Premenopausal women who have had a hysterectomy but who still have their ovaries intact won't even have a monthly period to tip them off.

To determine whether you are approaching menopause or are menopausal, your physician may periodically test your blood level of *follicle-stimulating hormone* (FSH), the pituitary hormone that helps govern the monthly release of an egg from your ovaries. The test is usually administered during the second half of your menstrual cycle, about a week before your anticipated period. (Women taking oral contraceptives can take the test during the pill-free week.) Levels above 40 mIU/ml (except at the time of ovulation) indicate that you are menopausal. If FSH levels are lower than 40 mIU/ml, further that you are menopausal. If FSH levels are lower than 40 mIU/ml, further diagnostic tests may be required to help find other causes for any possible symptoms and to make a definitive diagnosis.

• **Baseline bone-density test:** Bone-density measurements are one of the best ways we have of determining who is at greatest risk of developing osteoporosis later in life. One study of ours involving 859 women over age forty-five showed that *bone-mass measurements were much more accurate than any of the traditional risk factors, such as fair skin, small bones, family history, low-calcium diet, and lack of exercise, at predicting osteoporosis risk.*

A baseline bone-density measurement taken before menopause will be useful as a gauge in determining how rapidly you are losing bone mass after menopause, what kind of treatment you should receive to slow down bone loss, and how well the treatment is working.

There are several methods now available for determining bone density, but one of the quickest, safest, and most reliable screening tests for osteoporosis involves having a portion of your wrist scanned with a *dual energy X-ray absorptiometry* (DEXA) scanner. The test, which involves placing your wrist under a specialized X-ray scanner, takes just a few minutes to perform and exposes you to a fraction of the X-ray radiation of an ordinary arm X ray.

Another simple and reliable screening test is *radiographic densitometry*, in which your hand is placed alongside a standardized aluminum wedge and a routine X ray is taken. The X ray is then scanned by a computer and the bone density of your finger is compared with that of the aluminum wedge.

Yet another screening test involves the use of *single photon absorptiometry* (SPA) to measure the bone density of your wrist or heel.

Your bone-density measurement is then compared with that of the average woman (see Table A.2 on page 475) to determine your risk of developing osteoporosis later on.

If your bone density is found to be low during a screening with DEXA, radiographic densitometry, or SPA, additional tests may be necessary to determine the bone density of the more vulnerable "fracture zones," such as the hip and spine. (Your physician also has several blood and urine tests that can help determine the rate at which you are losing bone; for more on these tests, see Chapter 17.)

You should have your bone density tested once as a baseline in your mid-thirties, when bone mass is at its peak, and once every five years until menopause. (See The Postmenopausal Check-Up, on page 39 for recommendations for postmenopausal women.)

The technology for bone-density testing is fairly new and may not yet be available from your physician. If your doctor cannot provide a referral, contact the National Osteoporosis Foundation (Suite 500, 1150 Seventeenth Street NW, Washington, D.C. 20036) for a list of physicians, hospitals, and clinics near you that offer bone-density testing.

• **Baseline blood lipids:** Menopause is associated with a rise in blood lipids (fats) and in the risk of developing heart disease. This menopause-related change in blood lipids can often be offset by eating a low-fat diet, exercising, and, when necessary, taking medications (see Chapter 16). For this reason, you should have a full lipid profile before menopause to serve as a baseline in

TABLE 3.3 *Average Size of Breast Lump Detectable by Mammography and by Hand*

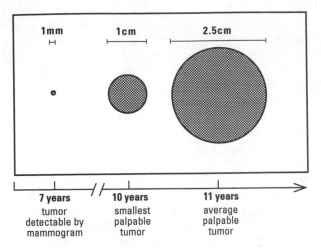

7 years	10 years	11 years
tumor detectable by mammogram	smallest palpable tumor	average palpable tumor

Note: Table adapted with permission from M. D. Wertheimer, M. E. Costanza, T. F. Dodson, C. D'Orsi, H. Pastides, and J. G. Zapka, "Increasing the Effort Toward Breast Cancer Detection." *Journal of the American Medical Association* 255, no. 10, March 14, 1986, 1311–15. Copyright © 1986 by the American Medical Association.

determining how the drop in estrogen associated with menopause affects your blood-cholesterol levels. The lipid profile includes measures of a variety of blood fats, such as total cholesterol, very low-density lipoproteins (VLDL cholesterol), low-density lipoproteins (LDL cholesterol), high-density lipoproteins (HDL cholesterol), and triglycerides. The test also provides the ratio of HDL cholesterol to total cholesterol, which is particularly important, since high levels of HDL, the "good" cholesterol, believed to rid the body of excess cholesterol, appear to protect against heart disease. For greatest accuracy, the blood test must be taken after an overnight fast. (A guide to test results of the lipid profile can be found on page 312.)

• **Baseline mammogram:** One in nine American women will develop breast cancer at some point in her life. When caught early, however, 90 percent of breast cancers are completely curable. One of the best ways of detecting breast cancer in its earliest, most curable stages is with mammography, low-dose X rays of the breast. *Mammograms can detect a breast lump up to two years before it can be felt by hand* (see Table 3.3).

While, in the past, mammography screening was thought to be most useful among women over age fifty, more recent studies suggest that women in their forties may also benefit from regular mammograms. In an eighteen-year study involving more than 280,000 women, researchers at the National Cancer Institute found *24 percent fewer cancer deaths among women ages forty to forty-nine who were screened with mammography every year, compared with a control group of women who weren't screened.*

Some women worry that exposure of breast tissue to repeated X-ray examinations may in itself increase their risk of developing breast cancer. Don't let this concern become an excuse for not having regular mammograms. The two types of mammography screening tests used today, *film-screen mammography* and *xeromammography*, both emit very low doses of X-ray radiation, exposing you to less than 1 rad for an entire examination. In a study investigating the potential health hazards associated with X-ray radiation, Harvard University researchers estimated that only 0.7 percent of all cases of breast cancer that occur annually in the United States may be attributed to lifetime exposure to diagnostic X-ray radiation. However, *the actual risk is probably even lower,* say critics of the study, who point out that the Harvard scientists used an outdated method of determining the risk.

You should have a baseline mammogram between ages thirty-five and thirty-nine and a mammogram every two to three years between ages forty and forty-nine. If a suspicious lump is found, additional tests may be necessary to rule out cancer (for more on mammography and other diagnostic tests, see Chapter 18). Remember, too, that nine out of ten breast lumps *are not cancerous.*

The Postmenopausal Checkup

The fact that you've stopped menstruating doesn't mean you should stop seeing your physician (particularly your gynecologist). In fact, the end of your reproductive years signals a whole new beginning in terms of your reproductive health.

The objective of a postmenopausal checkup is to monitor many of the physical changes that occur as a result of menopause—some of them are "silent" ones that won't even be apparent to you—and to initiate preventive and therapeutic measures (for instance, changes in diet and exercise or hormone therapy) when necessary. The postmenopausal tests you should consider include the following:

• **Check for menopausal status:** Your physician will measure the level of *follicle-stimulating hormone* (FSH) in your blood to determine whether you have reached menopause (for more on this test, see page 36). Levels over 40 mIU/ml indicate that you are menopausal.

• **Check of pelvic organs:** The pelvic exam, which includes an inspection of the outer genitals and internal reproductive organs, remains an important part of your annual physical *even after menopause.* For the pelvic exam, you'll be asked to lie on an examining table and put your feet in the stirrups attached to the table. A sheet will be draped over your chest and abdomen. The examination itself should include:

Check for cancer of the vulva: Your doctor will visually inspect your genitals for lumps, sores, and discoloration or inflammation, all possible signs of infection or cancer. He or she may also apply a blue dye known as *toluidine blue* on the vulva to detect possible precancerous changes of the vulva. After the dye has been applied, it is washed away with a dilute vinegar solution. Since the dye is absorbed by potentially precancerous cells, any remaining blue coloration of the skin may be an early sign of cancer of the vulva. This cancer is 90 percent curable when caught early, and treatment in the early stages is rarely disfiguring.

Check for strength of pelvic-floor muscles: After examining your genitals, your physician may insert one or two fingers into your vagina and ask you to squeeze your pelvic-floor muscles to check their strength. Strong pelvic-floor muscles may help protect against some types of urinary incontinence (loss of bladder control). You can strengthen your pelvic-floor muscles with the pelvic-floor exercises described on page 427.

Check for cervical cancer: If you're under the impression that because you are postmenopausal you no longer need a Pap smear, think again. This simple screening test has reduced deaths from cervical cancer (which increase with age) by 70 percent since it was first introduced in the 1940s. Yet studies have shown that only 57 percent of women ages forty to seventy are regularly screened. Moreover, some women who have had a hysterectomy still have their cervix intact and should be regularly screened for cervical cancer. Even a woman who has had her cervix surgically removed can benefit from annual Pap smears: The test can pick up asymptomatic yeast, bacterial, and viral infections and can help determine whether the vagina is lacking in hormones. The Pap smear can also detect rare cases of vaginal cancer.

To perform a Pap smear, your physician will insert a finger, then a speculum into the vagina as you lie on an examining table with your feet in the stirrups. Using a cotton swab, your doctor will gently scrape a few cells from the inside of the cervix and smear them on a glass slide. He or she will use a small wooden spatula to obtain a cell sample from the outside of the cervix. The cells are fixed with a spray so they don't deteriorate, then shipped to a laboratory to be examined under a microscope. If a Pap smear reveals abnormal cells, further tests may be necessary. Keep in mind, too, that an abnormal Pap smear doesn't always mean cancer (see Chapter 18).

Check for atrophic vaginitis: By taking a sample of cells from the side walls of the vagina, your physician can determine the acid-base balance (pH balance) of the vagina. A pH of more than 5 suggests that you may be developing *atrophic vaginitis,* or vaginal dryness as a result of low estrogen levels after menopause, a condition corrected by taking postmenopausal estrogen. The sample can also be tested for the *maturation index* of the cells; that is, the ratio of the three main cell types of the vagina: parabasal (deep), intermediate, and superficial. If 20 percent or more of the cells are parabasal cells, you probably have atrophic vaginitis. (For more on the treatment of atrophic vaginitis, see Chapter 12.)

Check for prolapsed organs: Your physician will look for visual clues of prolapses of the uterus or bladder (*cystocele*) into the vagina, or for evidence of prolapse of the vagina itself.

Check for uterine or ovarian problems: After your doctor removes the speculum, he or she will perform a bimanual examination to detect any pelvic masses or pain you may be experiencing. (It is especially important that you try to relax your abdominal muscles during this part of the examination; if you feel tense, take a few deep breaths and concentrate on relaxing your abdominal muscles.) Your physician will insert one or two fingers into your vagina and gently lift the uterus. He or she will then place the other hand on your tummy to palpate the uterus and check its position, size, shape, and mobility. (This is why it is so important to relax your abdominal muscles). Your ovaries will be examined in the same way to check for cysts or other masses. Indeed, a regular pelvic exam is one of the few ways physicians have of detecting ovarian cancer, a relatively rare but often deadly cancer that usually causes no symptoms until it has spread. (For more on ovarian cancer, see page 398.)

• **Check of the rectum:** After the pelvic exam, your doctor will insert a finger into your rectum to check for prolapse of the rectum (*rectocele*) or intestines (*enterocele*) and for hemorrhoids. He or she will also check for any abnormalities that may be early signs of colon cancer.

• **Check for endometrial cancer:** Some physicians recommend that all post-menopausal women who have not had a hysterectomy undergo a test called the *progestogen challenge* once a year as a screen for early signs of endometrial cancer. Treatment of high-risk women with progestogen usually eliminates their risk of developing this cancer altogether.

The test involves taking a progestogen every day for ten to thirteen days. If you experience *no bleeding,* the test is negative and should be repeated annually, provided you are not using any hormones and remain symptom-free (that is, you experience no abnormal menstrual bleeding during the year). If you experience "withdrawal" bleeding after taking the progestogen, this is a sign that your uterine lining is being stimulated by estrogen and that you may be at an increased risk of developing endometrial cancer. Your physician may then recommend that you continue taking progestogen for ten to thirteen days each month for as long as withdrawal bleeding follows. (For more on the diagnosis and treatment of endometrial cancer, see page 391.)

• **Check for bone loss:** Several different tests can be used to help determine the impact your menopause has on bone density and the rate at which you are losing bone.

Bone-density test: You should have your bone density tested every year after menopause to determine the rate of bone-mineral loss and whether you could benefit from hormone therapy or other medical interventions. If you are found to have low bone mass, more definitive tests of the hip and spine are strongly recommended. (For more on bone density testing, see page 37.)

Calcium-to-creatinine ratio: This test measures the levels of calcium and creatinine (an end product of metabolism) in the urine, which tells roughly how efficiently your bone-remodeling cycle (the breakdown of old bone and the creation of new bone in your body) is working. Because the calcium in the food you eat can affect these values, the test is performed on the *second* voided sample of urine after an overnight fast. A ratio of less than 0.16 is normal. A ratio greater than 0.16 may be a sign that your bone-remodeling cycle is accelerated for some reason and that you are losing bone mass.

Blood test for bone remodeling: A blood test that measures levels of the enzyme *alkaline phosphatase* may be used in conjunction with other tests of the bone-remodeling cycle (such as the calcium-to-creatinine ratio) to determine whether this cycle has been activated and new bone is being formed. (Newer urine and blood markers are being developed and may soon become commercially available; see Chapter 17.)

• **Check for heart-disease risk:** To assess the impact of menopause on your blood-cholesterol levels and your risk of heart disease, you should undergo a lipid profile every other year after menopause (You should have a lipid profile every year if you have high cholesterol). This test involves having blood drawn from a vein in your arm after an overnight fast; it gives a much more accurate assessment of your risk of heart disease than the widely used screening test for total cholesterol only. (See page 312 for a guide to test results.)

If you are over fifty and have high blood cholesterol or other risk factors for heart disease (such as a family history of premature heart disease) or if you are beginning an exercise program, you should consider having an *exercise stress test*. This test involves monitoring your heart rate and its electrical activity with an electrocardiogram (ECG) while you exercise on a treadmill. The exercise stress test (described in more detail on page 107) can detect early signs of heart disease, such as narrowing of the arteries, which may not be apparent during a resting ECG. It's also the best way to determine your level of physical fitness and to develop a fitness routine tailored to your needs.

• **Check for breast cancer:** The incidence of breast cancer rises significantly after age fifty, which is why you should have a breast exam by your physician and a mammogram *every year* if you are fifty years or older. Mammograms can detect a cancerous breast lump up to two years before it can be felt by hand (either yours or your physician's). Early detection often translates into less disfiguring surgery and an increased survival rate. (See Chapter 18.)

• **Check for colon cancer:** Colon cancer is the third leading cause of cancer death, following lung cancer and breast cancer. It is most common in women over fifty. As with other cancers, early detection and treatment increase your chances of cure.

In addition to a digital rectal exam (see page 41), you should undergo a stool test once a year after age fifty. You will be provided with a take-home test kit and instructions on how to obtain a stool sample. Your doctor will check the sample for hidden (occult) blood in the stool.

Your doctor will also recommend that you undergo *sigmoidoscopy*, in which a flexible tube with a light on the end of it is inserted into the rectum so the doctor can see into the large bowel. The American Cancer Society recommends that women age fifty and over undergo a sigmoidoscopy for two years in a row, and every three to five years after that if the results from the first two exams are negative.

The Older Woman's Checkup (Age Sixty-five and Over)

The objective of this checkup is to keep you as independent and active as possible in your later years. A major focus of this exam is on helping you to prevent falls, an important cause of disability and death in women age sixty-five and older.

• **Vision check:** Everyone's vision declines with age, and these age-related changes in vision—decreased near vision (*presbyopia*), night vision, peripheral vision, glare tolerance, and color vision—are some of the most significant factors predisposing older women to falls. Many of these vision changes are easily remedied with proper eye wear and adequate lighting in and around your house.

Your physician can check for changes in visual acuity simply by having you read letters from a Snellen eye chart. (If you wear glasses, you'll be asked to read the chart with your glasses on to make certain your current prescription doesn't need to be changed.) Vision of 20/20 is considered "normal" vision. Vision of 20/40 means you can read at twenty feet what a person with normal vision can read at forty. Peripheral vision can be checked by asking you to cover one eye with your hand while your physician moves a pencil or another object from outside your field of vision to a position in front of you. You'll be asked to say *now* as soon as you can see the object.

By shining the light of an ophthalmoscope into your pupils, your physician can check the reflexes of your eyes. Your doctor can also look for evidence of any age-related diseases, such as *glaucoma, cataracts,* or *macular degeneration,* in which the macula (the part of the retina responsible for sharp, clear sight) degenerates.

If your eyes are generally healthy, you can help prevent falls by keeping your eyewear prescriptions up-to-date and ensuring that all rooms and outside porches in your house are well lighted. Make sure that light switches are positioned near the entrance to each room.

If you have cataracts (a condition in which the lens of the eye becomes less transparent, preventing light rays from reaching the retina and resulting in a gradual loss of vision), they can be surgically removed, although the surgery is usually voluntary. When making the decision, remember: If you have low bone mass, cataract surgery is far less traumatic and the recovery period much quicker than the trauma of a broken hip.

Glaucoma, a buildup of pressure in the eye that can lead to blindness, can be treated with special eye drops. Some types of macular degeneration, if caught early enough, respond well to laser treatment.

• **Hearing check:** The hearing loss that occurs with age may also precipitate a fall—for instance, when you can't hear the warning sounds of an approaching car and don't have enough time to avoid an accident.

Sometimes, hearing loss is as easy to correct as having your physician clean out any excess earwax that has accumulated in your ears. However, since hearing loss can have many different causes, or even a combination of causes, a hearing evaluation is a must. Your physician may perform a few office tests to get a rough estimate of your ability to hear, such as placing a vibrating tuning fork in the middle of your forehead and on the mastoid bone (just behind your ear). Normally, the vibrating sound is perceived as equally loud on each side. If you have conductive hearing loss (inadequate conduction of sound from the outer ear to the inner ear), the vibrations may sound louder on the affected side.

If you complain of hearing loss or if an abnormality appears during office screening tests, you will be referred to a hearing specialist for a more in-depth evaluation.

• **Blood-pressure check:** Your physician should check your blood pressure while you are seated and again while you are standing to determine whether you suffer from *postural,* or *orthostatic-hypotension.* This is a drop in blood pressure that occurs when blood pools in your legs while you're seated and doesn't rise quickly enough to supply your brain with sufficient blood and oxygen when you stand. The condition can cause dizziness and, in severe cases, fainting. It is a common cause of falls among older women.

Postural hypotension develops partly as a result of several age-related changes throughout your body. For instance, your veins lose some of their elasticity as you grow older, increasing the likelihood that blood will pool in the veins and decreasing their ability to push blood back up toward your upper body when you stand. Your heart's ability to pump blood efficiently also declines somewhat, and levels of certain hormones that help control blood pressure fall as you grow older. However, some medications, particularly certain antihypertensive medications, antidepressants, and some drugs used to treat *angina* (chest pain caused by narrowing of the coronary arteries) may also cause postural hypotension. Alcohol use can trigger episodes of postural hypotension, too.

Your physician will use a blood-pressure cuff and a stethoscope to take your blood-pressure reading first while you are seated or lying down and, a few minutes later, while standing. Your blood pressure is actually a combination of two numbers: *systolic pressure,* the top number, measures blood pressure while the heart contracts. *Diastolic pressure,* the bottom number, indicates blood pressure between heartbeats. A drop of twenty or more points in systolic pressure and ten points in diastolic pressure while standing indicates that you have postural hypotension. (For advice on coping with postural hypotension, see page 304.)

• **Check of your musculoskeletal system:** In addition to the preliminary tests for all women in midlife, you should have a thorough assessment of your musculoskeletal system, particularly if you suffer from back pain. Your physician can check for *kyphosis* (an outward curvature in the spine that may develop in women over age sixty), uneven shoulder height (a sign of an S-shaped curvature of the spine caused by *scoliosis*), and pelvic rotation. Your physician can also roughly assess your muscle strength and any muscle spasms or tenderness you may experience. Strong muscles (particularly the abdominal and lower back muscles) provide better support for joints and enhanced stability, which lessens your chances of falling. Your physician can get a general idea of your lower-body-muscle strength in a few ways. (See Figs. 3.5–3.8.)

• **Other checks for balance:** Your physician should ask you to perform other tasks to assess your sense of balance. For instance, you may be asked to close your eyes and place your finger on your nose; stand on one leg; stand on one leg while resting the heel of the other on your knee; or walk in a straight line by placing one foot in front of the other while looking forward (not down at your feet).

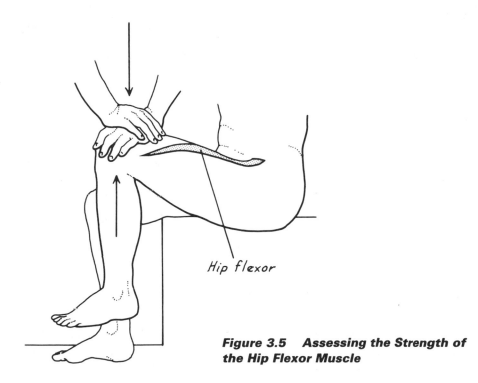

Hip flexor

Figure 3.5   Assessing the Strength of the Hip Flexor Muscle

1. While you are seated in a chair with your feet on the floor, your doctor will push down on your knee with both hands as you lift your knee.

2. As you lie on your stomach on an examining table with one knee bent, your physician will push down on your upper thigh as you raise your leg, to test the strength of the muscles in your buttocks and the back of the upper thighs.

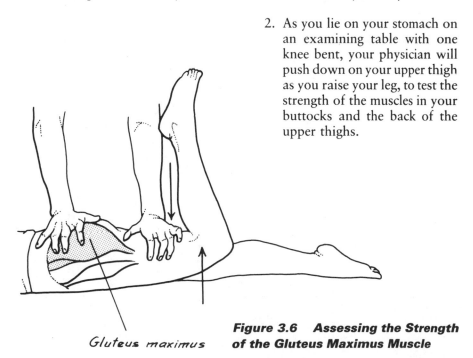

Gluteus maximus

Figure 3.6   Assessing the Strength of the Gluteus Maximus Muscle

45

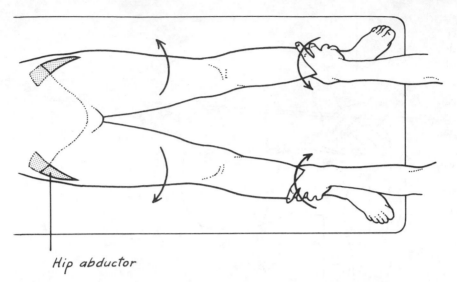

Hip abductor

Figure 3.7   Assessing the Strength of the Hip Abductor Muscle

3. While you are lying on your back on an examining table, your doctor will grasp your ankles and push in as you push your legs out, to determine the strength of your hip and outer thigh muscles.

4. Again while you are lying on an examining table, your physician will grasp both ankles and push outward as you push your legs together, to test the strength of your hip and inner thigh muscles.

Figure 3.8   Assessing the Strength of the Hip Adductor Muscle

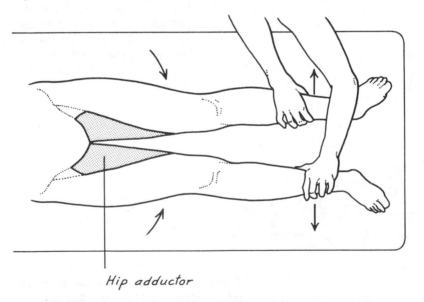

Hip adductor

• **Kidney check:** A urine test for *specific gravity* measures the kidney's concentrating ability and can pick up signs of kidney disease, diabetes, or dehydration. For this test, you'll be asked to collect an early-morning sample of urine and bring it to your doctor's office for laboratory analysis.

• **Pelvic exam and Pap smear:** You're never too old for these tests, which can help detect early signs of cancers of the reproductive organs—cancers whose incidence rises with age (see The Postmenopausal Checkup, starting on page 39, for more details on the pelvic exam and Pap smear).

What You Can Do

When you see your doctor, bring a list of medications you are taking. Many drugs, particularly barbiturates and other drugs used to treat anxiety or depression, can cause dizziness or a loss of balance and are associated with an increased risk of falling. The longer-acting drugs that remain in your bloodstream for up to twelve hours, such as tricyclic antidepressants and antipsychotics, increase the risk of falling by 80 percent or more.

Other drugs may influence the bone-remodeling cycle (the breakdown of old bone and creation of new bone) and can accelerate bone loss. For instance, thyroid medications and the commonly used diuretic furosemide are associated with excessive calcium loss in the urine.

Two Lifesaving Self-Exams for All Women In Midlife

In addition to the annual physical by your doctor, there are two self-examinations that you can and should perform on a regular basis in the comfort of your home.

Breast Self-Examination: Once a Week

Your physician examines your breasts once a year. However, breast self-examination (BSE) is something you can—and should—do for yourself, especially during the middle and later years, when the incidence of breast cancer rises. Women detect 85 percent of breast lumps themselves through BSE. And studies have shown that women who practice BSE are diagnosed at an earlier stage of the cancer's development than those who don't. This translates into improved survival rates: Breast cancer patients who practice BSE have a 15 percent increased survival rate over those who don't.

Of course, BSE is most effective when it's done correctly—and regularly. If you don't routinely practice breast self-examination, ask your doctor to show you how, or follow the guide here. While most major health organizations recommend that you examine your breasts once a month, we recommend that you perform BSE once a week. Weekly BSE not only gets you into the habit of performing this essential examination but also makes you more proficient at it. So make a habit of practicing BSE "always on Sundays."

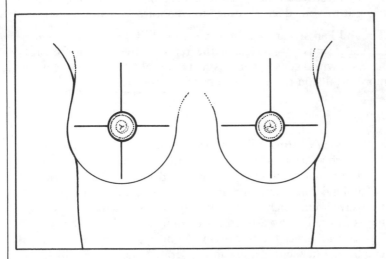

Figure 3.9   Diagram for Recording Breast Self-Examination Results

When examining your breasts, you may notice that your breast tissue naturally feels lumpy. You may be wondering how to differentiate between "normal" lumpiness and a lump you should report to your doctor. Once you've made BSE a regular habit, you'll be better able to tell the difference between what's normal and what's not. One way to keep track is to record "troublesome" areas on a diagram, much as your physician does. We've provided a diagram here for you to use (see Figure 3.9). As you examine your breasts, make a note of any areas that feel *soft, firm, thick,* or *grainy* (or choose another term that best describes what you feel). The next time you examine your breasts, you can refer back to the diagram and compare what you feel with your previous BSE.

Visual examination: Stand in front of the mirror and look at your breasts. They should be about the same size and shape. (Many women have one breast that is slightly larger than the other.)

Place your hands on your hips and push down. Do you notice any changes? A pulling in one area? Next, lean over slightly and continue to look for any differences in the two breasts.

Now raise your hands above your head and press your palms together. Again, look to see whether there is any difference between the two breasts. Look for dimpling of the skin, abnormal bulges or pulling, areas of redness, or what is called "orange peel" skin. Look at the nipple. Does it pull inward? If you see any of these abnormal signs, make a note of it on your diagram and have your breasts checked by your physician.

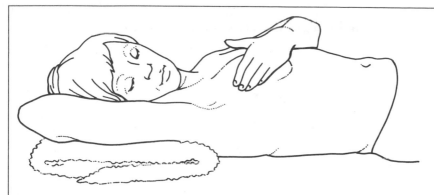

Figure 3.10

Manual Examination: Lie down and place a small pillow or folded towel behind your back on the right side (see Figure 3.10). Raise your right arm over your head or place your right hand behind your head. Using one of the BSE patterns shown in figures 3.11A and B (below and next page), examine your right breast with your left hand. Use the flat part of your fingers to examine your breast, *not* your fingertips (see Figure 3.12). Now, moving your fingers in a circular motion, feel the breast tissue lightly, then more deeply. Be sure to feel the upper chest areas, the area just under the breasts, and the area under

Figure 3.11A

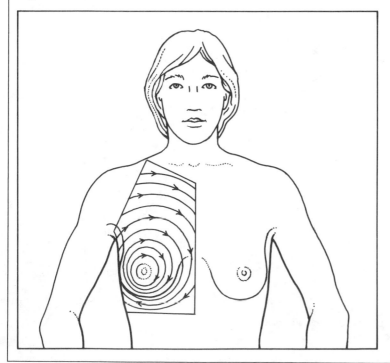

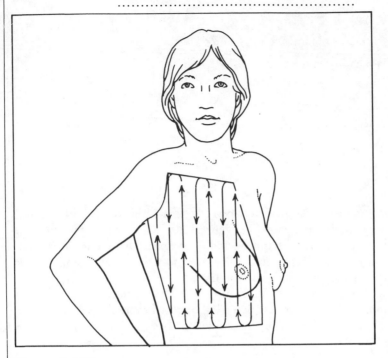

Figure 3.11B

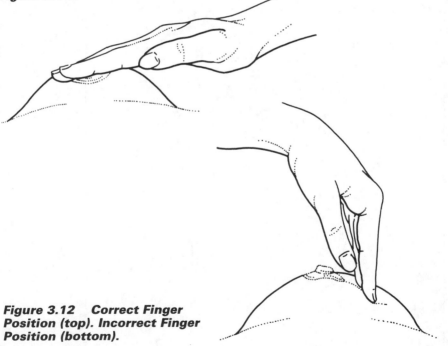

Figure 3.12   Correct Finger Position (top). Incorrect Finger Position (bottom).

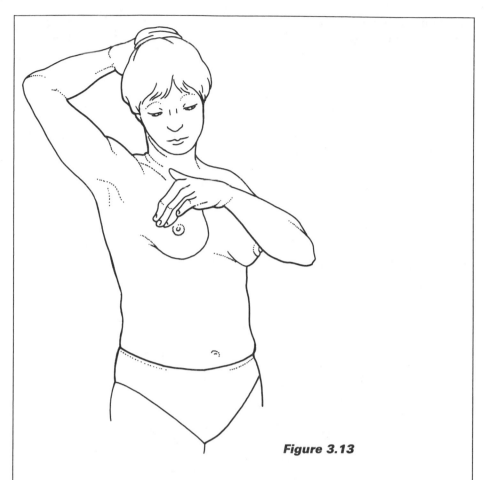

Figure 3.13

your arms just as carefully as you have examined the breast itself. When you have completed the examination on one side, repeat the procedure on the other, remembering to move the pillow or towel to the other side.

Repeat the examination while standing or sitting upright (see Figure 3.13). You are looking and feeling for lumps that are not normal. Remember, every woman's breasts have some areas that may feel thickened or grainy. This is especially true as you grow older. A lump that is not normal may be any size. It may move around freely or be fixed. If you find something unusual, see your physician.

Genital Self-Examination: Once a Month

Since cancerous and precancerous conditions of the vulva have risen sharply over the last ten years, many doctors now recommend that you examine your own genitals once a month using a technique called genital self-examination (GSE). Vulvar cancer often produces some visible signs, making it possible to spot during self-examination. Genital self-exam may also help alert you to other conditions that need medical attention, such as a vaginal infection or a sexually transmitted disease.

How To Perform a Genital Self-Exam

To examine the vulva, you'll need good lighting and a hand-held mirror. You may need to experiment to find the best position, one that is comfortable but allows you to have a good view of your vulvar area. Try sitting on your bed, facing a bedside lamp, with your knees drawn up. Or you may be more comfortable standing, with one leg propped up on a stool (see Figure 3.14).

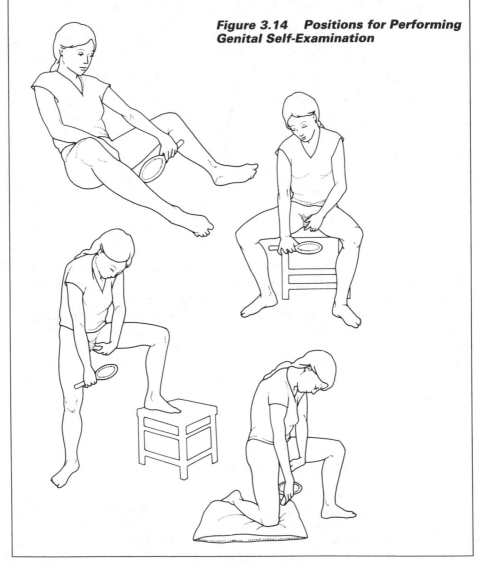

Figure 3.14   Positions for Performing Genital Self-Examination

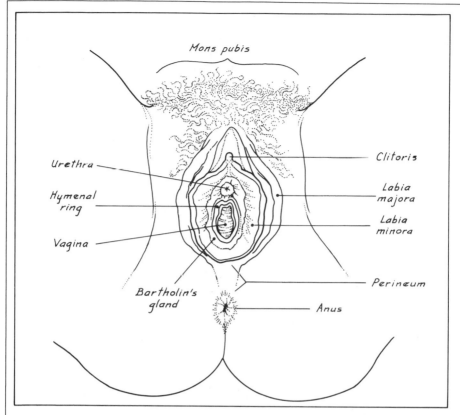

Figure 3.15   Anatomy of the Genital Area

To start the exam, spread your legs apart, hold the mirror in one hand, and use the other hand to separate the pubic hair of the mons and outer lips (See Figure 3.15). Look carefully at the skin beneath for warts, sores, bumps, moles, and ulcers. Also, feel the area for any bumps. Then check for changes in skin color—reddish or white patches. Any of these changes could be early stages of an abnormal condition that requires medical attention.

Now spread apart the outer lips and look closely around the clitoral hood and inner lips for the same signs. Then gently pull back the clitoral hood and examine the clitoris. Next, spread apart the inner lips and examine the area around the vaginal opening. Finish the exam by looking at your anus (rectal opening or rectum) and perineum (the region between the vagina and anus) for the same signs.

Perform the genital self-exam once a month. In most cases, the suspicious bump or other lesion is not due to cancer, but it will require prompt evaluation by your physician.

Note: Instructions for genital self-examination reprinted with permission from "A Patient Guide to External Genital Exam for Women," prepared in consultation with R. Allen Lawhead, Jr. *Medical Aspects of Human Sexuality.* New York: Cahners Publishing Company, 1990.

A Final Word

No midlife physical examination is complete without an evaluation of your diet and exercise habits and at least an inquiry as to whether you smoke cigarettes, drink alcohol, or take over-the-counter or prescription medications on a regular basis. The overall level of stress in your life can affect your health, too, and your physician will want to know what your home and work environments are like. In the chapters that follow, we'll discuss the impact that these lifestyle habits and environmental influences can have on your health, and offer ways to improve your health by making a few adjustments in your lifestyle.

Chapter 4

....

A Healthy Diet for Your Prime Years

The foods you eat are much more than sustenance to get you through the day. Many of the ailments associated with the middle and later years, including premenstrual syndrome, heart disease, osteoporosis, and cancer, can be at least partially remedied by making a few changes in your eating habits. Many can be prevented altogether! In the pages that follow, you'll learn how to strike a healthy balance between calories and good nutrition.

Calories

One of the biggest nutritional traps for women in the middle years is *overeating*, which often leads to creeping obesity or middle-age spread. In your later years, getting enough to eat to meet your daily need for protein, vitamins, and minerals may become a problem.

In your premenopausal years: The battle of the midlife bulge will likely begin now, just as the metabolic changes associated with aging set in. At about age thirty, your body's metabolic rate (the rate at which you burn calories) starts to slow—by about 2 percent each decade, by some estimates. So by age eighty, you should eat two hundred calories fewer per day than you ate in your thirties. Two hundred calories may not seem like much, but, if you're like most women, your level of activity declines, too. Some studies show that a more sedentary lifestyle in the middle and later years combined with this "metabolic slide" means that you'll need about four hundred fewer calories per day at age eighty than you needed at age thirty. If you don't adjust your calorie intake to your reduced energy needs, you will inevitably gain weight.

As you are probably aware, obesity is associated with an increased risk of heart disease, high blood pressure, noninsulin-dependent diabetes (the kind that usually develops in adulthood), and certain types of cancer (notably breast, endometrial, and colon cancers). Moreover, the pounds you put on in the middle years may be more hazardous to your health than any extra weight you may have carried with you from childhood. Studies have shown that women who gain weight in the middle years are more likely to develop heart disease than those who had been overweight all their lives.

If you *do* gain weight, crash dieting or yo-yo dieting can actually make matters worse. When you go on a crash diet, your body—in an effort to keep you from starving to death—sets in motion a number of adaptive changes that tend to conserve energy. The more often you diet, the more efficient your body becomes at conserving energy, which is why it becomes progressively harder to lose weight with each new diet you undertake. You'll also *regain* the weight more rapidly after you go off your diet. Crash dieting also often causes you to lose muscle mass, which can slow your metabolism even more, because muscle is metabolically more active than fat.

In your postmenopausal years: By the time you reach age fifty, maintaining normal weight by watching your calorie intake becomes even more critical, since your risk of many obesity-associated illnesses—heart disease; hypertension; endometrial, breast, and colon cancer; and diabetes—naturally rises with age.

In your later years: By age sixty-five, the average woman won't need more than sixteen hundred calories a day to maintain her weight. Yet your need for protein, vitamins, and minerals remains unchanged. So the challenge is to eat nutrient-rich foods without consuming too many calories.

Sometimes, the problem for older women may not be eating too much but eating too little. Many older women are at increased risk of developing malnutrition. Often, the age-related diminished senses of taste and smell make eating less enjoyable. Chronic illness or medication use plays a part, as well. Difficulty chewing or swallowing, poor-fitting dentures, or gastrointestinal upsets may also contribute to the problem. Psychological and social factors, such as living alone, loneliness, or depression, may alter an older woman's appetite and eating habits, too. Sometimes, the problem is compounded by physical disabilities that make food shopping and meal preparation difficult.

How Many Calories Do You Need?

Your age, body size, genetic makeup, the amount of muscle and fat you have, your activity level, basal metabolic rate, and other factors all play into how many daily calories you need.

Begin by comparing your weight with the ideal weight in the standardized height-weight table on page 472. These tables are meant to give you a *general idea* of what your ideal weight should be. Keep in mind that you may feel fine and look great above the recommended weights. Or you may feel fat at the weight the tables say is ideal for you. (We've included both the 1959 and 1983 Metropolitan tables and the more recent USDA table, which allows you to weigh a little more in your middle years.)

As we mentioned in Chapter 3, a better gauge of your weight, particularly for predicting possible obesity-related health risks, is your body composition; that is, your percentage of fat, muscle, and bone. Use the instructions for determining your body-mass index (a rough indicator of your percentage of body fat) on page 29. Or have a health professional determine your body composition using one of the other methods described in Chapter 3. Use Table A.1 on page 474 to determine your percentage of body fat now, as well as the ideal percentage you should aim for.

Obviously, your level of activity helps determine the amount of calories you require each day. The more active you are, the more you can eat. To estimate the number of calories you use daily, check Calories Burned During Common Exercises and Activities on page 480. When determining your level of physical activity, consider only regular exercise or other strenuous activities that you participate in for more than thirty minutes per day.

Finally, you'll want to know your basal metabolic rate, the amount of calories your body uses at rest. Probably the most accurate way to do this is using a new high-tech method called *indirect calorimetry*. This method has been used mostly in hospitals in the past and is quite simple. You will be told to come to the hospital or clinic first thing in the morning, before having anything to eat or drink. You simply lie on an examining table and breathe through a mouthpiece for twenty minutes. The machine measures the amount of oxygen you inhale and the amount of carbon dioxide you exhale. From these measurements, the machine calculates your basal metabolic rate. Studies at our clinic have found that indirect calorimetry is much more accurate than the standard way of estimating total daily calories—the Harris-Benedict equation. However, it may be years before indirect calorimetry becomes more available to the public. In the meantime, you can do what many dietitians do and estimate your total daily calories using the Harris-Benedict equation. We've simplified and adapted the equation for you here.

If you are overweight, use your desirable weight to calculate your total daily calories.

Weight _____ (lbs.) × 0.45 = _____ (kg) × 9.563 = _____ (A)
Height _____ (in.) × 2.5 = _____ (cm) × 1.850 = _____ (B)
Age   _____ × 4.676 =   _____ (C)

Now use the figures you have obtained to find your basal metabolic rate and total daily calories in the equation here:

        655.1
+ _____ (A)
+ _____ (B)
− _____ (C)
= _____ Your basal metabolic rate
×   1.2
= _____ Total daily calories (sedentary lifestyle)
+ _____ Calories used during daily exercise or
                strenuous activity (see page 480)
= _____ TOTAL DAILY CALORIES

If you're worried about *overeating* in the middle years, relax. You won't have to start eating like a rabbit once you hit age forty. By *gradually* reducing the amount you eat over the years rather than dieting in fits and starts, you'll be more likely to keep your weight in check and your risk of numerous obesity-related illnesses down. Increasing your level of physical activity helps, too. In fact, regular exercise may be the most overlooked recommended dietary allowance for women in midlife.

Older women can help offset the risk of malnutrition from a reduced calorie intake by eating nutrient-rich foods and, if necessary, taking a multivitamin supplement. Try the suggestions here for balancing your calorie intake with your midlife nutritional needs.

How to Cut Calories Without Skimping on Nutrition

• **If you haven't already done so, start by determining how many calories you'll need to eat each day to maintain your ideal weight.** (See How Many Calories Do You Need? on page 56.)

• **Eat less fat.** Fat contains more calories per gram than protein or carbohydrate, so by cutting the fat out of your diet you're cutting out the most calorie-rich foods. (See Getting the Fat Out of Your Diet on page 60.)

• **Eat more satisfying high-fiber foods.** Several studies suggest that high-fiber diets aid in weight loss by increasing feelings of satiety. Fiber-rich foods, such as whole-grain breads, brown rice, fruits and vegetables, and dried peas and beans, take longer to digest, making you feel full longer and reducing the temptation to eat foods strictly because you're hungry. These foods are also chock-full of vitamins and minerals and, best of all, are naturally low in fat, so they make excellent substitutes for high-fat fare.

• **Eat the majority of your calories before 5:00 P.M.** *When* you eat your meals during the day may be almost as important as how much you eat. Some studies have shown that when you eat a single large meal during the day, certain enzymes undergo changes that encourage your body to store the calories as fat. These changes don't occur among women who eat several small meals per day. So if you starve yourself all day and splurge with a big dinner at night, you may be programming your body to store fat.

In addition, studies by cardiologist Robert Superko at the University of California at Berkeley have shown that blood-triglyceride (fat) levels gradually rise after a meal, reaching their highest point about four hours after you've eaten—what we call the "triglyceride bulge." If you eat a big meal in the evening, fats circulating in your bloodstream (blood lipids) reach their peak in the early-morning hours, while you're sleeping, and triglycerides are more likely to be stored as fat. Eating a big meal early in the day still causes your blood lipids to rise, but the triglycerides are more likely to be used as energy to fuel your daily activities than to be stored as fat. For these reasons, it's better to eat your biggest meals early in the day, an eating pattern we call the "PPP Principle"—that is, you should eat like a potentate for breakfast, a princess for lunch, and a pauper for dinner.

• **Increase your level of physical activity.** Remember: A gradual reduction in physical activity accounts for a big portion of the reduced calorie needs of women in the middle and later years. Raising your level of physical activity not only helps you burn more calories (and hence allows you to eat more food) but also slows the metabolic slide of the middle years by preserving muscle mass. (To start an exercise program, see Chapter 5.)

Fat

Your body needs a certain amount of dietary fat, which aids in the absorption of fat-soluble vitamins. Fat stored in your adipose tissues is a portable storehouse of energy and water that your body can draw on when food is scarce. Dietary fat also makes food taste good. And because fat takes longer to digest, it provides a pleasant feeling of satiety after a meal.

Most of the fats in your diet are *triglycerides*, or chains of carbon, hydrogen, and oxygen molecules. The building blocks of triglycerides are *fatty acids*, each with a different chemical makeup. *Saturated* fatty acids, found mostly in meat and dairy products, are "saturated" with hydrogen atoms and contain no double bonds of carbon atoms. *Polyunsaturated fats*, found in fish, as well as in corn, soybean, and safflower oils, have several double bonds. *Monounsaturated fats*, found in olive and peanut oils (and some meats) have only one double bond. Dietary fats contain all three kinds of fatty acids; when a fat contains a large percentage of, say, saturated fatty acids, it's said to be a "saturated fat." *Cholesterol* isn't a fat, per se, but a fatty substance found in meats and dairy products (such as eggs, milk, and butter.)

In terms of its contribution to health problems, excess dietary fat (and its cousin cholesterol) is *nutrition enemy number one.*

In your premenopausal years: Fat is the most concentrated source of energy in your diet. One gram of fat contains nine calories, compared with four calories per gram of protein or carbohydrate. Dietary fat appears more likely to turn into body fat than proteins or carbohydrates, too. Too much fat in the diet is a major cause of obesity. Cutting back on dietary fat is one of the most sensible ways of reducing calories to maintain your weight.

In your postmenopausal years: Dietary fat plays a key role in many of the serious illnesses that often develop in the postmenopausal years. For instance, the drop in estrogen levels after menopause appears to increase blood-cholesterol levels, which naturally rise with age. One of the best ways to counter rising cholesterol levels after menopause is to lower the amount of saturated fat and cholesterol in your diet, both of which elevate blood-cholesterol levels. New studies show that a very low-fat diet (along with other changes in lifestyle habits) can actually *reverse* narrowing of the arteries caused by atherosclerosis.

Fatty foods are also believed to be a major cause of colon and breast cancers. A study by Harvard physician Walter C. Willett, M.D., found that women who ate red meat (beef, pork, or lamb as a main dish) on a daily basis were two and a half times more likely to develop colon cancer than those who ate red meat less than once a month. When you eat fat, bile acids are secreted from the liver to help break down the fat in the colon. Some scientists think bacteria in the colon transform bile acids into bile salts, believed to be cancer promoters that fuel the growth of existing precancerous or cancerous cells.

Most of the evidence linking diet and breast cancer comes from population studies showing an increased incidence of breast cancer in countries such as the United States, where the diet is high in fat. When Japanese women (who eat a low-fat diet and have a low incidence of breast cancer) move to the United States, their rate of breast cancer rises, presumably along with the increased fat in their diets. The role of dietary fat in the development of cancer is still controversial, however. In the Nurses Health Study at Harvard University, Dr.

Willett and his colleagues concluded that a *moderate* reduction in fat intake (to 30 percent of total daily calories) by women doesn't result in a substantial reduction of breast-cancer risk. However, the researchers didn't rule out the possibility that dietary fat intakes of less than 30 percent might reduce risk. Animal studies suggest that dietary fat must be cut to less than 20 percent of total calories to reduce the risk of breast cancer. This is about the amount of fat in the diets of Japanese women.

Remember, too, that dietary fat is a major contributor to obesity and its associated health risks, including heart disease, hypertension, and diabetes.

In your later years: Since older women require less energy than younger women, reducing calorie-rich dietary fat is a good way to cut calories without skimping on nutrition. Many older women have problems digesting fat, anyway, as a result of an age-related decrease in the secretion of bile by the liver.

Getting the Fat Out of Your Diet

Most major health organizations, including the U.S. government, urge you to reduce fat in your diet to less than 30 percent of total calories. However, based on early reports on breast-cancer prevention, we recommend that you aim for a diet in which you limit fat to *no more than 25 percent of your calories.* Of your total fat calories, about a third should come from saturated fats. The remaining two-thirds should be about equally divided between monounsaturated and polyunsaturated fats. You should limit cholesterol to no more than 300 milligrams a day (one large egg contains 213 milligrams of cholesterol— about two-thirds of the recommended amount).

Counting Fat Grams
There are several ways to get the fat out of your diet. One way is to calculate the amount of fat, in grams, that you can eat based on your total daily calories. All you have to do is keep track of the fat you eat in the same way you count calories on a diet. To do this, check food labels or Nutritional Values of Selected Foods on page 485. (When calculating your fat intake, don't forget to count the oil you use in cooking, the mayonnaise you spread on your sandwich, and the salad dressing you pour onto your fresh greens.) Here's a general guide:

	.... **Fat Intake Guidelines**	
If your total calories are approximately	*Your total fat calories should be*	*Which converts to (grams of fat)*
1,000	250	28
1,200	300	33
1,400	350	39
1,500	375	42
1,600	400	44
1,800	450	50
2,000	500	55

Counting Fat Calories
The U.S. Food and Drug Administration's new food-labeling guidelines are bound to make it easier for you to determine the amount of fat in packaged foods. According to the new regulations, food manufacturers are now required to tell you the percentage of calories in a product that comes from fat, or the product's "fat calories." Although the new regulations became effective in January 1993, it may be some time before *all* food labels adhere to the guidelines. For this reason, it may be helpful for you to know how to calculate fat calories. To do this, you'll need to know the total number of calories and grams of fat in a serving size (check the label). The percentage of calories from fat can be calculated as follows:

(grams of fat per serving × 9) ÷ total calories per serving × 100

For instance, a two-ounce serving of chunk white tuna fish (water-packed) contains 2 grams of fat and 70 calories. So the percentage of fat calories is 2 (grams of fat) × 9 (calories per gram of fat) = 18 (fat calories) ÷ 70 (total calories) = .25 × 100 = 25 percent of calories from fat.

As a general rule, you should look for foods with an *overall average* of 3 grams of fat for every one hundred calories. Of course, some foods will have more than this; others will have less. Your goal is to eat more foods low in fat and fewer foods with a high fat content, but not necessarily to cut every gram of fat out of your diet.

Cutting Back on Fat Without Counting
By following a few simple guidelines, you'll automatically cut back on fat—without having to count fat grams or calculate fat calories.

• **Choose lean meats and the leanest cuts of meat.** Poultry (with skin removed), fish, and veal are the leanest meats. Also look for lower grades of meat; choose "select" and "choice" grades over "prime" meats, which contain the most fat. Most shoppers usually purchase their meat by cut, not grade, however. When selecting cuts of meat, keep in mind the following guidelines:

Poultry: Choose light meat over dark; it contains about half the fat of dark meat. Always remove the skin before cooking.

Fish and shellfish: Most fish is low in saturated fat and high in polyunsaturated omega-3 fatty acids, which are believed to help protect against heart disease (see page 321). While shrimp and squid are relatively high in cholesterol, they're extremely low in fat, so you can still include them in your diet.

Veal: All trimmed cuts of veal (except chopped) are relatively low in fat, but somewhat high in cholesterol, so eat veal sparingly.

Beef: Round, sirloin, and loin are lowest in fat. Ground beef is high in fat. If you do use ground beef, choose ground round and ground sirloin.

Pork: Tenderloin and leg contain the least fat; bacon and sausage the most.

Organ meats: Liver, kidney, brain, tongue, and other organ meats are low in fat but high in cholesterol, so limit your consumption of these meats to about once a month.

61

Processed and luncheon meats: These are notoriously high in fat *and* sodium. Look for low-fat luncheon meats, such as boiled ham, honey loaf, and turkey breast. Beware of purportedly low-fat turkey and chicken products (bologna and franks). Most contain less fat than all-beef products, but not much less.

• **Choose low-fat and no-fat milk and dairy products over whole dairy products.** An eight-ounce glass of skim milk contains virtually no fat, compared to 8 grams of fat in a glass of whole milk (3.3 percent milk fat).

• **Limit your consumption of high-cholesterol foods.** Eggs, butter, and other whole dairy products, red meats, and organ meats (liver, kidney, and brain) are highest in cholesterol. (Check Nutritional Values of Selected Foods on page 485 for more high-cholesterol foods.)

• **Use monounsaturated and polyunsaturated oils instead of saturated fats whenever possible, especially in cooking.** Vegetable, olive, and peanut oils should be your first choice, since they're unsaturated fats. Use margarine and spreads sparingly, since the *trans fatty acids* (created when unsaturated fats are hydrogenized, or hardened) may raise blood-cholesterol levels.

• **Eat smaller portions of high-fat foods.** This is especially true of meats. You can get all the protein you need each day from just two two- to three-ounce portions of meat plus protein from milk (for more on protein, see page 71). A three-ounce portion of meat is about the size of a deck of playing cards or the palm of your hand.

• **Use reduced-fat cooking methods.** Making a few simple changes in the way you prepare and cook foods (particularly meats) can reduce their fat content by up to one-half. For instance, a fried chicken breast with skin has 12.2 grams of fat. The same chicken breast roasted with the skin removed contains just 4.5 grams of fat.

Trim all visible fat from the meats you buy and remove the skin from poultry before cooking. Try broiling, roasting, stir-frying, and stewing, which require the least amount of fat. When possible, cook meat on a rack so the fat drips down. Avoid panfrying or deep-frying.

• **Use fat substitutes sparingly.** Fat substitutes may seem like a boon for those who want to cut the fat but not the flavor out of their diets. However, many health professionals worry that the fat substitutes may encourage poor eating habits. High-carbohydrate foods, with their complement of protein, vitamins, and fiber, are still a better stand-in for fat-laden foods—even those made with fake fat.

• **Avoid cream sauces and creamy salad dressings.** Use lemon juice and herbs rather than butter to season foods.

• **Stay away from fast foods.** Between 40 to 55 percent of the calories in fast-food meals comes from fat. Even such seemingly low-fat fare as chicken nuggets and chicken-patty sandwiches often contain ground chicken skin, which increases their fat content. If you do find yourself in a fast-food restaurant, order a salad, low-fat milk, grilled chicken breast, and other low-fat fare that's finally making its way onto the menus of many fast-food chains.

• **Consider the no-meat option.** Meat is one of the primary sources of fat in the American diet. Many people find that eliminating meat (and sometimes dairy products) from their diets altogether is the easiest way to cut back on fat and cholesterol. (For more on vegetarianism, see page 92.)

Meal	Total daily calories				
	1,000	1,200	1,500	1,800	2,000
Afternoon (cont.)					
Whole-wheat bread	1 slice	2 slices	2 slices	2 slices	2 slices
Turkey breast	2 oz.	2 oz.	3 oz.	3 oz.	4 oz.
Low-fat mayonnaise	1 tsp.	1 tsp.	1 tsp.	1 tsp.	1 tsp.
Evening					
Broccoli	1 cup	1 cup	1 cup	1 cup	1 cup
Fruit cup	½ cup	½ cup	½ cup	½ cup	½ cup
Baked potato	1	1	1	1	1
Dinner roll	—	1	2	2	2
Lean beef	1 oz.	2 oz.	2 oz.	3 oz.	3 oz.
Margarine	2 tsp.	2 tsp.	2 tsp.	2 tsp.	2 tsp.
Snack					
Popped popcorn	—	—	—	3 cups	3 cups
Morning					
Skim milk	8 oz.	8 oz.	8 oz.	8 oz.	8 oz.
Orange juice	6 oz.	6 oz.	6 oz.	6 oz.	6 oz.
100% bran cereal	—	—	—	½ cup	½ cup
Whole-wheat toast	1 slice	1 slice	2 slices	2 slices	2 slices
Margarine	1 tsp.	1 tsp.	1 tsp.	1 tsp.	1 tsp.
Afternoon					
Chef's salad made with:					
Mozzarella cheese	1 oz.	1 oz.	1 oz.	1 oz.	1 oz.
Lettuce	1 cup	1 cup	1 cup	1 cup	1 cup
Tomato	½	½	½	½	½
Potato salad	—	½ cup	½ cup	1 cup	1 cup
Roast beef	1 oz.	1 oz.	1 oz.	1 oz.	1 oz.
Ham	1 oz.	1 oz.	1 oz.	1 oz.	1 oz.
Turkey breast	—	—	1 oz.	1 oz.	2 oz.
Salad dressing	1 tsp.	1 tsp.	1 tsp.	1 tsp.	1 tsp.
Saltine crackers	4	4	4	4	4
Evening					
Tossed salad	1 cup	1 cup	1 cup	1 cup	1 cup
Mashed potato	½ cup	1 cup	1 cup	1 cup	1 cup
Green peas	—	—	—	½ cup	½ cup
Baked chicken	1 oz.	2 oz.	2 oz.	3 oz.	3 oz.
Dinner roll	—	—	1	1	1
Margarine	1 tsp.	1 tsp.	1 tsp.	1 tsp.	1 tsp.
Snack					
Fruit, your choice	1 piece	1 piece	1 piece	1 piece	2 pieces

Meal	Total daily calories				
	1,000	1,200	1,500	1,800	2,000
Morning					
Skim milk	1 cup	1 cup	1 cup	1 cup	1 cup
Whole-wheat bagel	½	1	1	1	1
Cheerios	—	—	½ cup	1 cup	1 cup
Margarine or cream cheese	1 tsp.	1 tsp.	1 tsp.	1 tsp.	1 tsp.
Afternoon					
Pizza made with:					
Mozzarella cheese	1 oz.	1 oz.	1 oz.	1 oz.	1 oz.
Tomato sauce					
Pizza crust	1 slice	1 slice	1 slice	1 slice	1 slice
Tossed salad	1 cup	1 cup	1 cup	1 cup	1 cup
Salad dressing	1 tsp.	1 tsp.	1 tsp.	1 tsp.	1 tsp.
Evening					
Peas and carrots	1 cup	1 cup	1 cup	1 cup	1 cup
Brown rice	½ cup	1 cup	1 cup	1 cup	1 cup
Baked seafood	3 oz.	4 oz.	5 oz.	6 oz.	7 oz.
Margarine	1 tsp.	1 tsp.	1 tsp.	1 tsp.	1 tsp.
Snack					
Fruit salad	1 cup	1 cup	1 cup	1 cup	2 cups
Morning					
Orange juice	6 oz.	6 oz.	6 oz.	6 oz.	6 oz.
French toast	1 slice	1 slice	2 slices	3 slices	3 slices
Margarine	1 tsp.	1 tsp.	1 tsp.	1 tsp.	1 tsp.
Syrup	1 tbsp.	1 tbsp.	1 tbsp.	1 tbsp.	1 tbsp.
Afternoon					
Cottage cheese	½ cup	½ cup	½ cup	½ cup	½ cup
Tossed salad	1 cup	1 cup	1 cup	1 cup	1 cup
Baked potato	1	1	1	1	1
Chili	4 oz.	8 oz.	8 oz.	8 oz.	8 oz.
Evening					
Broccoli and cauliflower	1 cup	1 cup	1 cup	1 cup	1 cup
Shrimp	1 oz.	2 oz.	3 oz.	4 oz.	5 oz.
Fried rice	½ cup	1 cup	1 cup	2 cups	2 cups
Dinner roll	—	—	1	1	1
Snack					
Fruit salad	1 cup	1 cup	1 cup	2 cups	2 cups

	Low-Fat Living				
	Total daily calories				
Meal	1,000	1,200	1,500	1,800	2,000
Morning					
Eggs	1	2	3	3	3
Grits	½ cup	½ cup	1 cup	1 cup	1 cup
Pancakes	1	2	2	3	3
Orange juice	6 oz.	6 oz.	6 oz.	6 oz.	6 oz.
Afternoon					
Fruit salad	1 cup	1 cup	1 cup	1 cup	2 cups
Yogurt	8 oz.	8 oz.	8 oz.	8 oz.	8 oz.
Grapenuts	—	—	—	¼ cup	¼ cup
Evening					
Tossed salad	1 cup	1 cup	1 cup	1 cup	1 cup
Baked beans	½ cup	½ cup	½ cup	½ cup	½ cup
Corn on cob	—	1	1	1	1
Potato salad	—	—	½ cup	1 cup	1 cup
BBQ chicken	2 oz.	2 oz.	2 oz.	3 oz.	3 oz.
Salad dressing	1 tsp.	1 tsp.	1 tsp.	1 tsp.	1 tsp.
Snack					
Fruit salad	1 cup	1 cup	1 cup	1 cup	2 cups

Menus reproduced with permission from Kathryn Parker, R.D. Copyright © 1992 Kathryn Parker, R.D.

Complex Carbohydrates

Complex carbohydrates are chiefly starches, such as potatoes, rice, pasta, bulgur, couscous, millet, corn, dried peas and beans, as well as fruits and vegetables. When consumed mainly in their unrefined state, these foods provide protein, dozens of vitamins and minerals, and plenty of dietary fiber. Fiber—the indigestible part of fruits, vegetables, and grains—has been found to confer numerous health benefits, including protection against colon cancer and possibly heart disease. There are two kinds of fiber: *water-insoluble fiber,* found predominantly in whole-wheat products, wheat bran, and fruit and vegetable skins, and *water-soluble fiber,* found in oat-bran cereals, oatmeal, dried peas and beans, and barley. Here's how a diet high in complex carbohydrates can help improve your health and well-being in your middle and later years:

In your premenopausal years: Complex carbohydrates may hold promise for women suffering from premenstrual and menopause-related mood swings and anxiety. New research on food and mood suggests that some of these problems may be partly managed by eating foods high in complex carbohydrates.

Foods containing proteins, and carbohydrates are instrumental in the formation of several central-nervous-system neurotransmitters believed to influence your moods. For instance, a meal high in carbohydrates raises brain levels of an amino acid called *tryptophan,* which in turn is converted into the neurotransmitter *serotonin.* Serotonin controls hormone secretions, sleep patterns, and perception of pain and has an overall calming effect. Low levels of serotonin have been associated with depression.

Protein, on the other hand, contains large amounts of the amino acid *tyrosine,* which competes with tryptophan for entry into the brain. Once tyrosine enters the brain, it increases levels of *dopamine* and *norepinephrine,* two neurotransmitters that make you feel more alert. At the same time, tryptophan levels fall, decreasing the brain's production of serotonin and its calming effect.

At least one study by Judith Wurtman, Ph.D., of the Massachusetts Institute of Technology in Cambridge has shown improvement of premenstrual symptoms with the intake of certain foods. In that study, nineteen PMS sufferers and nine control subjects lived at an MIT research center for three to five days during the premenstrual phase of their menstrual cycles and for two days in the postmenstrual weeks of their monthly cycles. For one part of the study, the women took standardized psychological tests to measure such moods as depression, anxiety, and anger. An hour later, they ate a large bowl of high-carbohydrate cornflakes together with low-protein artificial milk. An hour after eating the meal, the psychological tests were readministered to the women. During the premenstrual phase of the study, the PMS sufferers reported 43 percent less depression, 38 percent less confusion, 47 percent less fatigue, 42 percent less tension, and 69 percent less anger after eating the cornflakes. Moreover, these dramatic results occurred only among the PMS sufferers in the study and only during the premenstrual phase of the study. The control group of women reported no change in their mood after eating the cereal. Neither did the PMS sufferers when they ate cornflakes at other times during their menstrual cycle.

In other studies, men have reported feeling more drowsy after eating a high-carbohydrate meal compared with a high-protein meal. Their reaction time and motor performance was slower after the high-carbohydrate meal, too. In another study, women had more difficulty concentrating after a high-carbohydrate meal compared to a protein meal.

Keep in mind that the effects of food on your mood are subtle, and it's too early to tell whether diet alone can be used as a mood-enhancing drug. Some experts dispute the theory altogether, pointing out that other factors may be responsible for any changes in mood or mental performance. Even your body's biological (*circadian*) rhythms may influence you. For example, short-term memory peaks around 11:00 A.M. and reaches a low around 8:00 P.M. And stress stimulates hormones that reduce brain levels of tryptophan and serotonin.

Obviously, more research needs to be conducted before we fully understand the effects of certain foods on your mood. But if the theory proves to be valid, it soon may be possible to manage one of the most prevalent emotional complaints of women in the middle years—anxiety—through diet and exercise instead of tranquilizers.

In your postmenopausal years: The dietary fiber in complex carbohydrates takes on new importance in your postmenopausal years. Insoluble fiber is believed to help protect against colon cancer. This type of fiber is thought to dilute bile acids in the colon that are suspected of promoting cancer. And soluble fiber appears to reduce blood-cholesterol levels, in turn, reducing your risk of heart disease. In a Northwestern University study, volunteers on a low-fat diet who ate 35 grams of oat bran a day (equivalent to a bowl of oat-bran cereal and one or two oat-bran muffins), experienced a 3 percent drop in blood cholesterol, which translates into a 6 percent reduction in the risk of heart disease. Studies on men with *hypercholesterolemia*, dangerously high blood-cholesterol levels, showed that they experienced an even greater drop (about 19 percent) in blood-cholesterol levels by adding foods high in soluble fiber to their already low-fat diet. The University of Florida's James Cerda, M.D., found that pectin, a soluble fiber found primarily in citrus fruits, such as grapefruit, also lowers blood-cholesterol levels.

In your later years: Constipation becomes more problematic for older women as the muscles in the colon wall weaken with age and *gastrointestinal motility* (the transit of feces through the large intestine) declines. Water-insoluble fiber bulks up the stool and speeds its passage, helping to relieve constipation. Fiber also helps prevent hemorrhoids (swollen blood vessels in the rectum) and *diverticular disease*, a common problem among adults over age sixty caused by abnormal pouchlike sacs in the colon.

The National Cancer Institute and the American Dietetic Association recommend that you eat between 20 to 30 grams of fiber a day from a variety of foods to protect against colon cancer and other illnesses. No recommendations have been made for soluble fiber, since its value in lowering blood cholesterol is still being debated. And of course, the research on food and mood is too tentative to make any strong recommendations. However, complex carbohydrates are excellent nutrient-packed, low-fat substitutes for the fatty foods in your diet. By eating more of these foods, you simply can't go wrong.

Simple Ways to Increase Complex Carbohydrates

You can easily eat four or more servings of complex carbohydrates a day from whole-grain foods, fruits, and vegetables, and dried peas and beans. Stick with breads, cereals, rice, pasta, crackers, and other baked goods made from whole grains, which contain the most nutrients. One-half cup cooked cereal, pasta, rice, or beans, one cup ready-to-eat cereal, or one slice of bread equals one serving. Raw fruits and vegetables contain the most fiber, especially when you eat the skins, peels, pulp, and edible seeds.

Don't feel obligated to load up on special oat-bran products that promise to lower your blood-cholesterol level. More research needs to be conducted before any oat-bran products can make such claims. Besides, some of these products contain enough fat to cancel out any possible cholesterol-lowering effect, so check the label before you buy. As a general rule, eat a variety of foods rich in both soluble and insoluble fiber.

Again, as with most nutrients, more fiber isn't necessarily better. Too much fiber can bind to and hinder the body's absorption of calcium and other vitamins, minerals, and trace elements, so limit fiber to no more than 35 grams per day.

When increasing the fiber in your diet, do so gradually (a gram or two per day) and drink plenty of fluids to help prevent indigestion and gas.

Coping with Constipation

Constipation, characterized by small, hard stools, may well be the most common digestive complaint in the United States. Constipation is more common in the middle and later years, partly because as you grow older the turnover rate of cells lining the colon wall slows down. This slows the time it takes waste to pass through the colon, allowing more water to be absorbed through the colon wall and resulting in smaller, harder stools. In addition, the muscular wall of the colon begins to weaken, resulting in less of an urge to defecate. But many experts now believe that such lifestyle factors as a low-fiber diet, a sedentary lifestyle, and stress may contribute much more to constipation than normal aging.

Ironically, the over-the-counter laxatives sold to solve the problem often make it worse. Laxatives may empty the bowel so completely that it takes days before enough waste accumulates to trigger the urge to defecate. By then, you may be tempted to take more laxatives. Regular use of laxatives can also permanently weaken the natural muscular action of the bowels, making defecation more difficult. (For more on laxatives, see page 152.) Instead of relying on laxatives, try these remedies to help prevent common constipation.

• **Eat plenty of fiber-rich foods.** Fiber holds water and adds bulk and softness to the stool, allowing it to pass more easily and quickly through the colon.

• **Drink six to eight glasses of water a day.** Water helps keep stools soft and easy to pass.

• **Tune into prunes.** Eat three to four prunes before bedtime. Prunes are a natural laxative. By taking them at night, you'll help prepare your body for a morning bowel movement.

• **Schedule a regular time for a bowel movement every day.** This helps train your bowels to become more regular. In the beginning, you should make time for a bowel movement even if you don't feel the urge.

• **Increase your activity.** Walking, jogging, and bicycling are ideal exercises for stimulating the bowels.

• **Take laxatives only on your doctor's recommendation.**

What are the best sources of dietary fiber? Here are some likely choices.

	Serving portion	Total fiber (grams)	Soluble fiber (grams)
Cereals			
All Bran (Kellogg)	½ cup	12.9	2.1
Fiber One (General Mills)	½ cup	11.9	0.8
40% Bran Flakes	½ cup	4.3	0.3
Grapenuts (Post)	½ cup	5.6	1.6
Heartwise (Kellogg)	½ cup	2.8	1.4
Oat bran, cooked (Quaker)	¾ cup	4.0	2.2
Oat bran cereal, cold (Quaker)	¾ cup	2.9	1.5
Oatmeal, uncooked	⅓ cup	2.7	1.4
Raisin bran	¾ cup	5.3	0.9
Shredded wheat	⅔ cup	3.5	0.5
Breads			
Bagel, plain	½ bagel	0.7	0.3
Pita bread	½ pocket	0.5	0.2
Pumpernickel bread	1 slice	2.7	1.2
White bread	1 slice	0.6	0.3
Whole-wheat bread	1 slice	1.5	0.3
Fruits			
Apple, fresh (with skin)	1 medium	2.8	1.0
Blackberries, fresh	¾ cup	3.7	1.1
Cranberries, fresh	½ cup	1.6	0.5
Figs, dried	1½	2.3	1.1
Grapefruit, fresh	½ medium	1.4	0.9
Peaches, fresh (with skin)	1 medium	2.0	1.0
Pears, fresh (with skin)	1 small	2.9	1.1
Plums, red, fresh	2 medium	2.4	1.1
Prunes, stewed	¼ cup	1.6	0.9
Prunes, dried	3 medium	1.7	1.0
Raisins	2 tbsp.	0.4	0.2
Raspberries, fresh	1 cup	3.3	0.6
Strawberries, fresh	1¼ cup	1.8	0.6
Vegetables			
Asparagus, cooked	½ cup	1.8	0.7
Beets, canned, cooked	½ cup	2.2	0.7
Broccoli, cooked	½ cup	2.4	1.2
Brussels sprouts, cooked	½ cup	3.8	2.0
Cabbage, fresh	1 cup	1.5	0.6

	Serving portion	Total fiber (grams)	Soluble fiber (grams)
Vegetables			
Carrots, sliced, cooked	½ cup	2.0	1.1
Carrots, fresh	1 medium	2.3	1.1
Cauliflower, cooked	½ cup	1.0	0.4
Corn, whole kernel, cooked	½ cup	1.6	0.2
Kale, cooked	½ cup	2.5	0.7
Okra, frozen, cooked	½ cup	4.1	1.0
Peas, freen, frozen, cooked	½ cup	4.3	1.3
Potatoes, white, cooked (with skin)	½ cup	1.5	0.8
Spinach, cooked	½ cup	1.6	0.5
Sweet potato, cooked (flesh only)	⅓ cup	2.7	1.2
Zucchini, cooked	½ cup	1.2	0.5
Legumes (dried peas and beans)			
Butter beans, cooked	½ cup	6.9	2.7
Chickpeas, cooked	½ cup	4.3	1.3
Kidney beans, cooked	½ cup	6.9	2.8
Lima beans, cooked	½ cup	4.3	1.1
Lentils, cooked	½ cup	5.2	0.6
Pinto beans, cooked	½ cup	5.9	1.9
Split peas, cooked	½ cup	3.1	1.1

Note: Table excerpted with permission from James W. Anderson, *Plant Fiber in Foods*. Lexington, KY: HCF Nutrition Research Foundation, Inc., 1990. Copyright © 1990 by James W. Anderson, M.D.

Protein

The word *protein* comes from a Greek word meaning "of first importance." Indeed, proteins are the most abundant organic compounds in the body. Most of the protein in your body is in your muscles. Protein is also a major component of soft tissues, bones, teeth, blood, and other body fluids. Hormones and enzymes are proteins.

Amino acids are the building blocks of protein. Your body can produce adequate amounts of most of the amino acids it needs to function normally. But nine amino acids are considered "essential" because your body can't produce them by itself; they must be supplied by food. This is why a certain amount of protein in your diet is essential.

In your pre- and postmenopausal years: The problem for most women in the menopausal years isn't a lack of protein but, rather, an overabundance. Diets high in protein cause you to excrete calcium in your urine. A 50 percent increase in protein above the recommended 15 percent of your total daily calories is associated with a net calcium loss of 32 milligrams per day. Another concern: The two main sources of protein in the typical American diet—meat and dairy products—are also major sources of fat, which, as you know, can increase your risk of obesity, heart disease, and certain cancers.

In your later years: Some women over sixty-five may not get enough protein in their diets. Too little protein can compromise your immunity and can slow wound healing, which can be serious, particularly if you are hospitalized for surgery or other medical problems. Studies have shown that older women (and men) who don't eat enough calories and protein remain hospitalized longer and experience a higher rate of medical complications than well-nourished patients.

Since animal proteins (meat and dairy products) are also good sources of calcium, iron, B vitamins, and trace minerals, older women who don't eat enough protein risk developing deficiencies in these nutrients, as well.

How to Get Enough (but Not Too Much) Protein

About 15 percent of your total daily calories should come from protein (67 grams of protein for someone on an 1,800 calories-a-day diet). The meat group, which includes beef, poultry, fish, eggs, cheese, and milk, is a primary source of protein in our diet, as well as an excellent source of iron, niacin, thiamine, vitamin B_{12}, and some trace minerals. Animal proteins are also considered "complete"—that is, they contain most or all of the nine essential amino acids you need. The downside is that meat and whole dairy products also contain a lot of fat and cholesterol, so choose low-fat meats and dairy products (see page 61).

Protein: Meeting Your Daily Need

If you eat meat . . .

3 8-ounce glasses skim milk (8.4 g protein × 3)	= 25.2
2 ounces water-packed tuna	= 16.7
3.5 ounces chicken (½ breast)	= 26.7
TOTAL	= 68.6

If you are a vegetarian (lacto-ovo):

3 8-ounce glasses skim milk (8.4 g protein × 3)	= 25.2
Salad topped with 1 boiled egg and 2 ounces feta cheese	= 14.1
1 cup cooked lentils with ½ cup cooked brown rice	= 26.8
TOTAL	= 66.1

If you are a strict vegetarian (vegan):

2 tbsp. peanut butter on 2 slices whole-wheat bread	= 12.5
½ cup tofu	= 10.0
1 cup cooked split peas with ½ cup cooked brown rice	= 25.3
Salad topped with ½ cup cooked chickpeas and 1 ounce sunflower seeds	= 13.7
½ cup lentil soup	= 8.9
TOTAL	= 70.4

Certain vegetables, particularly dried peas and beans, are excellent stand-ins for meat because they are high in protein *and* low in fat. A cup of lentils, for instance, contains slightly more protein than two ounces of ground beef and virtually none of the fat and cholesterol. Remember, though, that protein from vegetables is "incomplete" and usually must be eaten together with other vegetables and/or grains to ensure that you're getting the full complement of amino acids. (For more on protein complementation and vegetarianism, see page 92.)

How much protein do you need? If you're healthy, two two- to three-ounce servings of lean meat or a meat substitute (such as tofu or dried peas and beans), together with protein from milk, is all the protein you'll need each day. If you eat meat, choose fish and chicken with the skin removed over red meat, and lean cuts of red meat over fatty ones (see page 61). Also choose low-fat or nonfat milk and dairy products. If you're a strict vegetarian (no meat, fish, dairy products, or eggs), you should increase the number of protein servings to three or four.

Sodium

Sodium, a main component of table salt, is needed to maintain your body's blood volume and fluid balance. Your cells need sodium to help exchange nutrients and waste across the cell walls. Sodium also aids in the transmission of nerve impulses. But too much sodium can cause problems. Here are some good reasons to cut back on sodium now:

In your premenopausal years: Too much sodium may contribute to fluid retention (including breast swelling and tenderness, bloating, and possibly even premenstrual irritability), particularly just before your period. Decreasing the sodium in your diet—especially in the week or two preceding your period—can be just as effective as taking a diuretic, with none of the side effects associated with the use of diuretics (see page 153).

Even if you don't experience premenstrual fluid retention, there's another reason to cut back: Sodium can cause your body to excrete calcium in the urine—the more sodium you consume, the more sodium and calcium you excrete.

In your postmenopausal years: A low-sodium diet can reduce your risk of developing high blood pressure, heart and vascular disease, and kidney disease. A diet low in salt-cured and smoked foods (such as pickles, hot dogs, and cold cuts) appears to lower your risk of stomach cancer, as well. And, because high-sodium diets may cause you to excrete calcium, reducing your sodium intake will make it easier for you to maintain positive calcium balance.

In your later years: Women over age sixty-five are even more prone to develop hypertension than younger women. Many people find that simply cutting back on sodium is enough to keep blood pressure in check.

According to the recommended dietary allowances, you can get by with a minimum of 500 milligrams of sodium a day (the amount in a pinch of table salt). However, most Americans consume from 3,000 to 6,000 milligrams of sodium a day, not just from the salt shaker but from hidden sodium in processed snacks, prepackaged foods, and fast foods.

How to Decrease the Sodium in Your Diet

1. **Substitute herbs and spices** or a salt substitute for salt when cooking.

2. **Omit salt in recipes** and instead sprinkle a little on the food on your plate. Studies show that you'll use considerably less salt this way.

3. **Use yeast in baking** instead of baking powder or soda.

4. **Avoid processed and fast foods,** which are usually high in sodium. If you must buy processed foods, look for low-salt or no-salt versions. (Check the label before you buy!)

5. **Avoid smoked, processed or cured meats and fish,** such as ham, bacon, corned beef, hot dogs, pickled herring, and anchovies.

6. **Buy unsalted potato chips, nuts, and other snack foods**. Better yet, have a piece of fruit or raw vegetables.

Calcium

Your bones, which contain 99 percent of the calcium in your body, need calcium for *mineralization* (the process by which newly formed bone becomes hard). The other 1 percent of calcium that circulates in your bloodstream is critical for muscle contraction, blood clotting, blood pressure regulation, and nerve-impulse transmission. Indeed, if you don't get enough calcium from your diet to maintain adequate levels of calcium in your bloodstream, your body will take it from your bones. Calcium becomes even more important to your diet as you grow older and biological changes increase your need for this mineral.

In your premenopausal years: Around age thirty-five, you reach skeletal maturity, also known as *peak bone mass*. After that, you begin losing skeletal bone faster than your body can build it back up, a process called *bone remodeling*. The bone-remodeling process is complex, and calcium is just one of many factors that influence bone health (see page 339). But one way to help offset this gradual loss of bone mass is to get enough calcium in your diet.

If you're over thirty-five, you need as much calcium as you needed as a teenager—possibly more. For reasons that aren't entirely understood, it becomes more difficult for you to maintain calcium balance (that is, take in and absorb more calcium than your body excretes) as you grow older. Whereas children absorb up to 75 percent of calcium—particularly during growth spurts—adults absorb only 30 to 50 percent of the calcium they take in.

In your postmenopausal years: Calcium becomes even more critical to your bone health after menopause, when declining estrogen levels make it even more difficult for you to maintain positive calcium balance. (Estrogen helps your body absorb calcium.) In addition, aging skin produces less vitamin D, which also aids in calcium absorption.

As we mentioned earlier, calcium isn't the *only* contributor to strong bones, but it is an important part of maintaining bone health. One Tufts

University study showed that menopausal women whose calcium intake was fewer than 400 milligrams a day significantly reduced bone loss by increasing their calcium intake to 800 milligrams a day. A 1993 study by New Zealand researchers demonstrated that even postmenopausal women whose calcium intake before taking supplements is close to the 800-milligram recommended dietary allowance can slow bone loss by taking a 1,000-milligram calcium supplement.

There are two other good reasons to get the calcium you need in your postmenopausal years. There's evidence that calcium may protect against both high blood pressure and colon cancer. Population studies from the National Center for Health Statistics showed that the incidence of hypertension was less than one percent among people who consumed more than 1,000 milligrams of calcium a day. People in the study who had hypertension, on the other hand, consumed an average of 18 percent less calcium than healthy people.

In your later years: Even older women need plenty of calcium in their diets to maintain bone health. Older women are susceptible not only to osteoporosis but also to *osteomalacia*, a condition of decreased bone mineralization caused by a severe lack of vitamin D. When not enough calcium and vitamin D are available for normal bone maintenance, the bones gradually weaken and fractures frequently result.

The recommended dietary allowance for calcium is 800 milligrams per day. However, most experts now recommend that *all* women in midlife consume even more calcium than this. To protect your bones, you'll need 1,000 milligrams of elemental calcium per day if you are premenopausal, 1,200 milligrams per day if you are perimenopausal (forty-five to fifty-five years old), and 1,400 milligrams per day if you are postmenopausal.

Most women *don't* get enough calcium in their diets. Among one hundred postmenopausal women we studied, more than half did not meet the 800 milligram RDA for calcium. Only 12 percent met the desired RDA of 1,400 milligrams of calcium that most experts now recommend for postmenopausal women. According to government studies, the average woman consumes a mere 450 milligrams of calcium a day—just a third of what she needs. This creates a *negative calcium balance* of 40 milligrams per day, which translates into a bone loss of 1.5 percent per year. At this rate, a woman who experiences menopause at age fifty will have lost 15 percent of her bone mass by the time she is sixty.

How to Get More Calcium in Your Diet

It doesn't matter *where* your calcium comes from—only that you get enough of it every day. (To find out how much dietary calcium you're consuming now, fill out the Calcium Questionnaire on pages 78–82. Use the questionnaire as a guide to calcium-rich foods, as well.) Contrary to the belief that calcium from dairy products is better absorbed than calcium in supplements, several studies now show that it's the *amount* of calcium and not the source that determines whether you maintain calcium balance. Some types of calcium supplements may even be absorbed *better* than food. The important thing is to *take in enough calcium on a regular basis to create a positive calcium balance.*

Increasing your calcium intake by eating high-calcium foods should still be your first priority. Food provides other valuable nutrients not found in supplements. Moreover, high doses of almost *any* supplement can cause nutrient imbalances. (Large doses of calcium supplements may interfere with iron absorption and can slow the bone-remodeling cycle.)

Low-fat dairy products, such as skim milk, low-fat yogurt, and nonfat dry milk, are excellent sources of calcium. A single eight-ounce carton of low-fat yogurt contains 452 milligrams of calcium—nearly half of a perimenopausal woman's requirement. Plus, the lactose in milk appears to help your body absorb calcium better.

Dairy products are by no means the only good source of calcium, however. Green leafy vegetables (except spinach, chard, sorrel, beet greens, parsley, and rhubarb, whose calcium is bound up and not very available), shellfish, almonds, Brazil nuts, tofu (made with calcium sulfate), and small fish (such as sardines with their bones) are high in calcium. Added to these natural sources are many fortified foods, including orange juice (Minute Maid), calcium-fortified breads, and even calcium-fortified milk (Calcimilk). There are a few simple things you can do to increase the amount of calcium in your food, as well.

Some foods hinder calcium absorption or cause your body to excrete it. Watch out for the following calcium robbers in your diet:

Fiber: Dietary fiber binds calcium and prevents its absorption, so limit your fiber intake to no more than 35 grams per day. If you are using calcium supplements, take them at least one hour before or two hours after eating a high-fiber meal.

Protein: Remember, a high-protein diet causes you to excrete calcium in your urine (see page 71).

Phosphorus: No one is sure what effect phosphorus has on calcium absorption. Early reports stating that too much phosphorus inhibits calcium absorption proved to be untrue. However, excessive consumption of phosphorus-containing foods (particularly soft drinks, red meat, and processed foods containing phosphorus additives) may contribute to an increase in bone-dissolving parathyroid hormone (see page 354) and in an indirect way may lead to the development of low bone mass. Until we know more, it would be wise to keep your phosphorus intake down. (One way to reduce the phosphorus and increase calcium in your diet is to substitute milk for high-phosphorus soft drinks.)

Sodium: High-sodium diets cause your body to excrete calcium. Unfortunately, many dairy products contain substantial amounts of sodium, and women advised to cut back on sodium inadvertently also cut back on some of the best sources of calcium in their diets. If you're concerned about sodium in dairy products, choose low-sodium cheeses.

Caffeine: Drinking more than five cups of coffee per day makes it harder for you to maintain positive calcium balance; a high caffeine intake causes you to excrete calcium. So limit your consumption of coffee and other caffeinated beverages and foods.

How to Boost the Calcium Content of Foods

1. **Make your own soup.** By adding a small amount of vinegar when preparing stock from bones, the vinegar will dissolve the calcium from the bones, making a single pint of your homemade soup equal to a quart or more of milk in calcium content. The vinegar also tenderizes the meat and reduces the cooking time. As the stock is boiled, the calcium combines with the vinegar and the vinegary taste disappears.

2. **Use vinegar to tenderize bone-containing meats before cooking.** Again, cooking time is reduced and the vinegary taste disappears after cooking. Pour the remaining meat juices (which contain most of the dissolved calcium) over the meat as a light gravy.

3. **Sprinkle shredded or grated cheese over vegetables instead of butter.** Parmesan cheese is especially good for adding both calcium and taste.

4. **Garnish soups or salads with cubes of cheese or tofu** to enhance their taste and nutritional value.

5. **When making a salad, use deep-green lettuce leaves,** which are richer in calcium and vitamins A, C, E, and B, folic acid, and other minerals than pale lettuce leaves.

6. **When pickling fruits or vegetables, use calcium chloride instead of sodium chloride** (table salt). Calcium chloride is more effective and more nutritious.

7. **Add powdered nonfat, dry milk to everything you can.** It makes skim milk, coffee, and tea "thicker" and creamier, and enhances the flavor of cream soups and casseroles. Every teaspoon you use gives you 50 milligrams of calcium and no fat.

8. **When baking bread, cakes, cookies, or muffins, add powdered nonfat milk** (about ¼ cup) to the recipe to boost the calcium content. No one will be the wiser.

9. **When choosing a brand of tofu, make sure its ingredient label includes calcium sulfate rather than sodium chloride.**

Note: Text in list above adapted with permission from Morris Notelovitz and Marsha Ware. *Stand Tall: The Informed Woman's Guide to Preventing Osteoporosis.* Gainesville, FL: Triad Publishing Company, 1982. Copyright © 1982 by Morris Notelovitz, M.D., Ph.D.

For each of the following foods you consumed in the last three days, estimate the total amount for each day and write it in columns 1, 2, and 3 (e.g., ½ cup, 6 oz., 5 tbsp., etc.). Then calculate your total calcium intake for the three days by multiplying the amount of calcium in a single serving by the number of servings you had. Add up the total amount of calcium you ate, then divide that number by 3. This will give you an estimate of your daily calcium intake. Compare your daily intake with the recommended intakes for women at the end of the questionnaire.

....
Dairy Products
....

	Serving size	Calcium (mg)	1	2	3	Total
Milk						
Whole	1 cup	288				
Low-fat (2%)	1 cup	352				
Skim and Buttermilk	1 cup	296				
Nonfat, dry	¼ cup	220				
Chocolate	1 cup	278				
Condensed, sweetened	1 cup	802				
Evaporated	1 cup	635				
Lactimilk	1 cup	300				
Cheese						
Swiss	1 oz.	262				
Cheddar and Provolone	1 oz.	213				
Edam	1 oz.	207				
Monterey Jack and Mozzarella	1 oz.	200				
Muenster	1 oz.	200				
American and Gouda	1 oz.	198				

Dairy Products

	Serving size	Calcium (mg)	1	2	3	Total
Cheese (cont.)						
Brick	1 oz.	191				
Velveeta (cheese food) 2 tbsp. =	1 oz.	162				
Romano	1 oz.	156				
Blue	1 oz.	150				
Parmesan	1 oz.	136				
Feta	1 oz.	100				
Ricotta (skim)	1 oz.	84				
Ricotta (whole)	1 oz.	65				
Brie	1 oz.	52				
Camembert	1 oz.	30				
Cottage (low-fat)	1 cup	204				
Cottage (regular)	1 cup	131				
Other						
Ice cream (hard)	1 cup	194				
Ice cream (soft)	1 cup	253				
Ice milk (hard)	1 cup	204				
Pudding (instant)	1 cup	374				
Pudding (cooked)	1 cup	265				
Custard (baked)	1 cup	297				
Yogurt (low-fat, plain)	1 cup	452				
Yogurt (low-fat, fruited)	1 cup	313				
Yogurt (whole-milk)	1 cup	275				
Yogurt (frozen)	1 cup	220				

Seafood

	Serving size	Calcium (mg)	1	2	3	Total
Clams, canned (solid/liquid)	8 oz.	121				
Mackerel, canned (solid/liquid)	8 oz.	552				
Oyster stew (milk, 6 oysters)	1 cup	274				
Salmon, sockeye, canned (solid, liquid w/bones)	8 oz.	587				
Sardines, canned (w/bones)	4 med.	69				

Vegetables and Nuts

	Serving size	Calcium (mg)	1	2	3	Total
Broccoli (frozen, chopped, cooked)	1 cup	100				
Bok choy (chopped, cooked)	1 cup	250				
Collards (frozen, chopped, cooked)	1 cup	299				
Kale (frozen, chopped, cooked)	1 cup	157				
Mustard greens (frozen, chopped, cooked)	1 cup	156				
Turnip greens (frozen, chopped, cooked)	1 cup	195				
Beans, all types (dry, cooked, canned, solid/liquid)	1 cup	80				
Almonds (shelled, chopped)	1 cup	304				
Brazil nuts (8 med. nuts)	1 oz.	50				

Vegetables and Nuts

	Serving size	Calcium (mg)	1	2	3	Total
Pecans (shelled, chopped)	1 cup	86				
Peanuts (shelled)	1 cup	104				
Mixed nuts and dry-roasted peanuts	1 cup	96				
Tahini (sesame butter)	1 tbsp.	64				
Walnuts, English (shelled, chopped)	1 cup	119				

Miscellaneous

	Serving size	Calcium (mg)	1	2	3	Total
Tofu	1 oz.	36				
Soybeans, sprouted (steamed)	1 cup	54				
Sunflower seeds (hulled)	1 cup	174				
Cream soups (made with milk)	1 cup	184				
Macaroni and cheese (homemade)	1 cup	362				
Pizza (frozen w/cheese)	4.5-inch arc	89				
Carob flour	1 cup	480				
Molasses, blackstrap	1 tbsp.	137				

Calcium-Fortified Foods

	Serving size	Calcium (mg)	1	2	3	Total
Minute Maid orange juice	1 cup	320				
CalciMilk	1 cup	500				

Total Calcium   _____

Average Daily Calcium Intake   _____
(Divide Total Calcium by 3)

RECOMMENDED CALCIUM INTAKE FOR WOMEN

Age	Recommended daily intake (mg)
Children (ages 1–10)	800
Adolescents (age 11–18)	1,200
Pregnant/lactating women over age 20	1,200
Premenopause (to age 35, with functioning ovaries)	800–1,000
Perimenopause (age 35–50, with functioning ovaries)	1,000–1,200
Postmenopausal (natural or surgical menopause)	1,400–2,000

Note: Calcium Questionnaire copyright © 1993 by Morris Notelovitz, M.D., Ph.D. This form may not be duplicated without the written permission of Morris Notelovitz, M.D., Ph.D.

Iron

Iron helps your red blood cells deliver oxygen to your body's tissues. If you don't get enough iron in your diet, you risk developing iron-deficiency anemia, a condition marked by low energy, fatigue, and increased susceptibility to infection. On the other hand, there's evidence to suggest that *high* levels of stored iron—what's known as *ferritin*—may increase your risk of heart disease (see page 326), so, again, more isn't necessarily better.

In your premenopausal years: You're more likely to develop an iron deficiency in the years just preceding menopause than after menopause, particularly if you experience heavy, irregular bleeding.

In your postmenopausal years: Our research has shown that iron deficiency isn't a problem for most postmenopausal women (see Table 3.2, on page 35).

In your later years: Iron-deficiency anemia may become a problem for some older women, usually because they fail to get enough iron in their diets.

Although the recommended dietary allowance (RDA) for iron has been reduced from 18 milligrams to 15 milligrams (before age fifty-one), most premenopausal women still don't get enough. Nutrition surveys suggest that women consume just 10 to 11 milligrams of iron a day. And from 15 to 20 percent of older women have lower than normal iron levels, even though the RDA for iron among women age fifty-one and older drops to 10 milligrams.

How to Increase the Iron in Your Diet

If you are premenopausal or over sixty-five, you can increase the amount of iron in your diet by following these guidelines:

Iron-Rich Foods

	Serving size	Iron (mg)
Meat (heme) sources		
Beef liver, cooked	3.5 oz.	6.7
Beef, lamb, pork, veal, cooked	3.5 oz.	2.8
Chicken or turkey, cooked	3.5 oz.	1.5
Eggs	1 whole	1.0
Yolk	1	.9
Clams	3 oz.	11.8
Oysters	6 medium	5.6
Vegetable (nonheme) sources		
Baked beans	1 cup	5.0
Black beans, boiled	1 cup	3.6
Chickpeas, boiled	1 cup	4.7
Lentils, boiled	1 cup	6.5
Lima beans, cooked	1 cup	4.5
Apricots, dried	10 halves	1.6
Figs, dried	5	2.0
Prunes, dried	5	1.0
Bread, enriched or whole-grain	2 slices	1.7
Greens, all types, cooked	½ cup	1.5
Peas, fresh or frozen	½ cup	1.5

• **Eat foods rich in iron.** Iron comes in two forms: *heme* and *nonheme*. Heme iron, found mostly in meat, is more readily absorbed by the body than nonheme iron, the chief type of iron in vegetables. From 2 to 10 percent of the iron in vegetables is absorbed by the body, compared with 10 to 30 percent of the iron in animal protein. Good sources of heme iron include lean red meat, pork, liver, and the dark meat of poultry. Foods high in nonheme iron include dried fruits, beans, nuts, iron-fortified cereals and breads, and blackstrap molasses.

• **Eat vitamin C–rich foods with every meal.** One way to enhance your body's absorption of both types of iron is to eat foods high in vitamin C along with iron-rich foods. These include citrus fruits, tomatoes, strawberries, melons, peppers, potatoes, and green leafy vegetables (broccoli, kale, mustard greens).

• **Use cast-iron skillets when cooking acidic foods such as tomato sauce and vegetable soup.** Small amounts of iron from the pan dissolve in the acids during cooking and add iron to the food.

• **Avoid substances that decrease iron absorption.** These include the food preservative ethylenediamine tetraacetic acid (EDTA) in soft drinks, and tannic acid in tea and coffee. Substances containing carbonate or phosphate, such as certain calcium supplements, may also inhibit iron absorption, so wait an hour or two after eating an iron-rich meal to take calcium supplements.

If your doctor finds that you have low iron stores (see page 34) or iron-deficiency anemia, you may need to take an iron supplement, as well (see page 89).

Vitamins

Certain vitamins take on increasing importance in your middle and later years.

In your premenopausal years: If you experience premenstrual mood swings, *pyridoxine,* more commonly known as vitamin B_6, may have a positive effect on your mood. Vitamin B_6 is instrumental in the formation of serotonin, and serotonin levels fall in people suffering from a vitamin B_6 deficiency. This may explain why some women who have other signs of a vitamin B_6 deficiency also report feeling depressed. When these women are treated with B_6 supplements (20 to 40 milligrams a day), the depression subsides.

In experimental animals, researchers have noticed interactions between vitamin B_6 and estrogen receptors, suggesting that vitamin B_6 may be somehow related to the hormonal fluctuations of the menstrual cycle. Estrogen in birth-control pills affects the body's metabolism of vitamin B_6, creating an increased need for vitamin B_6 among oral-contraceptive users. Indeed, low levels of vitamin B_6 may explain why some women who take oral contraceptives experience depression. Some studies suggest that the mood swings associated with PMS may also be helped by taking vitamin B_6.

In your postmenopausal years: Vitamins A, C, E, and the trace mineral selenium are *antioxidants,* which may help protect against what many experts believe to be a major cause of aging and disease: oxygen-free radicals. Free radicals are highly charged particles that are missing one electron. They occur naturally in the environment and are formed in your body as a by-product of metabolism. These unstable molecules literally bombard the cells in your body in an attempt to pair up with another electron to make up for the missing one. The force of the collision can damage cell membranes, impairing the cell's ability to function properly. Free radicals can also damage DNA, the genetic blueprint in every cell, crippling the cell's ability to reproduce, or creating a carcinogenic mutation that is passed down to new cells when the damaged cell divides.

Liver spots, skin wrinkles, and hardening of the arteries may be partly due to the damaging effects of free radicals on collagen and other connective tissues. Much of the tissue damage after a heart attack is believed to be caused by the release of free radicals around the heart muscle. Tissue damage from inflammatory diseases, such as rheumatoid arthritis, may also be caused by free radicals. And, of course, the uncontrolled growth of cancer cells may be touched off by cell damage due to free radicals. New research is linking *oxidized LDL cholesterol* (LDL cholesterol that has been damaged by free radicals) to the formation of artery-clogging plaques that can lead to a heart attack (see page 310).

Antioxidants bind to and neutralize free radicals, rendering them harmless. Vitamin E is probably the most effective antioxidant. This fat-soluble vitamin, present in all cell membranes, soaks up free radicals before they can attack the cell membrane and disrupt the cell's function or damage its DNA. Vitamin E has been found to delay the development of liver spots. Animal studies have shown that Vitamin E can increase resistance to cancer cells and protect against tissue damage caused by inflammation. It has also been found to protect against the tissue damage apparently caused by free radicals that form when the blood supply to the heart is disrupted. When blood flow is restored after bypass surgery, tissue damage is reduced when vitamin E is given at the same time.

Vitamin A and its derivatives—particularly *carotenoids*—pigments in green and yellow vegetables that are converted to vitamin A in the body—are thought to protect against cancer of the lung, colon, breast, pancreas, stomach, bladder, prostate, uterus, and cervix. Several population studies have suggested that people with high blood levels of *beta carotene* (the most common carotenoid) are at a lower risk of developing lung cancer and melanoma, a deadly form of skin cancer. Beta carotene may protect against heart disease, too. In a six-year study of 333 male physicians with heart disease, those who took 50 milligrams of beta carotene supplement every other day had a 50 percent lower rate of heart attack and stroke. The researchers suspect beta carotene may neutralize the damaging effects of oxidized LDL cholesterol on the artery wall.

Vitamin C appears to short-circuit free radicals. For instance, ascorbic acid blocks production of *nitrosamines,* powerful cancer-promoting compounds formed by nitrates in foods (such as hot dogs) and acids in the digestive tract. Vitamin C also works together with vitamin E to break the chain reaction that free radicals have on fats, particularly oxidized LDL cholesterol in the bloodstream.

Although it is *not* an antioxidant, another vitamin of increasing importance in your postmenopausal years is vitamin D. Vitamin D is probably best known for its role in keeping bones strong. Vitamin D helps regulate calcium levels in your body by increasing absorption of calcium in the intestines and increasing the reabsorption of calcium through the kidneys. In addition, high levels of vitamin D—like calcium—have been associated with possible protection against colon cancer. New evidence suggests that vitamin D may play a role in reducing the risk of breast cancer, as well. Breast-cancer patients with vitamin D receptors in their breast tissue have been found to survive longer than those without vitamin D receptors. When vitamin D is added to breast-cancer cells in a culture dish, the cancer's growth is inhibited. Frank Garland, Ph.D., and his colleagues at the University of California at San Diego have now correlated a decreased incidence of breast cancer among women who live in areas that receive more exposure to ultraviolet light. Cities with the lowest levels of ultraviolet light also had the highest mortality rates from breast cancer. The lowest mortality rates from breast cancer were in the sunny South and Southwest United States (17 to 19 per 100,000); the highest were in the Northeast (33 per 100,000). While the researchers concede that there are many different causes of breast cancer, they suspect that vitamin D may somehow play a protective role.

In your later years: The reduced energy needs of older women, together with age-related changes in the absorption and metabolism of nutrients, may contribute to an increased risk of developing marginal deficiencies of vitamins

C, D, the B vitamins, folic acid, and the trace mineral zinc. Many of the so-called "normal" vision changes associated with aging, such as deteriorating night vision (slow adaptation of the eyes to darkness) improve when vitamin A supplements are taken. And mental and behavioral changes, such as depression, anorexia, and irritability, may be partially caused by vitamin B deficiencies. Folic-acid deficiency, common among older women, can result in a vitamin-deficiency anemia known as *hyperchromic megaloblastic anemia.*

Older women also have a much harder time getting enough vitamin D, particularly those living at higher latitudes during the winter months, when sun exposure is limited. One study of ours, which compared blood levels of vitamin D among women living in Finland and in Florida, found that the women living in Florida had twice the levels of vitamin D in the springtime as the Finnish women. Another study of a group of postmenopausal women in Boston showed that one-half of them became vitamin D–deficient during the winter months. Vitamin D deficiency is also partly due to an age-related decline in the skin's production of vitamin D. As we mentioned earlier, a vitamin D deficiency can compromise bone health and increase your risk of developing both osteoporosis and osteomalacia.

Should You Be Taking Vitamin and Mineral Supplements?

With the exception of calcium, vitamin D, iron, and, for some premenopausal women, Vitamin B_6, most healthy women *won't* need to take vitamin supplements. Your first line of action should be to increase your intake of vitamins and minerals through foods (particularly fruits and vegetables), since food also provides other nutrients not found in supplements, such as fiber and water. Also, the protective effects attributed to certain nutrients, such as beta carotene, may be the result of other nutrients in foods. Another problem with supplements is that taking high doses of one vitamin or mineral may interfere with the body's use of another. For instance, large doses of vitamin E can hinder the body's absorption and use of vitamin K, which aids collagen formation in bones and helps blood clotting.

Calcium

Even the most calcium-conscious women will find that it's almost impossible to get the amount of calcium they need from food alone. And calcium supplements provide an excellent, calorie-free way to close the gap between your calcium intake from food and the daily amount you need to maintain positive calcium balance. Supplements may be the only way to assure adequate calcium intake for women with *lactose intolerance.* These women lack the stomach enzyme *lactase*, which helps break down the milk sugar lactose. As a result, they often suffer cramps, gas, and bloating when they eat dairy products.

There are several types of calcium supplements, but not all contain the same amount of calcium. For instance, 500 milligrams of calcium carbonate contains just 200 milligrams of elemental calcium (see A Guide to Calcium Supplements on the next page). What's more, not all supplements are equal in terms of "bioavailability," so you should submit your supplements to the acid test on page 90. Here's a sampling of some of the more common types of calcium supplements:

Calcium citrate: (Citracal) The quickest to dissolve and best absorbed of the most common types of supplemental calcium. It is most quickly absorbed when taken on an empty stomach.

Calcium carbonate: (Tums, Os-Cal 500) The most widely used ingredient in calcium supplements, calcium carbonate is usually the least expensive

A Guide to Calcium Supplements

Generic name (brand names appear in parentheses)	Total calcium per tablet (mg)	Elemental calcium (mg)	Number of tablets to provide 1,000 mg of calcium
Calcium carbonate	625	250	4
(BioCal, Calcarb 600,	650	260	4
Calci-Chew, Calciday 667	750	300	4
Calcilac, Calcium 600	835	334	3
Calglycine, Caltrate 600	1,250	500	2
Chooz, Dicarbosil,	1,500	600	2
Gencalc, Malamint, Nephro-Calci, Os-Cal 500, Os-Cal 500 Chewable, Oysco, Oscyo 500 Chewable, Oyst-Cal 500, Oyst-Cal 500 Chewable, Ostercal 500, Rolaids Calcium Rich, Super Calcium 1200, Titralac, Tums, Tums E-X)			
Calcium citrate (Citracal)	950	200	5
Calcium gluconate (Kalcinate)	500	45	22
	650	58	17
	1,000	90	11
Calcium lactate	325	42	24
	650	84	12
Calcium phosphate, dibasic	500	115	9
Calcium phosphate, tribasic (Posture)	800	304	4
	1,600	608	2

Note: Table adapted with permission of the publisher from "Calcium Supplements," in *The Complete Drug Reference*, Yonkers, N.Y.: Consumer Reports Books, 1991. Copyright © 1991 by Consumers Union of U.S., Inc., Yonkers, N.Y. 10703-1057.

and contains the highest amount of calcium per tablet. It dissolves quickly, as well. For better absorption, take with foods containing citric acids and/or a glass of orange juice. Studies suggest that citric acid may react with calcium carbonate to form calcium citrate in the stomach.

Calcium phosphate: (Posture) One of the least soluble and least bioavailable preparations, according to laboratory studies.

Calcium lactate: Dissolves more reliably than calcium carbonate. Since it has less elemental calcium (only 13 percent elemental calcium), you may need to take more tablets.

Calcium gluconate: Again, more soluble than calcium carbonate but less concentrated (only 9 percent elemental calcium), so you'll need to take more tablets to get the same amount of calcium.

Calcium chloride: Good for pickling but bad as a supplement, calcium chloride tends to irritate the stomach.

Chelated calcium: Although chelated supplements are supposed to improve absorption, there's no evidence that they're better absorbed than nonchelated supplements.

Bonemeal and dolomite: High in calcium, but in the past have been found to be contaminated with toxic metals.

Calcium levulinate, calcium ascorbonate, and **calcium orotate:** Other forms of calcium on the market.

Vitamin D

Your primary source of vitamin D is the sun; about 75 percent of the vitamin D in your body is produced in the skin with the help of ultraviolet radiation from the sun, then activated in the liver and kidneys (hence the name the "sunshine" vitamin). The only problem is that there's no way to measure how much you are getting. The amount of vitamin D you receive depends on the length of time you are exposed to the sun, the sun's intensity, atmospheric conditions, and whether you use a sunscreen, which blocks the ultraviolet rays your body needs to manufacture vitamin D. Some experts estimate that a Caucasian woman needs between fifteen minutes to one hour of unprotected sun exposure daily to meet her vitamin D requirement. Keep in mind that overexposure of your skin to the sun can increase your risk of skin cancer (see page 401). You are probably the best judge of whether or not you are getting enough sunshine on a regular basis.

Vitamin D in the diet is fairly limited: fatty fish, butter, eggs, liver, and fortified milk are the best sources.

Most multivitamin preparations contain the 400 units you need each day. But don't overdo it, as too much vitamin D can stimulate bone loss. You should avoid amounts in excess of 1,000 units per day.

Iron

You'll need an iron supplement only if you're found to have an iron deficiency. The most widely used iron supplement is a form of iron called *ferrous sulfate*. It is best absorbed on an empty stomach; however, this often causes stomach upsets. Taking your supplement with a glass of vitamin C–rich orange juice and a little food will both increase your body's absorption of the iron and reduce the likelihood of stomach irritation.

Iron supplements sometimes cause constipation. However, a number of nonconstipating supplements are now available, including Dual Action Ferro-Sequels, Slow FE, Ferancee-HP tablets, Mol-Iron tablets, and Tabron.

You can expect to feel better and have more energy after just three weeks of taking iron supplements. However, your doctor will probably recommend that you continue taking the supplements for six to twelve months to help replenish your iron stores.

Vitamin B$_6$

Premenopausal women who take birth-control pills or who experience premenstrual mood swings may want to consider taking a vitamin B$_6$ supplement. You should be aware, however, that large doses of vitamin B$_6$ (more than 1 gram per day over a period of months) can cause nerve damage, including a tingling sensation or numbness in the hands and feet and an unsteady gait. If you take vitamin B_6, limit your dose to no more than 50 milligrams daily. Better yet, take vitamin B_6 as part of a vitamin B complex, since taking high doses of one B vitamin can result in imbalances of others.

Fluids

Fluids aren't listed in the recommended dietary allowances for women, but they're essential to maintaining your health in the middle and later years. Water is a major part of every cell and is crucial in transporting nutrients to all the cells in your body and in carrying away wastes. It also helps you maintain an even body temperature. Indeed, you can live without food for weeks, but you'd die in a matter of days without water.

Drinking plenty of fluids is especially important in your later years, when inadequate fluid intake, decreased kidney function, and use of drugs that enhance water loss, such as diuretics, all increase the risk of dehydration. Drinking plenty of fluids (five to eight glasses a day) actually improves kidney function, aids digestion, and helps control constipation, which so frequently plagues older women.

Caffeine

Caffeine is not a nutrient; it's a powerful stimulant to the central nervous system and is found in hundreds of foods, beverages, and drugs (see Caffeine Content of Some Common Foods, Beverages, and Drugs on page 91). While caffeine can make you feel more alert and, according to some people, less anxious, there are several reasons to consider cutting back on caffeine in your middle and later years.

In your premenopausal years: Caffeine can aggravate mood swings and breast tenderness associated with premenstrual syndrome. Caffeine can also interfere with your body's absorption of calcium and iron—two minerals that are hard enough to consume in adequate amounts in the middle and later years. If you suffer from anxiety, depression, or panic disorder (see Chapter 6), caffeine can trigger or exacerbate episodes of these psychological disorders.

In your postmenopausal and later years: At a time when hot flashes and other menopausal symptoms may be robbing you of sleep, there's little room for caffeine in your diet. The effects of caffeine on sleep are indisputable:

Caffeine Content of Some Common Foods, Beverages, and Drugs

Item	Caffeine (mg)
Coffee, 5-ounce cup	
Brewed, drip method	115
Instant	65
Decaffeinated, brewed	3
Decaffeinated, instant	2
Tea, 5-ounce cup	
U.S. brands, brewed	40
Imported brands, brewed	60
Instant	30
Iced (12-ounce glass)	70
Chocolate	
Cocoa beverage, 5-ounce cup	4
Chocolate milk, 8-ounce glass	5
Milk chocolate, 1 ounce	6
Dark, semi-sweet chocolate, 1 ounce	20
Soft drinks	
Cola or Pepper	30–45
Decaffeinated cola	trace-0.18
Caffeine-free cola	0
Orange	0
Other citrus*	0–54
Ginger ale, root beer, tonic water, soda, seltzer, sparkling water	0
Prescription drugs	
Cafergot (for migraine headaches)	100
Fiorinal (for tension headaches)	40
Darvon Compound, pain reliever	32.4
*Over-the-counter drugs**	
Analgesic/Pain relief	
Anacin and Anacin Maximum Strength	32
Excedrin	65
Midol	32.4
Vanquish	33
Diuretics	
Aqua-Ban	200
Permathene H2 Off	200

* Soft drinks containing caffeine are so labeled.

** More than 100 over-the-counter drug products contain caffeine. Caffeine is often found in weight-control aids, alertness tablets, headache and pain relief remedies, cold products and diuretics. When caffeine is an ingredient, it is listed on the label.

Source: U.S. Food and Drug Administration, October 1983.

Consuming caffeine just before bedtime makes it more difficult for you to fall asleep, decreases the total amount of time you sleep, and worsens the quality of your sleep. Since your body takes from four to seven hours to clear caffeine from the bloodstream, even an afternoon caffeine "perk" may deprive you of sleep at night.

Remember, too, that caffeine interferes with calcium absorption, which becomes even more critical after menopause. Also, women who take postmenopausal estrogens may experience breast tenderness that sometimes can be dissipated by cutting back on caffeine. Finally, caffeine acts as a diuretic, which may overload the bladder with urine and trigger or exacerbate urinary incontinence (loss of bladder control). Because it is a stimulant, caffeine may also cause involuntary bladder contractions, another cause of urinary incontinence.

Breaking the Caffeine Habit

A wide variety of decaffeinated coffees and teas are available for those who just can't give up their morning cup of java. Most major brands of cola now come in a decaffeinated form, as well. (Better yet, switch to carbonated water or fruit juices; these beverages are just as refreshing and contain no phosphorus, which may affect bone health. Fruit juices supply vitamins, too.)

If you're a heavy coffee, tea, or cola drinker and you try to quit cold turkey, you can expect to experience such withdrawal symptoms as irritability, nervousness, restlessness, lethargy, nausea, and headaches. To minimize these symptoms, gradually reduce the amount of caffeine you consume. For instance, drop down to two cups of coffee per day for a few days. Once you've adjusted to two cups, gradually reduce your daily intake a quarter of a cup at a time until you're down to one cup and then to none. Or switch to a half-caffeinated/half-decaffeinated brew and gradually increase the amount of decaffeinated coffee you use until the coffee is 100 percent decaffeinated.

Should You Become a Vegetarian?

Even if you don't give up meat for religious or ethical reasons, you may want to consider the vegetarian way of life simply for its health benefits. A vegetarian diet is low in fat (after all, you forgo meat, one of the top contributors of fat in the American diet), high in fiber (the vegetarian staples—whole grains, fruits, and vegetables—are loaded with both soluble and insoluble fiber), and rich in vitamins (fruits and vegetables are top sources of most vitamins, too). Vegetarianism appears to be good for your bones, as well. In one study, older Caucasian women who ate meat regularly lost 35 percent of their bone mass between the ages of fifty and eighty-nine, while lacto-ovo vegetarians (who eat eggs and dairy products but no meat) lost a mere 18 percent—even though both the meat eaters and the vegetarians had similar amounts of calcium in their diets. Another study showed the average bone density of vegetarians in their seventies was greater than that of meat eaters in their fifties.

One of the biggest concerns most women have about vegetarianism—getting enough protein—isn't really a problem, particularly if you supplement your diet with (low-fat) diary products and eggs. Remember, most Americans consume far more protein than they need (see page 71). You will, however, have to plan your meals more carefully to include the full complement of essential amino acids. Usually, this means simply eating vegetable proteins together with other vegetables, beans, grains, or nuts—for instance, serving lentils over brown rice, or eating peanut butter on whole-grain bread, together with a glass of milk.

Of greater concern will be ensuring that you get your fair share of calcium, vitamin B_{12}, and iron. Generally speaking, the more strict your vegetarian regimen is, the more difficult it will be to get adequate amounts of these nutrients. *Lacto-ovo vegetarians,* whose diet includes milk, cheese, and eggs but no red meat, chicken, or fish, and *lacto vegetarians,* who eat milk and cheese but no eggs or other animal proteins, are least likely to suffer a calcium or vitamin B_{12} deficiency. But iron may still be a problem. (Remember, meat contains the more readily absorbed *heme* iron.) *Vegans,* who eat no animal products, are most vulnerable to calcium, vitamin B_{12}, and iron deficiencies.

To ensure that you're consuming enough calcium, first fill out the Calcium Questionnaire on pages 78–82 and then follow the suggestions for getting more calcium in your diet beginning on page 75. Even if you include dairy products in your vegetarian diet, you may want to consider taking a calcium supplement, since most women generally don't get enough calcium in their diets (see page 74).

The recommended dietary allowance for vitamin B_{12} is 1.2 milligrams a day. If you include dairy products in your vegetarian diet, you shouldn't have a problem meeting the RDA, as some of the best sources are milk and dairy products. If you are a vegan, you will need to take a multivitamin or a supplement of B complex.

The best vegetable sources of iron include dried peas and beans (lentils, lima beans, soybeans) dried fruits (apricots, raisins, peaches, prunes), soy flour, and dried brewer's yeast. Since iron in vegetables isn't as readily absorbed as that in meat, be sure to follow the tips on pages 82–84 to ensure adequate iron absorption.

Finding a Qualified Nutritionist

If you have a hard time making dietary changes on your own, you may want to seek the help of a qualified nutritionist with the experience and equipment to conduct a more through evaluation of your dietary needs. A dietitian can often perform a computer analysis of your diet. You'll be asked to keep a food diary for five to seven days, logging what you eat and in what amounts. This information is fed into a computer, which calculates the number of calories and nutrients in your diet and produces a graphic printout showing the excesses and deficiencies. A nutritionist can also advise you on how to correct any nutritional problems you may have.

When searching for a nutrition specialist, be aware that no special license is required to give nutritional advice, so anyone can claim to be a dietitian or nutritionist. Look for a nutritionist who holds a Ph.D. or a master's degree in nutrition from an accredited university, or one who is a registered dietitian (R.D.) Ask your physician for a referral, contact a local university nutrition department or community hospital, or look in the Yellow Pages of the phone book. The American Dietetic Association (ADA) will provide a list of Registered Dietitians in your area. For a referral, write to the ADA's National Center for Nutrition and Dietetics (Suite 800, 216 West Jackson Blvd., Chicago, IL 60606-6995) or call the ADA's consumer nutrition hotline: (800) 366-1655.

A Final Word

In your middle and later years, changes in your body make the balancing act between calories and nutrients a little more difficult. The trick is to get more nutritional mileage from less food, chiefly by cutting back on fat in your diet and loading up on nutrient-packed complex carbohydrates, including fruits, vegetables, and whole grains.

Resources and Support

National Center for Nutrition and Dietetics of the American Dietetic Association, 216 West Jackson Blvd., Chicago, IL 60606-6995. Phone: (800) 366-1655. Call the consumer nutrition hotline to speak to a registered dietitian, listen to recorded nutrition messages, or be referred to a dietitian in your area.

Suggested Reading

GENERAL NUTRITION, HEALTH, AND FITNESS

American Dietetic Association. *Nutrition and Fitness: What Women Should Know*. Chicago: American Dietetic Association, 1986.

Bailey, Covert. *Fit or Fat?* Boston: Houghton Mifflin Co., 1984.

Brody, Jane. *Jane Brody's Nutrition Book*. New York: W. W. Norton Co., 1981.

Herbert, Victor, M.D., and Genell J. Subak-Sharpe, eds. *The Mount Sinai School of Medicine Complete Book of Nutrition*. New York: St. Martin's Press, 1990.

Pennington, Jean, Ph.D., R.D., and Helen Church. *Food Values of Portions Commonly Used*, 15th ed. New York: Harper & Row, 1989.

West Suburban District of the Illinois Dietetic Association, *Nutritive Values of Convenience and Processed Foods*. Chicago: American Dietetic Association, 1986.

COOKBOOKS FOR HEALTHY EATING

Becker, Gail, R.D., and Dalia A. Hammock, M.S., R.D. *Eat Well, Be Well Cookbook*. New York: Simon & Schuster, Inc., 1987.

Brody, Jane. *Jane Brody's Good Food Book*. New York: W. W. Norton & Co., 1985.

Brody, Jane. *Jane Brody's Good Food Gourmet*. New York: W. W. Norton & Co., 1990.

Gilliard, Judy, and Joy Kilpatrick, R.D. *The Guiltless Gourmet: Low in Fat, Cholesterol, Salt, Sugar, Calories*. Minnetonka, MO: Chronimed Publishing, 1987.

VEGETARIANISM AND VEGETARIAN COOKING

Atlas, Nava. *American Harvest: Regional Recipes for the Vegetarian Kitchen*. New York: Fawcett Columbine, 1987.

Lappé, Frances Moore. *Diet for a Small Planet*. New York: Ballantine Books, 1991.

Robertson, Laurel, Carol Flinders, and Brian Ruppenthal. *The New Laurel's Kitchen*. Berkeley, CA: Ten Speed Press, 1986.

Shulman, Martha Rose. *Fast Vegetarian Feasts*. New York: Doubleday, 1986.

———. *The Vegetarian Feast*. New York: Harper & Row, 1979.

NEWSLETTERS

Berkeley Wellness Newsletter. University of California at Berkeley, P.O. Box 10922, Des Moines, IA 50340.

Diet & Nutrition Letter. Tufts University, P.O. Box 2465, Boulder, CO 80322.

Nutrition Action Healthletter. Center for Science in the Public Interest, Suite 300, 1875 Connecticut Ave., NW, Washington, D.C. 20009-5728.

C h a p t e r   5

....

A No-Excuses Exercise Program for Your Prime Years

Excuses, excuses. There must be a thousand and one reasons to put off exercising for another day. "It's too cold." "It's too hot." "It's too dark." "It's too hard." "I'm too tired." "I'm too old for that!"

There may be no better time in your life to get (or stay) in shape than the prime of your life, however. And with the exercise program outlined here, it's almost more difficult to come up with excuses than it is simply to get up and get fit.

Generally speaking, as you grow older, your workouts should be a little easier on your cardiovascular system and less jarring on your joints than the all-out workouts recommended for younger people. Our program emphasizes enjoyable low-impact activities (such as walking and bicycling) that can fit into almost any lifestyle (even yours!). Your program should also include an element you may have previously overlooked: muscle strength and endurance.

We hope that you'll find our approach to midlife fitness so enjoyable that you'll want to exercise every day. Even if you don't exercise daily, the program here will help you make increased physical activity a regular habit—as routine a part of your life as brushing your teeth, and a habit that you can continue for the rest of your life.

Why Exercise?

Some say laughter is the best medicine. We're inclined to believe that exercise is even better. Here are some convincing arguments to start an exercise program *now*.

In Your Premenopausal Years

• **To build bone.** Why wait until you start *losing* bone mass after menopause to start exercising? A better strategy is to start early and build up as much bone as you can *before* bone loss accelerates. The more bone you have to start out with, the more bone you can stand to lose after menopause without compromising skeletal health. Moreover, exercise builds bone more readily in premenopausal than in postmenopausal women.

• **To control weight.** Increasing your level of physical activity is a far better (and in the long run a more successful) way to get a handle on middle-age spread than chronic dieting. When you exercise, you burn calories. If you exercise long enough in a single session, you burn fat. Regular exercise also helps you retain vital muscle mass. Some studies suggest that exercise raises your metabolism for several hours after you stop. If you combine exercise with a sensible diet, you're far more likely to succeed at controlling or losing weight, because you won't have to cut calories so severely as when you only diet, and you won't feel so deprived.

• **To reduce stress.** Regular physical activity relieves muscle tension and enhances the activity of the adrenal glands, creating a reserve of hormones to counter stress. Exercise also has been shown to help relieve some of the stressful symptoms of premenstrual syndrome, so common among premenopausal women.

And don't forget the runner's high. This is a feeling of well-being experienced by exercisers that's believed to be caused by a rise in the levels and activity of neurotransmitters in the brain known as *beta-endorphins*. Experts theorize that the rise in beta-endorphins may explain why exercise has been found to help alleviate anxiety and depression.

In Your Postmenopausal Years

• **To reduce your risk of heart disease.** Sedentary living is now considered a major risk factor for heart disease, along with high blood cholesterol, hypertension, and cigarette smoking. One excellent way to offset your increased risk of a heart attack after menopause is to exercise. University of North Carolina researchers have found that sedentary women are three times more likely to die prematurely of heart attacks than physically active women. Another major study by Steven Blair and associates at the prestigious Institute for Aerobics Research in Dallas found that regular physical activity was associated with lower death rates from all causes (including cancer, accidents, and so forth). But the biggest decline was in deaths caused by heart attacks. The researchers concluded that even if you have another risk factor for heart disease—high blood cholesterol, for instance—you could reduce your risk of dying of a heart attack *by almost 50 percent simply by becoming physically fit.*

• **To reduce your cancer risk.** Several studies have suggested a decreased cancer risk among exercising women. A landmark study involving more than five thousand women ages twenty to eighty from Harvard University's School of Public Health showed that *athletes have 50 percent less breast cancer and 60 percent less cancer of the uterus, ovaries, cervix, and vagina, than nonathletes.*

• **To slow or reverse the bone loss associated with menopause and reduce your risk of osteoporosis.** As we mentioned earlier, exercise not only halts bone loss but also *actually stimulates the formation of new bone.* This is particularly true of younger women who have not yet attained peak bone mass. But *even* *postmenopausal women can slow the rate of bone loss and sometimes build bone mass with a regular program of physical activity.* Our research showed that naturally menopausal women who participated in aerobic (walking on a treadmill or riding a stationary bicycle) and muscle-strengthening exercises (Nautilus) lost significantly less bone mass over a one-year period than women who didn't exercise.

Other researchers have found substantial *increases* in bone density among postmenopausal women who exercise. A study from Washington University School of Medicine in St. Louis found that menopausal women who exercised (walking, jogging, and climbing stairs) three times a week increased their bone mass 5.2 percent, while the sedentary women lost an additional 1.2 percent of bone mass. After twenty-two months, the exercisers' bone mass had increased by 6.1 percent from the start of the study, while women who didn't exercise continued to lose bone mass.

• **To ease menopausal symptoms.** Exercise may help relieve hot flashes. Swedish researchers have found that physically active menopausal women who were not taking hormones reported fewer and less severe hot flashes than inactive women. Only 6 percent of the active women had severe hot flashes, compared to 25 percent of the sedentary women. The researchers suspect that hot flashes may be partly caused by lower levels of *beta-endorphins* (discussed in Chapter 12). Exercise raises the level and activity of beta-endorphins in the brain.

As for the common belief that menopause causes fitness levels to decline, we found the evidence to be lacking. Among women ages forty-five to fifty-five in a study we conducted, there was no difference in the fitness levels of those who were still menstruating and those who had already experienced menopause. In effect, any drop in physical fitness is a result of *aging*, not menopause. And this age-related decline in physical fitness can be reversed by a program of regular physical activity.

• **To improve sleep.** While your need for sleep declines as you grow older, the number of sleep problems increases, particularly around the time of menopause (see page 246). Daily exercise has been shown to be extremely effective in tiring out your body, leaving you ready for a good night's sleep. (Exercise before 8:00 P.M., however; late-night workouts can have the opposite effect, overstimulating your body and contributing to insomnia.)

• **To help guard against constipation.** Physical activity stimulates the bowels, reducing your risk of constipation.

• **To reduce your risk of adult-onset diabetes.** Our research and that of others has shown that exercise improves your ability to use blood sugars (glucose tolerance). (Most of the studies so far have involved men. We demonstrated that this was also true for women.) Thus, exercise may help offset insulin resistance, which naturally increases as you age and in some people leads to adult-onset, or Type II, diabetes. Indeed, a recent study published in the *New England Journal of Medicine* has found that middle-aged men who exercise regularly were much less likely to develop diabetes than nonexercisers.

• **To help prevent joint stiffness and arthritis.** Contrary to popular belief, exercises that stress the joints, such as jogging, don't lead to osteoarthritis.

What's more, flexibility exercises, in which joints are moved through their full range of motion, *may actually counter the joint stiffness associated with aging and help protect against arthritis.*

•   **To prevent low back pain.** Low back pain affects up to 80 percent of us at some point in our lives. Many orthopedists believe the main causes of back problems are muscle weakness (especially abdominal muscles) and poor joint flexibility in the back and legs. Muscle-strengthening and flexibility exercises can both help rehabilitate "bad" backs and prevent this common malady altogether.

•   **To counter many of the changes of aging.** Regular physical activity may be one of the best-kept antiaging secrets around. Exercise slows the age-related decline in the functioning of the heart and lungs, and slows or reverses the loss of muscle and bone mass associated with aging. Physically fit people appear to be buffered from certain aging changes in the central nervous system, as well. Reaction time is quicker among exercisers than nonexercisers. And exercise increases blood flow to the brain, which in some studies has translated into improved performance on tests of mental capacities (see Table 5.1).

Exercise improves your overall health and may give you a slight longevity edge, as well. Steven Blair's study showed that death rates from all causes fell as the levels of physical fitness rose. Death rates for women declined from thirty-nine per ten thousand persons per year among the least fit to eight per ten thousand persons per year among the most fit.

In Your Later Years

•   **To help prevent falls.** One of the most compelling reasons to stay physically active in your later years is to keep your muscles strong. Muscle weakness makes older women more prone to falls, the most common cause of accidents, disability, and death in people over sixty-five. Exercise improves posture and balance, too, helping to prevent accidents and keeping you independent and active well into your later years.

Are You Ever Too Old to Exercise?

If you're in relatively good health and have no medical or physical disabilities that would prevent you from exercising, the answer is almost always no! We found that even seventy-year-old women who participated in a regular program of physical activity could improve their overall physical fitness. After six months, exercisers in our study increased their fitness level by 8.4 percent, compared to a 6.1 percent decline in fitness among their sedentary counterparts. Muscle endurance of the seventy-year-old exercisers improved a whopping 25.4 percent, while nonexercisers' muscle endurance fell 5.4 percent over the course of the six-month study.

What's more, *even ninety-year-old nursing-home residents can improve their muscle strength by lifting weights.* Participants in a remarkable study at Tufts University experienced a three- to fourfold increase in muscle strength in just eight weeks of weight training.

The exercise principles involved in achieving physical fitness are essentially

TABLE 5.1 *Why You Shouldn't Take Aging Sitting Down*
Exercise can actually *reverse* some of the
physical changes associated with normal
aging.

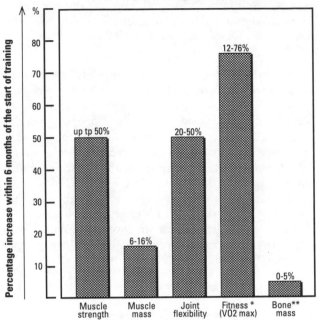

Active woman over age 30 (improvement)

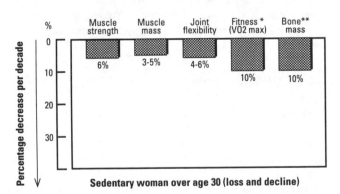

Sedentary woman over age 30 (loss and decline)

* VO2 max is a measure of how efficiently your heart and lungs can deliver
oxygen to your working muscles.

** Bone mass declines an average of 10% per decade after menopause; bone
loss from age thirty-five until menopause averages about 2 to 3 percent per
decade.

the same whether you're nine or ninety-two. The only difference is that you may not exercise as strenuously (or lift as much weight) as you did when you were younger.

What Kind of Exercise Is Best and How Much Is Enough?

What's best for you and how much you should exercise depends on your reasons for exercising and your overall fitness level. Generally speaking, a well-rounded program includes exercises that increase flexibility, muscle-strengthening exercises, and exercises for cardiovascular conditioning. You should try to include some of each in your fitness program.

Flexibility Exercises

As you grow older, connective tissue (cartilage, ligaments, and tendons) becomes stiffer and more rigid, which reduces joint flexibility. No one's certain how much of this reduced flexibility is a result of age-related biological changes and how much is caused by sedentary living or diseases that affect connective tissues and joints. We do know that *exercises that move joints through their full range of motion can improve flexibility by as much as 20 to 50 percent in men and women of all ages.*

Stretching exercises not only keep aging joints limber but also, when performed as a warm-up before a strenuous workout, keep your muscles supple, prepare you for movement by increasing blood flow to the muscles and joints, and help ease the transition from inactivity to more vigorous activity. Flexibility exercises may also improve coordination and help prevent such common injuries as shin splints and pulled muscles. Stretching is essential if you run, cycle, play tennis, or engage in other strenuous activity, because these types of activities promote muscle tightness and inflexibility. Finally, a good stretch can reduce muscle tension and help you feel more relaxed.

Flexibility exercises can be done virtually anywhere, anytime, and require no special equipment. You can complete our Stretches for Increased Flexibility, (page 116) in ten minutes or less. So why not take a few minutes every day for a good long stretch.

Muscle-Strengthening Exercises

Women tend to shy away from muscle-strengthening exercises for fear of developing the bulging muscles of professional bodybuilders. But our research and that of others now suggests that *you simply can't afford not to include muscle-strengthening exercises in your prime years fitness program.* Rest assured that, unless you choose to do so, you won't begin to look like a bodybuilder when you engage in muscle-strengthening exercises. Apparently, high levels of testosterone in men are what cause their muscles to bulk up. Here's why you should make muscle-strengthening exercises an integral part of your fitness routine:

• **Strong muscles protect your joints, and the increased strength helps prevent exercise-related injuries, such as sprains.** Injury prevention is especially important if you're a beginner, which is why you should start any fitness program with muscle-strengthening exercises before moving on to more strenuous aerobic activities.

•　**Strength training helps slow—and even reverse—the decline in muscle mass and muscle strength that comes with aging.** After age thirty, sedentary people begin to lose muscle mass at a rate of about 1 percent per year, replacing it with fat. While strength training generally doesn't reduce body fat, it can help you maintain muscle mass. You can regain strength lost to the aging process, too. Muscle strength declines by up to 30 percent between ages twenty and seventy if you're sedentary. Yet the nursing-home residents who participated in the Tufts University study mentioned earlier proved that you can not only slow the age-related loss of muscle mass but also *reverse* it.

•　**Strong abdominal muscles help prevent postural problems and low back pain.**

•　**Weight training may increase bone density.** In our research, postmenopausal women on hormone therapy experienced *an 8 percent increase in bone mass* when they performed muscle-strengthening exercises. A comparison group of women who took estrogen but didn't exercise neither gained nor lost bone mass.

•　**Strength training may boost immunity.** In a preliminary study of ours, women who experienced a natural menopause *and* participated in muscle-strengthening exercises for two years tended to have higher blood levels of immunoglobulin A (IgA), a major type of disease-fighting immune cell in the body. IgA, found in the blood and in the mucous membranes of the body, protects against such foreign invaders as yeast, bacteria, and certain viruses. Surgically menopausal women on estrogen therapy experienced a similar boost in immunity when they participated in a supervised program of muscle-strengthening exercises.

•　**You'll feel better about yourself.** You'll probably notice that your clothes fit better and you feel more trim as muscle tone improves—even if your overall weight doesn't change. This improvement in your appearance may enhance your self-esteem and your sense of well-being.

The fitness of your muscles can be measured in two ways. *Muscle strength* refers to the ability of your muscles to apply force (for instance, lift the heaviest weight you can just one time). *Muscle endurance* is the ability of your muscles to do a given amount of work over time (for example, lift a weight ten times).

There are several ways to increase muscle strength and endurance, but by far the safest and most effective way is to use weight machines that provide resistance, such as Cybex and Nautilus. This equipment can be found in fitness centers and gyms throughout the country. (See page 123 for information on how to choose a good fitness center or gym.)

If you can't manage two or three brief visits per week to a local fitness center, there are alternatives. Free weights (dumbbells and barbells) are fairly inexpensive to buy, and you can perform your exercises in your home at your leisure. Free weights, however, carry an increased risk of injury and are not recommended for beginners and older women. Free weights also should not be used without a spotter to monitor and assist you in lifting the weights (should you need help).

Home gyms are an option, too. But since proper form and technique are essential when performing muscle-strengthening exercises, your initial training should be under the supervision of a qualified instructor.

Calisthenics, such as leg lifts, which are featured in muscle-toning classes and home-exercise videos, may also be used to develop muscular strength, but it's often difficult to work out strenuously enough to achieve major gains in muscle strength. The low-intensity, high-repetition nature of calisthenics makes them more appropriate for the development of muscle endurance than muscle strength. Calisthenics are often incorporated into aerobic dance routines. Several home-exercise videos feature the muscle-toning exercises of calisthenics, as well.

What About Isometric Exercises?

Isometric strength training—exerting force against an immovable object, such as a wall (see Figure 5.1)—is a quick and easy way to strengthen muscles, because it requires no equipment or special skills. But this type of strength training has several drawbacks. To begin with, there's no way to measure your progress. You can't tell how much force you're exerting or whether you're straining your muscles by exerting too much force. Another problem is that

Figure 5.1   Isometric Exercise

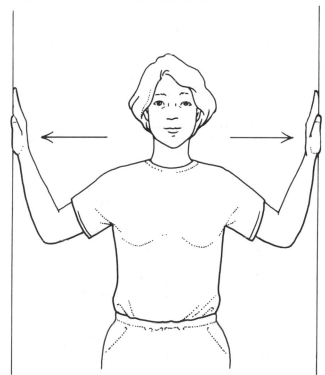

since your muscles aren't moved through their full range of motion (indeed, they don't move at all), the strength increases are limited to the particular angle at which you apply force.

Because the alternatives are not as safe or as effective as weight machines, we strongly urge you to consider using resistance weight-training equipment, particularly if this is all new to you. Properly trained staff at the better fitness centers can supervise you as you learn how to use the equipment. It's also easier to monitor your progress with this equipment as your strength improves.

How much time is involved? Most muscle-strengthening routines can be completed in *thirty minutes or less*. If you're beginning to exercise for the first time, or if you've been sedentary for more than a year, we recommend that you participate in a full range of muscle-strengthening exercises three times per week for a month or two before you take on more strenuous activities. Thereafter, twice a week is sufficient to maintain and gradually improve your muscle strength. That's not a lot of time when you consider the benefits to your health and well-being.

Cardiovascular Conditioning

When you think of exercise, what most likely comes to mind are activities that improve cardiovascular fitness. These are rhythmic exercises that use the large muscles in your body and raise your heart rate and breathing, such as brisk walking, jogging, bicycling, swimming, and aerobic dance.

If you groan at the idea of repeatedly jogging around a track or keeping up with an aerobic dance instructor who's half your age, it's time to reprogram your thinking about aerobic exercise. The problem with these high-impact, high-exertion activities is that they carry a greater risk of injury, particularly muscle strains, knee injuries, and stress fractures. This is particularly true as you grow older. Michael Pollock, Ph.D., director of the Center for Exercise Science at the University of Florida in Gainesville, found that the rate of injuries among beginning joggers increases with age, from about 18 percent among those ages twenty to thirty-five to 41 percent among those ages forty-nine to sixty-five. It's no wonder: When you jog or run, your feet literally collide with the ground from fifty to seventy times per minute at a force of two to four times your body weight.

You're much more likely to become discouraged and drop out of an exercise program that's too strenuous for you. Instead, we recommend enjoyable, low-impact activities such as walking, bicycling, and swimming. Walking is one of the easiest and most convenient exercises you can do, because you can walk practically anywhere and walking requires no special skills or equipment, just comfortable loose-fitting clothes and a good pair of walking shoes (for guidelines to buying shoes, see Special Gear on page 123). Walking is less likely to cause injury than jogging or running because it's a low-impact activity that doesn't put too much strain on your muscles and joints.

Bicycling is another good choice for women in midlife. Like walking, bicycling doesn't strain your joints. Better yet, invest in a stationary bicycle. Indeed, *stationary bicycling may well be the ideal workout for women in midlife*. A stationary bicycle allows you to exercise even in poor weather or after dark. If you're pressed for time, you can catch the evening news while you work out, or read a book or business documents while exercising. Moreover, you don't need any special skills to ride a stationary bicycle—not even good balance, which you *do* need to ride a regular bicycle or to walk on a treadmill. You can buy a good stationary bicycle for roughly the amount of money you'd spend on a regular bicycle. (See Special Gear, page 123, for tips on buying a stationary bicycle).

Swimming is another excellent activity, particularly for older women who have lost a considerable amount of bone mass. The buoyancy of the water helps protect your bones and joints, and the water's resistance to your movements gives you a great cardiovascular workout. (You should note, however, that if you don't have osteoporosis and your goal is to build bone, weight-bearing activities, such as walking and cycling, may be more appropriate. While one study showed that swimming increased overall bone density in men, the same wasn't true for the women in the study.)

As far as cardiovascular fitness is concerned, it appears that *any* activity is better than none. Even leisure-time activities, such as gardening and bowling, have been shown to reduce the risk of heart attacks (at least among men). However, most experts agree that you'll get better results by making a regular (if not daily) habit of exercising.

How much exercise you need depends on your goals. (Remember, these are goals toward which you gradually work; *Don't* try to start out at these levels.)

Cardiovascular fitness: You'll need to exercise at your target heart rate (see page 108) for twenty minutes three to four times a week to keep your body's most important muscle—your heart—in shape.

Weight control: If your goal is to lose weight, you should exercise at your target heart rate for *at least* forty to forty-five minutes at a time. During the first thirty minutes of exercise, your body relies mainly on glycogen (stored sugars in the muscles) for energy. Only after glycogen stores are depleted does your body start drawing on fat reserves for energy.

Bone building: We still don't know how much exercise is sufficient to build bone mass. One of our studies suggests you need to exercise at least forty-five minutes per session to maintain bone mass after menopause if you don't take postmenopausal estrogen.

Stress reduction: While endurance athletes report that the runner's "high" comes only after one or two hours of strenuous activity, you don't have to run a marathon to reduce stress and relieve anxiety. Even thirty to forty minutes of brisk walking is sufficient.

At first glance, it may seem that physical fitness involves a lot of time and energy. Again, the trick is to choose activities that you *enjoy*, like walking or cycling. (The beauty of these exercises is that they're a cinch to work into an already busy schedule and lifestyle.) Another key to success is gradually to work your way up to the levels here (see our beginner's programs for walking and cycling beginning on page 120). Before you know it, you'll be hooked! (Interestingly, many athletes claim they experience *withdrawal* symptoms a few days after they stop working out. Exercise is one healthy addiction you can feel good about!)

Before You Begin

A medical examination is a must before you launch an exercise program. Some women may have certain asymptomatic health conditions (hypertension, heart disease, or asthma, for instance) that could be aggravated by a sudden burst of vigorous exercise. Other physical conditions may limit the amount of exercise you can do or may require that you exercise only under a doctor's supervision. If you have *angina* (chest pain), or other cardiovascular conditions (such as *cardiomyopathy* or *thrombophlebitis*—blood clots in the legs), uncontrolled diabetes, or musculoskeletal problems that interfere with exercise, you may be advised not to exercise.

The examination should include a comprehensive medical history (including a personal and family history), measures of blood pressure, blood cholesterol, and blood sugar, and a review of your current health habits, including cigarette smoking, alcohol consumption, medications, and diet. If you're over sixty, you should have your bone density tested before beginning an exercise program.

Women who have one or more of the following risk factors for heart disease may need to undergo additional tests before beginning an exercise program:

- family history of heart disease
- high blood cholesterol
- high blood pressure
- diabetes

Women over fifty should also undergo an exercise stress test, which involves monitoring your heart rate and its electrical activity with an ECG while you exercise on a treadmill. The grade of the treadmill (similar to the slope of a hill) is gradually increased as the test progresses. This type of exercise stress test can detect early signs of heart disease (such as narrowing of the arteries) that may not be apparent during a resting ECG.

If you're under age fifty and are serious about beginning a meaningful exercise program, you should consider having an exercise stress test to detect any potential problems and to determine your fitness level.

How Fit Are You?

Along with a medical examination, it's a good idea to undergo a fitness evaluation to determine your current fitness level and to help tailor an exercise program suited to your needs and abilities. Knowing your fitness level now also helps you set realistic goals and gives you a baseline from which to measure your progress.

A typical evaluation includes measures of cardiorespiratory fitness, body composition, flexibility, and muscle strength. If you're generally in good health, have had a recent medical evaluation, and are under age fifty, you can get a rough idea of your fitness level yourself using some of the field tests described here. If you're over fifty, if you smoke, or if you're at increased risk of heart disease, you should undergo a more in-depth evaluation at your doctor's office.

Measuring Your Cardiorespiratory Fitness

Measuring Your VO₂ Max
(Maximal Oxygen Consumption)
So important is oxygen to your workout (it helps release energy stored in your muscles and fat tissues) that the single most important measure of your fitness level is VO_2 max. Simply put, VO_2 max is a gauge of how efficiently your heart and lungs deliver oxygen to your working muscles and how effectively your muscles use that oxygen. Scientifically speaking, VO_2 max is the point at which your body's consumption of oxygen levels off in spite of an increase in physical activity. VO_2 max is influenced by your age, sex, heredity, and the amount of oxygen-carrying red blood cells (hemoglobin) you have. The following list describes various ways to measure VO_2 max.

• **Graded exercise stress test:** One of the most accurate ways of measuring VO_2 max is using the *maximal exercise stress test*, a graded exercise stress test in which your breathing, heart rate, and blood pressure are monitored as you walk on a treadmill. This test, however, is relatively expensive, fairly uncomfortable, and impractical for use in a physician's office. Moreover, the test was designed for use by men. At the Women's Medical and Diagnostic Center, we developed a modified version of the maximal exercise stress test specifically for use by women in the middle years. The test is less complicated, easier on the person being tested, and simple enough to perform in a doctor's office. Like the maximal GXT, you'll walk on a treadmill that gradually increases your speed and the slope of your walk while an electrocardiogram monitors your heart rate. Generally, the test lasts from six to fifteen minutes. (The test will end sooner if you experience chest pains, dizziness, nausea, or exhaustion, or if the electrocardiogram indicates abnormalities in your heart rate or rhythm at any time during the test.) Your VO_2 max can be calculated using an equation that factors in the amount of time you spend on the treadmill. (Your doctor or other interested health care professionals can write to the authors for more information about the modified GXT, including the formula used to determine your VO_2 max.)

The modified GXT is recommended for all women over fifty and for younger women who have one or more risk factors for heart disease.

• **Bicycle test:** Healthy women under age fifty may take an exercise stress test on a stationary bicycle. During the test, you'll ride the bicycle at a certain speed and adjusted tension for about six minutes. Your heart rate will be monitored by an electrocardiogram, or by a health professional, who will take your pulse several times during the test. The test ends when you reach a specific heart rate or work load, when you feel too fatigued to continue, or when you suffer symptoms such as chest pains, dizziness, or nausea. The test results are then used in a formula to estimate your VO_2 max.

If you undergo one of the above exercise stress tests, have your physician or other health care professional help interpret the results, and write your VO_2 max in the fitness profile form on page 113. Use this score as a baseline to measure your progress. To see how your fitness level compares with that of other women your age, check your score with the Fitness Norms for Women in Midlife (Maximal Oxygen Uptake) on page 476 and indicate your fitness level in the left-hand column of the form on page 113.

• **Walking field test:** Several field tests have been developed to estimate your VO_2 max while you climb stairs, run, or walk. While these tests typically aren't as accurate as an exercise stress test in determining your cardiovascular fitness, they can give you a general idea of your fitness level, *provided you're under age fifty, you've had a medical checkup, and have your physician's approval for beginning an exercise program.*

One of the least taxing field tests is the one-mile walk test developed by researchers at the University of Massachusetts at Amherst and the Rockport Walking Institute. To take the test, you'll need a measured track or other *flat* surface on which you can walk for one mile and a watch with a second hand (or a digital watch that displays seconds). You'll need to know how to take your pulse, too (see page 109).

To take the test, simply note the time you start walking and walk as briskly as you comfortably can. When you've walked one mile, record the time (to the nearest second) it took you to cover the distance and check your heart rate *immediately*. Now find the tables for your age group on pages 478–479 to determine your fitness level.

Determining Your Maximum Heart Rate
and Target Zone
To get a good cardiovascular workout, you'll need to raise your heart rate to somewhere between 50 to 85 percent of its maximum capacity. An ideal training zone is between 60 to 80 percent of your maximum heart rate. This is known as your *target heart range*, or target zone. To find your target zone, use the following formula:

$$\text{Target zone} = (220 - \text{your age}) \times .60 \text{ to } .80$$

So if you're forty years old, your maximum heart rate would be 180 (220 minus 40), and your target zone would be between 108 (60 percent of 180) and 144 (80 percent of 180) pulse beats per minute. Write your target heart range in the fitness profile form on page 113. While working out, you should periodically take your pulse (see Measuring Your Resting Heart Rate, on page 109) to determine whether you have reached your target zone. If after 20 minutes of aerobic activity your pulse beats are still below your target zone, you should increase the intensity of your workout.

Note: Our research has shown that the equation for determining your maximum heart rate (220 minus your age) and target heart range is actually quite accurate among premenopausal women. The formula becomes increasingly inaccurate as you grow older, however: The equation underestimates your maximum heart rate by 9.6 percent in your sixties and by up to 16 percent in your seventies. Essentially, this means that many healthy older women may not be exercising to their full potential or reaping all the benefits of exercise on their cardiovascular system. This is another good reason for women over fifty to undergo an exercise stress test.

Measuring Your Resting Heart Rate

In addition to the cardiovascular evaluations above, you should measure your resting heart rate. Although your resting heart rate in itself is *not* a good way to predict your level of physical fitness, it can help gauge your progress in an exercise program. Generally, your resting heart rate goes down as you become more physically fit.

You can measure your resting heart rate any time of day, but the most accurate reading is taken first thing in the morning, before you get out of bed. To find your resting heart rate, you'll need to take your pulse: Place two fingers along your carotid artery (at the side of your neck) or on the thumb side of your wrist (see Figure 5.2). Count your pulse for six seconds. Multiply that number by ten to determine the beats per minute. Now check your resting heart rate with the Fitness Norms for Women in Midlife on page 476.

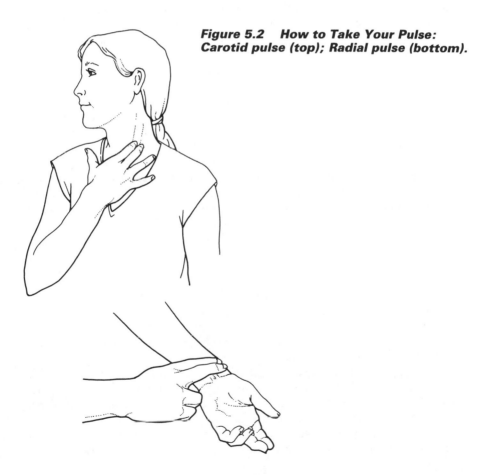

**Figure 5.2   How to Take Your Pulse:
Carotid pulse (top); Radial pulse (bottom).**

Measuring Your Body Composition

Generally speaking, the more muscle mass you have, the stronger and more fit you are likely to be and the easier it will be to exercise. People with excess body fat burn up to 30 percent more calories than normal-weight people doing the same amount of work.

Determining your body-mass index (see page 29) can give you a rough idea of your body composition. A health professional may use girth measurements, skin-fold calipers, or some of the newer high-tech methods for determining body composition discussed in Chapter 3.

Once you know what your percentage of body fat is, compare it with the Fitness Norms for Women in Midlife (Body Composition) on page 476 and make a note of it in your fitness profile form.

Measuring Your Flexibility

The best way to determine your flexibility is with a *goniometer,* a protractorlike device typically used by physical therapists to measure how far you can move each of your joints through their range of motion. However, a much more practical way to gauge your flexibility is the standard sit-and-reach test, in which you sit on the floor and try to touch your toes (or beyond). The test measures the flexibility of your legs and back, and gives you a general idea of your overall flexibility. (Note: *Do not* attempt this test if you have a curvature of the spine, such as *kyphosis* or *scoliosis,* or if you have suffered vertebral fractures as a result of osteoporosis; the test could put too much strain on your back.)

To perform the sit-and-reach test, place a yardstick on the floor (you may want to tape it in place). Sit down so that your legs are extended directly in front of you, the zero mark of the yardstick is pointing toward your trunk, and your heels are aligned with the 15-inch mark. Try to touch your toes a few times to warm up before actually performing the test. Make sure your knees are always touching the floor and *try not to bounce.* Now, reach forward slowly as far as possible, exhaling as you bend over. Make a note of the distance you reach on the yardstick; this is your flexibility score. Use the Fitness Norms for Women in Midlife (Sit and Reach Test) on page 477 to see how you measure up with other women your age.

Measuring Your Muscle Strength and Endurance

To get a clear picture of your muscle strength and endurance, the muscle groups of various parts of your body should be tested. As a rule, women have greater leg strength than upper body strength. (In fact, when differences in body size and percentage of body fat are equalized for both sexes, *women have equal or greater lower body strength than men.*)

Your physician can get a general idea of the strength of your arm and leg muscles during your physical examination. Muscle endurance can be estimated by tracking the length of time you remain active during an exercise stress test; the longer you exercise, the more muscle endurance you have.

If you're being evaluated by a trained exercise physiologist, you may have your muscle strength tested in any number of ways, including the use of weights (both free-standing and machines); mechanical or electronic instruments called dynamometers and cable tensiometers, which test such muscle functions as grip strength; and sophisticated isokinetic devices, which test muscle strength as you move your muscles (usually arms and legs) through their full range of motion.

It isn't necessary to undergo elaborate strength testing to get an idea of your muscle strength and endurance. In fact, sophisticated test equipment is not necessarily more accurate than some of the more mundane field tests commonly used. The field tests described here are easy enough for healthy women to perform by themselves and don't require any special equipment.

One-Repetition Maximum Test

Muscle strength can be assessed by the *one-repetition maximum test*, a test of how much weight you can lift correctly just one time. If you're not accustomed to lifting weights, you should not attempt this test on your own. Instead, take the test under the supervision of a trained specialist at your local YMCA, YWCA, or fitness club. A specialist can instruct you on proper form when lifting weights.

Push-Ups and Sit-Ups

Push-ups and sit-ups are the two standard tests for measuring muscle endurance. Push-ups gauge muscular endurance of the upper body, and sit-ups give an estimate of abdominal muscular endurance. The idea is to complete as many correct push-ups or sit-ups as you can in one minute. Proper form is essential; otherwise, you risk injuring yourself.

Push-ups: The modified knee push-up is recommended for women (see Figure 5.3). Lie on your stomach, supporting your weight with your hands and knees. Push your entire body, except for your hands and knees, off the floor until your arms are straight. Then lower your body until your chest touches the floor. Remember to keep your back straight while you do push-ups.

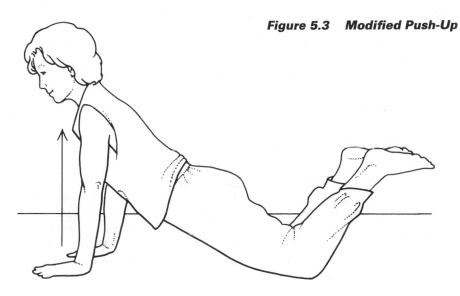

Figure 5.3   Modified Push-Up

111

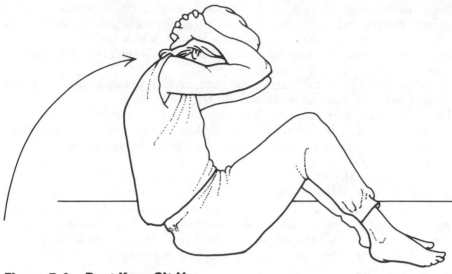

Figure 5.4   Bent Knee Sit-Up

Sit-ups: To test your abdominal muscle strength, a full sit-up is recommended. Lie on your back, with your knees bent, your feet flat on the floor, and your heels between twelve and eighteen inches from your buttocks. (You may want to have someone hold your ankles during this exercise.) Place your hands behind your neck with your fingers interlocking. Sit up, touching your elbows to your knees (see Figure 5.4), then return to a full lying position before starting the next sit-up.

If you decide to incorporate sit-ups into your fitness program, it's not necessary to do a full sit-up, since your abdominal muscles perform most of the work involved in this exercise as you lift your trunk the first thirty to forty degrees off the floor. Instead, try stomach crunches, which are a lot easier on your back. Again, lie on your back, with your knees bent and your feet flat on the floor. Cross your arms over your chest and pull your trunk up about thirty-five degrees off the floor, returning to a full lying position before starting the next stomach crunch.

Now find your fitness level by comparing your score with the Fitness Norms for Women in Midlife (Push-Ups and Sit-Ups) on page 477.

Putting It All Together:
Your Midlife Fitness Plan

When developing an individualized exercise program, specialists talk of writing an "exercise prescription" just as a physician would write a prescription for medication, including the dosage and the number of times per day you should take it. You've already seen that physical activity may be as important as many of the medications you may take (such as hormone-replacement therapy to protect your bones). After completing the following steps, you should be able to write an exercise prescription for yourself using the Midlife Fitness Planner that begins on the next page.

	Baseline	3 weeks	6 weeks	3 months	6 months
Weight	_____	_____	_____	_____	_____
Percent body fat	_____	_____	_____	_____	_____
Resting heart rate	_____	_____	_____	_____	_____
VO$_2$ max or one-mile walk	_____	_____	_____	_____	_____
Flexibility	_____	_____	_____	_____	_____
Sit-ups	_____	_____	_____	_____	_____
Push-ups	_____	_____	_____	_____	_____

....
Midlife Fitness Planner
....

LONG-TERM GOALS

_____

_____

_____

_____

_____

EXERCISE PRESCRIPTION

1. Calculate your target heart range (see page 000 for directions).

2. Using your long-term goals as a guide, choose the exercises best suited to your needs, abilities, and tastes. Write down the type of exercise you plan to incorporate into a routine and the number of repetitions (or distance or amount of time) for each exercise.

Target Heart Range   _____

Flexibility   _____

_____

_____

Muscle Strength   _____

_____

_____

Cardiovascular Conditioning _____

_____

WEEKLY WORKOUT PLANNER
Using the exercise prescription above, develop one or more exercise routines and schedule them into the weekly planner below. At the top of each column, indicate the time of day you plan to perform your routine(s). Then pencil in the actual exercises you intend to perform each day.

Weekly Goals _____

	Sun.	*Mon.*	*Tues.*	*Wed.*	*Thurs.*	*Fri.*	*Sat.*
Time							
Routine							

1. **Start with sensible goals.** Setting goals helps you choose the activities most suited to your needs and may help you stick with your exercise regimen by giving you something tangible to work toward. *Your ultimate goal is to make regular physical activity a permanent part of your life.*

Take a moment now to set your goals. Be as specific as possible. If your goal is to lose weight, how much weight do you want to lose? If you're exercising to prevent disease, write down which disease(s) you hope to avoid.

In addition to your long-term goals, take a few moments at the beginning of each week to set goals for the next seven days. Successfully achieving weekly goals may be just the incentive you need to continue exercising.

2. **Make a time commitment.** Fitting exercise into an already hectic schedule may be the biggest challenge you face. Rather than carving out three one-hour time slots for exercise (which is enough to keep any busy woman from exercising altogether), we recommend starting with a commitment of just ten or fifteen minutes a day (twice a day is preferable). Then add five minutes more to your workout each week. This strategy not only gradually conditions your body to an increased level of activity, it also helps make exercise a regular habit.

Some other tips for squeezing exercise into your lifestyle: Take a brisk walk during your lunch hour. Get up a half-hour earlier each morning and exercise before you go to work. Try splitting your workout into two or three shorter sessions during the day. (Two shorter daily exercise sessions—one in

114

A One-Hour Total Fitness Plan

(3 to 4 times a week)

Component	Activity	Time
Warm-up	Stretching, low-level calisthenics, walking	5 minutes
Muscular conditioning	Calisthenics, weight training, pulley weights	15 minutes
Cardiovascular conditioning	Fast walk, jog-run, swim, cross-country skiing, vigorous games, dancing, or climbing stairs	30 minutes
Cool-down	Walking, stretching	10 minutes

A Thirty-Minutes-a-Day Fitness Plan

(30 minutes, 4 to 5 times a week)

	Component	Activity	Time
Day 1:	Warm-up	Stretching	5 minutes
	Cardiovascular conditioning	Brisk walk, cycling, or swimming	20 minutes
	Cool-down	Stretching	5 minutes
Day 2:	Warm-up	Stretching	5–10 minutes
	Muscular conditioning	Calisthenics and weight training	15–20 minutes
	Cool-down	Stretching	
Day 3:	Warm-up	Stretching	5 minutes
	Cardiovascular conditioning	Brisk walk, cycling, or swimming	20 minutes
	Cool-down	Stretching	5 minutes
Day 4:	Warm-up	Stretching	5–10 minutes
	Muscular conditioning	Calisthenics and weight training	15–20 minutes
	Cool-down	Stretching	5–10 minutes

Note: Fitness Plans adapted with permission from Michael L. Pollock and Jack H. Wilmore, *Exercise in Health and Disease*, 2nd ed. Philadelphia: W. B. Saunders Company, 1990, p. 375.

the morning before you go to work and another after you return home—are ideal for reducing stress.) Another alternative is to combine your fitness routine with your daily activities: Ride your bicycle or walk to work three days a week, for example.

Or try the "30/60 timesaver": One way to shave a few minutes off of your exercise session is to make your warm-up and cool-down an integral part of your workout. This timesaver works particularly well with low-impact activities such as walking or bicycling, which are generally used as a warm-up to more strenuous activities, anyway. To save time, simply begin your exercise session by walking or bicycling slowly. Then gradually build up speed until you reach your target heart-rate zone. To cool down, spend the last five or ten minutes of your session walking or cycling at a slower pace. Before you know it, you'll be done.

3. Develop a program. Ideally, your midlife fitness program should include a combination of flexibility exercises, strength training, and cardiovascular-conditioning exercises. If you prefer a one-hour exercise session, you can work all three components into a single session. Otherwise, you can alternate activities, performing your muscle-strengthening routine on, say, Tuesdays and Thursdays, and getting a cardiovascular workout on Mondays, Wednesdays, and Fridays.

Getting Started: A Prime Years Program for Beginners

If you've been sedentary for more than a year, we recommend that you start with flexibility and muscle-strengthening exercises for the first month or two. After you've built up your muscle strength and flexibility, you can add aerobic activities to your routine.

Stretches for Increased Flexibility

Sustained static stretches are used to increase flexibility. When stretching, slowly elongate the muscle being stretched until you feel a mild tension. Hold the position between ten and thirty seconds, remembering to breathe slowly and fully. As tension is released from the muscle, slowly move a fraction farther again, until you feel tension. Hold the position for about thirty seconds more. Try the stretches here to improve overall flexibility.

Groin stretch (see Figure 5.5). Lie on your back with your knees bent and the soles of your feet together. Relax your legs, letting them gently fall toward

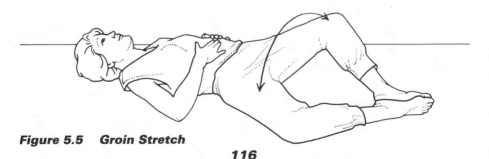

Figure 5.5   Groin Stretch

116

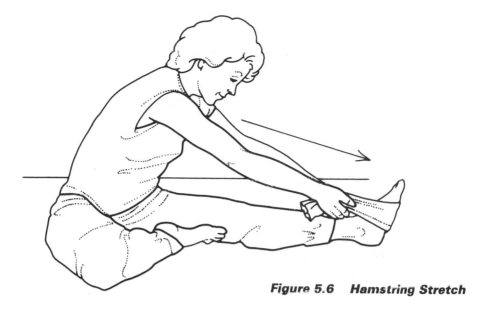

Figure 5.6 Hamstring Stretch

the floor. You should feel a stretch in the upper muscles of the inner thighs and the groin area.

Hamstring stretch (see Figure 5.6). Sit upright on the floor or a mat with your right leg positioned straight in front of you and your left leg bent so that your left foot touches your right thigh. Keeping your back straight, slowly bend forward from your hips toward your right foot until you feel a stretch in the hamstring muscle along the back of your thigh. Now stretch the hamstring muscle of the left leg in the same way. If you have difficulty reaching your foot, use a towel, as shown here.

Elongated stretch (see Figure 5.7). Lie on your back, bringing your arms straight up over your head and keeping your legs straight. Reach as far as you comfortably can with your arms and legs. Hold the position for thirty seconds. Relax.

Leg stretch (see Figure 5.8). Lying down with your knees slightly bent, pull your right leg up toward your chest, keeping your lower back and the back of your head on the floor. Repeat with the other leg.

Upper back, shoulder, and arm stretch (see Figure 5.9). While standing, interlace your fingers together above your head and reach up as far as you comfortably can.

Note: The time you spend holding the stretch is more important than the number of repetitions you do. *Never* try to rush through stretching exercises by bouncing or using fast, jerky movements. This can strain or tear muscles and may actually set up a reflex action that causes the muscle to resist stretching.

Figure 5.7 Elongated Stretch

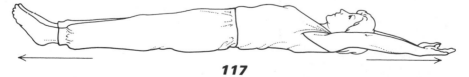

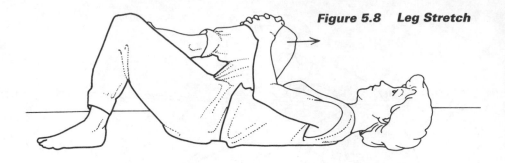

Figure 5.8   Leg Stretch

Exercises for Muscle Strength and Endurance

Muscle strength increases when the muscle is overloaded, either by lifting weights or by creating muscle tension. An all-around muscle strength—conditioning program includes exercises for the neck, arms, forearms, shoulders, abdomen, back, chest, buttocks, and legs. You can usually finish your routine within fifteen to twenty minutes.

If you're working out on equipment at a fitness center or gym (see Figures 5.10–5.13), your instructor will help you set up an optimal routine and help you find your starting weight. If your goal is to increase muscle strength, you'll use a little more weight, eventually working your way up to one set of ten repetitions. If your aim is to increase muscle endurance, you'll use lighter weights and perform two sets of ten repetitions.

Your workout should begin with a five to ten minute warm-up of simple stretches and calisthenics. A few minutes of the warm-up should be devoted to

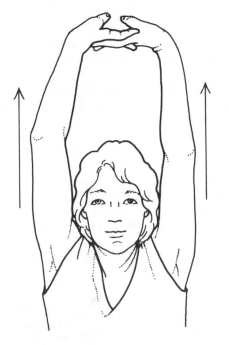

Figure 5.9   Upper Back, Shoulder, and Arm Stretch

118

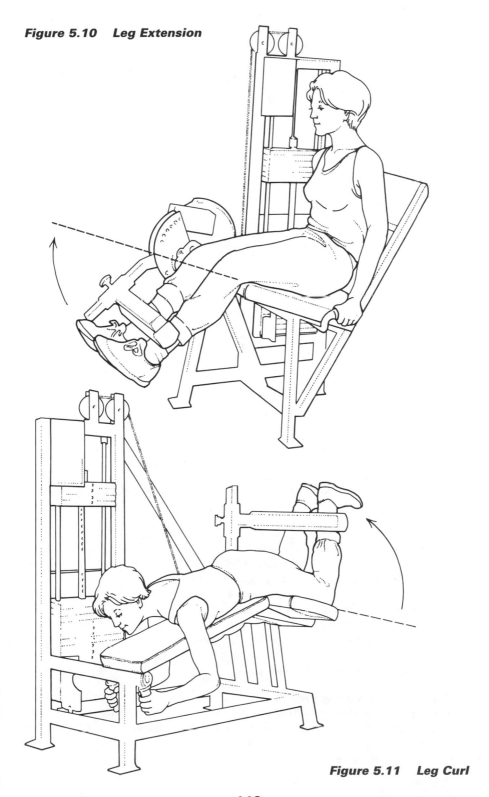

Figure 5.10 Leg Extension

Figure 5.11 Leg Curl

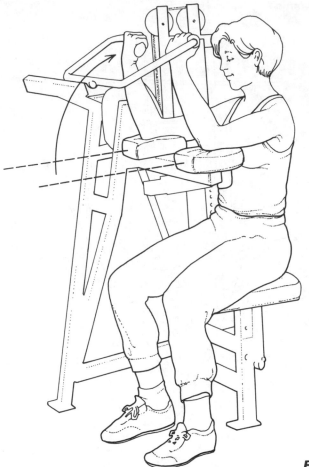

Figure 5.12   Arm Curl

brisk walking or some other rhythmic activity that elevates your heart rate somewhat and gets the blood flowing to your muscles. End your session by stretching the muscles you used during your workout.

To reduce muscle fatigue, vary your routine, changing the order of your exercises on consecutive workout days. Also, be sure to give your muscles a forty-eight-hour rest between these strength/endurance workouts (which means you should skip a day between exercise sessions).

Exercises for Cardiovascular Conditioning

•   **A beginner's walking program:** If you are in fair to poor physical condition, researchers at the Brookhaven National Laboratory recommend the following walking program: Begin with a five minute walk, preferably in an area with some slopes. Move along at a brisk pace. Add one minute each week, gradually building up to a thirty-minute brisk, nonstop walk.

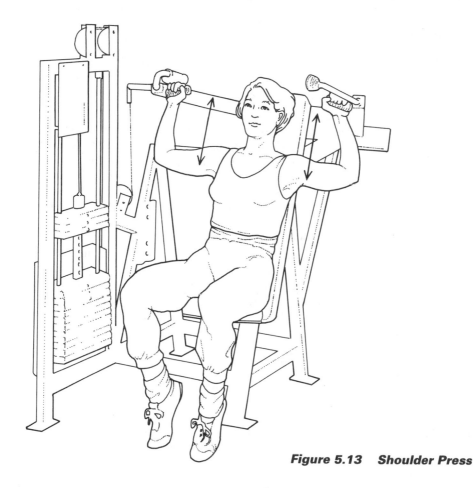

Figure 5.13 Shoulder Press

Your biggest concern will be ensuring that you walk briskly enough to get a cardiovascular workout. Monitor your heart rate while you walk and pick up the pace if your heart rate doesn't reach its working range after ten minutes or so. For a more intensive workout, swing your arms as you walk, or plan your walk along a hilly route.

• **A beginner's program for stationary bicycling:** Adjust the bicycle's resistance to the lowest setting. Adjust the seat height so that your knee is slightly bent and just over your toes when the pedal is at its lowest point and your foot is positioned horizontally in the stirrup. Now start pedaling.

During the first week, ride for ten minutes twice a day (in the morning before you go to work and in the evening when you come home, for example). Then increase the time you spend on the bicycle by five minutes each week. When you can ride for thirty minutes per session, gradually increase the resistance each week for a more intensive workout. (As you increase the bicycle's resistance, be sure to monitor your heart rate and exercise in your target range.)

Minimizing the Risks of Exercise

Virtually everything you do carries some risk, and exercise is no exception. However, your risks can be minimized by following the guidelines we've discussed throughout the chapter, as well as heeding the specific recommendations here.

• **Exercise-related injury:** Most exercise-related injuries occur to muscles and bones. Although injury may occasionally be traumatic, such as a torn ligament or bone fracture, by far the most common are minor overuse injuries: muscle strains, *tendinitis* (inflammation of the tendons), *synovitis* (inflammation of the synovial lining of the joint), *bursitis* (inflammation of the *bursa,* or fluid-containing membranes in the connective tissues surrounding the joints), and *stress fractures* (hairline fractures of bones).

If you follow the guidelines in this chapter, you will automatically minimize your risk of injury. You may experience sore muscles for the first few days (over-the-counter analgesics such as aspirin, acetaminophen, or ibuprofen can ease muscle soreness and stiffness; taking a hot bath before bedtime helps, too). But overall, if you start out slowly and warm up before exercising, you'll avoid the most common overuse injuries altogether. Don't forget to wear appropriate shoes (see page 123).

Your body has several ways of warning you that you may be overdoing it. Watch for these signs of trouble during your workouts:

• **Slow down:** If you experience any of the following symptoms, you may be working out too strenuously. Slow down by training at a lower heart rate and progressing to higher levels of activity more gradually. If symptoms persist even after you've taken the following measures, see your doctor.

persistent rapid pulse lasting throughout five to ten minutes of your cool-down

nausea or vomiting after exercise

extreme breathlessness lasting more than ten minutes after you stop exercising

prolonged fatigue lasting more than twenty-four hours after a workout

• **Stop:** If you experience any of the following symptoms, *stop your workout immediately and see a physician before resuming your exercise program:*

abnormal heart activity, including fluttering, jumping, or palpitations in the chest or throat; sudden burst of rapid heartbeats; or a sudden slowing of a rapid pulse rate

pain or pressure in the center of the chest, arm, or throat during or immediately after exercise

dizziness or light-headedness, sudden lack of coordination, confusion, cold sweats, glassy stare, pallor, or fainting

illness, particularly viral infections (if you exercise when you're ill, you risk developing myocarditis, a viral infection of the heart muscle)

Special Gear

Your exercise program is bound to be more enjoyable and less risky when you dress appropriately and use the proper equipment.

• **Clothing:** The clothes you wear will depend on the type of exercise you do and the environment you're in. If you exercise outdoors, wear comfortable, loose-fitting clothing that provides protection from the sun, heat, cold, and wind. As a rule, it's better to underdress than overdress, since the activity itself will warm you. If you have large breasts, you may want to wear an athletic bra that provides extra support.

• **Shoes and socks:** A good pair of athletic shoes may well be one of your biggest investments. The cost of a good pair of walking, running, or aerobic shoes ranges from $30 to $175 or more. But it's usually money well spent: Properly fitting shoes help prevent injuries and make your workouts more comfortable and enjoyable.

In general, look for an athletic shoe with a strong, highly supportive heel counter, a heel wedge and midsole, a good arch support, a comfortable inner-sole, a fairly pliable outer sole, and a comfortable toe box. Above all, buy a shoe that fits comfortably.

• **Stationary bicycles:** Look for a bike with *reliable resistance* that's constant and won't change as you work out (the bicycle's resistance controls the intensity of your workout). Choose a bicycle with an *adjustable seat and handlebars,* a *sturdy base,* and *free-swinging pedals* that stop when you stop pedaling. Stationary bicycles range in price from $250 to $2,000, but the differences in price usually reflect differences in the sophistication of the bicycle's computerization, which allows you to program the pace and timing of your workout. Some of the more sophisticated models will even tell you how many calories you're burning as you ride. Don't feel obligated to buy the most expensive bicycle you can find, however.

• **How to choose a good fitness center or gym:** The most important consideration you should keep in mind is whether the fitness center is staffed with qualified instructors. Look for instructors and trainers certified by the American College of Sports Medicine, the American Council on Exercise, the Aerobic and Fitness Association, or the Institute for Aerobic Research. The staff should also include at least some members certified in cardiopulmonary resuscitation (CPR).

Instructors at the better fitness centers will ask about your overall health, too (for instance, whether you have a bad back or weak knees, a heart condition, or hypertension), since certain health problems may affect the amount and type of exercises you can do.

Ask if you can try working out at the fitness center for a week or two at no charge (most will offer at least one free visit). This way, you can determine whether the programs offered, the staff, the atmosphere, and environment meet your needs.

Stick-to-itiveness

To reap the benefits of physical fitness, you have to keep exercising. Months of physical conditioning can be wiped out in a matter of weeks after you stop exercising. For example, 50 percent of the gains you make in an aerobic training program can be lost within four to twelve weeks of inactivity. Postmenopausal women who increase their bone mass while exercising begin to lose it again once they stop training. You can see, therefore, why regular exercise and improved physical fitness should be a lifetime goal. Here are a few ways you can help make exercise a regular part of your life.

• **Set realistic goals.** Setting goals is so important to the success of your exercise program that it bears repeating here. Successfully achieving a goal you set for yourself can be just the incentive you need to stick with your routine.

• **Start slowly.** Beginners often try to get fit in a day, then get discouraged when they develop sore muscles or, worse, suffer an injury. Starting out slowly will keep you from getting too sore or from suffering an injury in the early weeks of your program.

• **Choose activities you enjoy and that are convenient for you.** You're much more likely to exercise if you're doing something you find enjoyable. On the other hand, if you love to swim but don't have ready access to a swimming pool, chances are you won't swim as regularly as you should to keep fit. Try to augment swimming with another form of exercise as well.

• **Vary your routine.** Most exercise routines are repetitive, and can quickly become boring. To keep your interest high and to minimize burnout, choose more than one exercise and alternate your activity from one exercise session to the next. If your fitness program involves walking, jogging, or bicycling, vary your route from day to day or from week to week to break the monotony.

• **Exercise with a partner.** This way, if your enthusiasm wanes, your partner may provide the incentive you need to go on, and vice versa. Make sure you and your partner are well matched in terms of your fitness levels and abilities, however. It can be discouraging to try and keep up with a runner if you're more suited for a brisk walk around the block.

• **Monitor your progress.** Periodically taking a few simple tests (such as some of the self-evaluations described in this chapter) can also be motivating, since you'll be able to see your progress. By monitoring your resting pulse rate before you get up in the morning, for instance, you should see a decrease of about one beat per minute every two weeks for the first fifteen to twenty weeks of your exercise program.

• **Reward yourself.** After a month or two of exercising regularly, treat yourself to a movie, a new outfit, or some other reward. Do the same after six months and again after a year.

A Final Word

Fitting exercise into your life isn't so difficult as it may seem. Just choose activities you enjoy and take it one day at a time. Before you know it, you'll wonder how you ever got through the day *without* exercising.

Suggested Reading

Alter, Michael J. *Sport Stretch*. Champaign, IL: Human Kinetics Publishers,* 1990.

American College of Sports Medicine, *ACSM Fitness Book*. Champaign, IL: Human Kinetics Publishers, 1992.

Anderson, Bob. *Stretching*. Bolinas, CA: Shelter Publications, 1980.

Rippe, James M., M. D., and Ann Ward, Ph.D. *The Rockport Walking Program*. New York: Prentice Hall, 1989.

YMCA of the USA. *Y's Ways to a Healthy Back,* 3rd Ed. Champaign, IL: Human Kinetics Publishers, 1991.

*To order books from Human Kinetics Publishers, write to Human Kinetics Publishers, Box 5076, Champaign, IL 61825-5076, or call toll-free (800)747-4457.

Resources and Support

American College of Sports Medicine Fit Society. The American College of Sports Medicine, the world's largest association of professionals devoted to sports medicine and exercise science, now extends membership in its Fit Society to the general public. For a $20.00 membership fee, you will receive the organization's quarterly newsletter, *The Fit Society Page*, and benefit from discounts on books and other member services. For more information or to join, write to the ACSM Fit Society, P.O. Box 1440, Indianapolis, IN 46206-1440.

The YMCA of the USA, 101 North Wacker Drive, Chicago, IL 60606. The YMCA has provided community-based health programs for more than 140 years. Local Ys offer a wide array of health and fitness programs for family members of all ages, including strength training, aquatics, general exercise, walking classes, and classes for people with disabilities. The YMCA also offers programs in weight control, stress management, lifestyle assessment, fitness testing, and CPR and first-aid classes. For more information, contact your local YMCA.

"How are things at home?" This may seem like an odd question for your doctor to ask during a routine office visit or at your annual physical. But it arises from a growing recognition by the medical profession that emotional stress can have an impact on your physical health. Stress can make you more susceptible to the common cold, headaches, and minor gastrointestinal upsets. Mounting evidence now suggests that stress may play a role in the development of more serious illnesses, including heart disease, high blood pressure, arthritis, peptic ulcers, and possibly cancer. Stress has been shown to worsen disease in people who are already sick, such as those with multiple sclerosis or diabetes. Researchers say stress also makes people more accident-prone.

Stress is an inevitable part of life, the natural consequence of change. You can't escape it. But you *can* change the way in which you cope with it. In the pages that follow, we'll show you how.

What Is Stress?

When we talk about stress, we're actually referring to stressors—situations that require us either to adapt or to suffer undesirable consequences. A new job demands that you take on new responsibilities and adjust to a new work setting. If you've moved to a big city where traffic is congested, you may have to adjust to aggressive drivers and hazardous driving conditions.

Not all stress is negative. Getting married, for example, is stressful, even though it's a happy event. Getting a promotion, becoming a new parent, winning the lottery, and many other positive events are stressors because they require life-changing adjustments. Hans Selye, M.D., one of the world's foremost authorities on stress, has said that some degree of stress is essential if we're to live fulfilling, productive lives. Stress, he says, is the spice of life. It can motivate us to work harder, to accomplish more.

In the face of stress, you respond in one of two basic ways: with an *acute reaction*, in which your body prepares you to deal with an immediate threat (what's known as the "fight or flight" response) or, if stress continues for a long period of time, with a *chronic reaction*. During acute stress, the adrenal glands churn out two related "stress" hormones, *epinephrine* and *norepinephrine*. These hormones accelerate your breathing and pulse rate, raise your blood pressure, boost your blood-sugar levels, and release high-energy fats into the bloodstream to provide your body with quick energy. Chronic stress is associated with the release of cortisol from the adrenal glands. Excess cortisol raises blood cholesterol and triglyceride levels and causes your body to retain sodium.

These stress responses were well-suited for the hostile environment of primitive peoples, who may have had to fight or flee from a saber-toothed tiger in the jungle. Most of the time, however, the "fight or flight" response is not appropriate for the psychological stressors of our twentieth-century world, such as traffic jams, long lines, difficult bosses, and so on. This needless flooding of the body with stress hormones is precisely why stress has become suspect in the development of a wide range of serious and not-so-serious illnesses.

Studies suggest that the constant firing of the "fight or flight" response may lead to *permanent* increases in your heart rate and blood pressure, a risk factor for heart disease. Chronic stress may elevate blood-cholesterol levels, another risk factor for heart disease. In one classic study, certified public accountants whose cholesterol levels were monitored from January 1 to the April 15 tax deadline, experienced as much as a 100 mg/dl rise in cholesterol without a change in their diets. Other researchers have found that cholesterol levels may remain elevated for up to ten days after a stressful event.

Scientists have known for some time now that mental stress can trigger an attack of angina (chest pain) in people with atherosclerosis (narrowing of the coronary arteries). Researchers at Harvard University have found that in addition to raising your blood pressure and heart rate, mental stress (doing an arithmetic problem) can reduce blood flow to the heart in people who already have atherosclerosis. (The blood flow in people with healthy coronary arteries was unaffected.)

The immune system appears to be responsive to stress, too. Scientists have known for some time that there's an increase in disease and death among bereaved spouses, and that the stress of losing a loved one—believed to be one of the most stressful of all life events—temporarily suppresses immune function. Studies have also shown that people who are under stress have lower levels of tumor-and virus-fighting natural killer cells, decreased numbers of disease-fighting white blood cells, and other signs of weakened immunity. Although no one has proved that changes in the activity or levels of these or other immune cells invites disease and death, the implications are there. And evidence like this is why some researchers suspect that stress may play a role in the development of cancer.

Not only can stress take a toll on your health over the long haul, it can also take the joy out of your daily life. As your stress levels rise, physical complaints may emerge. You may experience headaches, nausea, constipation, diarrhea, loss of appetite, nervousness, breathlessness, obscure pains (usually in the abdomen), and heart palpitations. Stress can also contribute to insomnia, making you irritable and tired during the day. Stress can aggravate premenstrual and menopausal symptoms, as well. When stress gets the best of you, you may also experience emotional symptoms, such as a feeling of helplessness and powerlessness. You may even begin to withdraw from social situations. If stress continues unabated, it may lead to alcohol or drug abuse.

How Stressful Is Your Life?

As we mentioned earlier, it's difficult to measure stress because each of us has different stressors, and what's stressful to one person may not be stressful to another. Nevertheless, psychologists have developed stress scales that can give you an *overall* idea of how much stress you are under now. The Holmes and Rahe Stress Point Scale, developed by Thomas H. Holmes, M.D., and Richard H. Rahe, M.D., measures the relative impact of a variety of stressful events. Keep in mind, though, that this test is designed to show you how change affects you. Your particular lifestyle and the way in which you handle the adjustment to situations actually determines your level of stress.

Holmes and Rahe Stress Point Scale

Check off the events that have occurred to you within the last twelve months and then add up the figures next to the events. If your score is 300 or more, you probably run a major risk of incurring some kind of illness in the next year. If your score is 200 to 299, your risk of illness is moderate. And if your score is between 150 and 199, your risk is mild.

Life event	Value	Your score
Death of spouse	100	_____
Divorce	73	_____
Marital separation	65	_____
Jail term	63	_____
Death of a close family member	63	_____
Personal injury or illness	53	_____
Marriage	50	_____
Firing from work	47	_____
Marital reconciliation	45	_____
Retirement	45	_____
Change in health of family member	44	_____

Life event	Value	Your score
Pregnancy	40	_____
Sexual difficulties	39	_____
Gain a new family member	39	_____
Business adjustment (merger, bankruptcy, etc.)	39	_____
Change in financial status	38	_____
Death of a close friend	37	_____
Change to a different line of work	36	_____
Change in number of arguments with spouse	35	_____
Mortgage loan over $100,000	31	_____
Foreclosure of mortgage or loan	30	_____
Change in responsibilities at work	29	_____
Son or daughter leaving home	29	_____
Trouble with in-laws	29	_____
Outstanding personal achievement	28	_____
Spouse beginning or stopping work	26	_____
Beginning or ending school	26	_____
Change in living conditions	25	_____
Revision of personal habits	24	_____
Trouble with boss	23	_____
Change in work hours or conditions	20	_____
Change in residence	20	_____
Change in schools	20	_____
Change in recreation	19	_____
Change in church activities	19	_____
Change in social activities	18	_____
Loan for major purchase (car, etc.)	17	_____
Change in sleeping habits	16	_____
Change in number of family get-togethers	15	_____
Change in eating habits	15	_____
Vacation	13	_____
Christmas	12	_____
Minor violations of the law	11	_____
	TOTAL	_____

Note: Adapted with permission from Thomas H. Holmes and Richard H. Rahe, "The Social Readjustment Rating Scale." *Journal of Psychosomatic Research II*: 213–218. Pergamon Press, 1967.

Some Keys to Coping

Some people appear to be naturally adapted to dealing with stress. They're said to have "stress-hardy" personalities. In studies of business executives and lawyers, Suzanne Kobasa, Ph.D., and her colleagues at the City University of New York found that certain types of individuals were resistant to illness, apparently as a result of three important attitudes toward life: commitment, control, and acceptance of challenge. An attitude of commitment was seen in their approach to work and to life in general. Also, they leaned toward taking control over life events rather than passively accepting them. And they accepted challenges as opportunities for personal growth rather than as threats to be escaped.

Dr. Kobasa found that people with stress-hardy personalities tended to react to stressful situations by getting more involved, exploring possibilities, and learning in the process. In other words, when conflict surfaced, they embraced it rather than avoided it. Individuals who were more passive tended to react with an attitude of helplessness, an approach Dr. Kobasa calls "regressive coping."

Developing a Stress-Management Program

You don't have to be a stress-hardy soul who enthusiastically embraces every challenge in life to protect yourself from the ill-effects of stress. There are several ways you can reduce the negative impact of stress on your health. What's more, taking a few positive steps to counteract stress is, in effect, taking control.

1. **Eat right.** It's easy to neglect your nutritional needs when you're under stress, but this is when good nutrition is more important than ever. Stress increases your metabolism, so your energy needs rise.

Research on the food-mood connection also suggests that you may be able to counterbalance some of the anxiety associated with stressful living by what you eat. There's some evidence that eating foods high in carbohydrates has a calming effect, making you feel more relaxed. (For more on food and mood, see page 66.)

If you're losing sleep over a stressful situation, you may be tempted to stay alert during the day by consuming more caffeine. This may make you feel more anxiety-ridden, however, since caffeine's effect on the central nervous system is more exaggerated during times of stress. In addition, if you consume caffeine late in the day—after 5:00 P.M.—it may lead to a vicious cycle of nighttime sleeplessness and daytime drowsiness. For this reason, you should cut *back* on caffeine (see page 92) and find more constructive ways of coping with insomnia (see How to Get a Good Night's Sleep on page 131).

You should also eat foods high in fiber (see page 70) and drink plenty of fluids to ward off constipation that could be triggered by stress. (If you do become constipated, avoid taking laxatives, which can make the problem worse. See page 152.)

2. Exercise regularly. Engaging in regular physical activity is one of the most dependable ways to reduce stress. The energy that your body gets ready to pour into a "fight or flight" response finds an outlet in exercise.

When you exercise, your body produces and releases a group of hormones known as *beta-endorphins*—the same hormones that produce the "high" experienced by long-distance runners. When you've finished a workout, you're left in a state of natural relaxation. Your heart rate decreases, your blood pressure goes down, and your breathing slows down. Even your body temperature declines as your muscles relax, releasing their tension. The mind, too, participates in this relaxed state, leaving stress behind. Vigorous physical workouts also relieve insomnia and help counter constipation.

To alleviate stress, we recommend that you engage in some kind of aerobic exercise (walking, bicycling, swimming, etc.) twice a day: once in the morning and again in the evening (preferably before 8:00 P.M.) for at least thirty minutes

---

How To Get A Good Night's Sleep

Specialists in sleep disorders recommend that insomnia be remedied by altering your lifestyle and environment rather than by taking medication. This is known as improving your "sleep hygiene," and includes the following commonsense approaches.

• **Keep to a sleep schedule.** Go to bed at the same time every night and get up at the same time every morning. This sets your body clock so that these sleep and wake times become routine. If you haven't fallen asleep within thirty minutes or if you wake up in the middle of the night and can't get back to sleep, get up and do something relaxing, like reading or sewing. Don't lie in bed tossing and turning.

• **Control your sleep environment.** Sleep in a darkened room. If window shades don't make the room dark enough, wear an eye covering. Block out noise as much as possible by wearing earplugs, or mask the noise by running an air conditioner or fan. Keep the room cool. It's hard to sleep when you're uncomfortably warm.

• **Get regular exercise.** Daily workouts are extremely effective in tiring out the body and preparing it for a good night's sleep. Don't exercise shortly before bedtime, however. Late-night workouts can overstimulate your body, contributing to insomnia.

• **Use your bed for sleep (and lovemaking) only.** Don't work, eat, or watch television in bed.

• **Avoid caffeinated drinks and foods late in the day.** Caffeine is a well-recognized stimulant. If you're having trouble sleeping, stay away from coffee, tea, caffeinated soft drinks, or other caffeine-containing beverages in the late afternoon or evening.

per session. The effects of endorphins, like most drugs, tend to wear off after a while. By exercising twice a day, you get a double dose. (For more on midlife fitness and launching an exercise program, see Chapter 5.)

3. Set your priorities. Often, the stressors that do us in aren't so much life's major tragedies as they are a buildup of minor annoyances over the years. If this is the case for you, try dividing your tasks into three categories—essential, important, and trivial. Don't even bother with the trivial tasks. Delegate what you can of the important tasks and concentrate your time and energy on getting the essential things done. Above all, make *time for yourself* a priority. Spend a little time each day—even ten minutes or so—engaged in some kind of enjoyable activity.

4. Get plenty of rest. Fatigue can reduce your ability to cope with stress. But if stress is contributing to sleeplessness, your insomnia may become a source of stress in itself. *Don't* rely on over-the-counter or prescription sleep remedies to break the cycle. Instead, try improving your sleep habits. (See How to Get a Good Night's Sleep on page 131.)

5. Practice relaxation techniques. A number of relaxation techniques have been developed to reduce stress. Among them are deep breathing, progressive muscle relaxation, yoga, and meditation, to name just a few. Relaxation techniques help you achieve what Harvard cardiologist Herbert Benson calls the "relaxation response," a state of consciousness marked by decreased oxygen consumption, respiratory rate, heart rate, and blood pressure—exactly the opposite of what happens during the stress-induced "fight or flight" response.

You'll find a variety of books on relaxation methods in most bookstores; relaxation tapes can usually be bought in a bookstore, as well. Or try the simple method in the box below from Herbert Benson's *The Relaxation Response* (New York: Avon, 1976).

If you don't have the luxury of secluding yourself in a quiet place during the day to practice relaxation techniques, there are some on-the-spot methods for relieving tension when your day gets rough. One is to close your eyes and take several deep breaths. This method is often used by speakers who get stage

---

How To Elicit The Relaxation Response

• Sit quietly in a comfortable position.

• Close your eyes.

• Deeply relax all your muscles.

• Breathe in and out through your nose; repeat the word *one* silently. This helps clear your mind of extraneous thoughts.

• Continue this routine for ten to twenty minutes.

• When finished, sit quietly with your eyes closed for a few moments, then gradually open them.

fright just before mounting the podium. It helps counter the body's rising adrenaline levels. Another method is to run in place for a minute or two or do a few jumping jacks just before or after a stressful event. The beauty of these exercises is that you're putting your stress hormones to the use for which they were intended.

6. Seek out support. Just talking about what you find stressful may help. A steady stream of research over the past several years has shown that emotional support can help protect us against the ill effects of stress. Sandra Levy, M.D., and her colleagues at the Pittsburgh Cancer Institute found that breast-cancer patients who received plenty of psychological support from their physicians, nurses, family, and friends had higher levels of cancer-killing natural killer cells circulating in their blood than those who lacked sympathetic listeners. It still isn't clear whether the elevated levels of natural killer cells will translate into improved survival for these women. However, another study by Stanford University psychiatrist David Spiegel, M.D., has shown that psychotherapy appears to have lengthened the lives of women with breast cancer that had spread to the lymph nodes and beyond.

Social support comes in many different forms. One way to seek out support is simply to open up about your stresses and share your feelings with your family, friends, and, when appropriate, coworkers. If you have a problem that you feel is too private to discuss with even your closest friends and family members, you may want to consider seeing a professional counselor. (For tips on how to find a counselor, see page 137.) Sometimes, the most sympathetic and helpful listeners are those who share the same problem. In this case, support groups can be enormously helpful. Community hospitals, mental-health clinics, and area churches and synagogues often sponsor support groups for a variety of emotional concerns, such as divorce, single parenthood, or death of a spouse. (You'll find support groups for various health problems listed in chapters throughout this book, as well.) Or check your newspaper for a listing of local support groups and meeting times.

How Not To Deal With Stress

You may be tempted to reach for a quick fix when you're under stress. If you smoke, you take out a cigarette. If you drink, you may increase your alcohol consumption. In the long run, however, tobacco and alcohol only make matters worse. While cigarette advertisements may lead you to believe that smoking a cigarette allows you to relax, in reality, tobacco intensifies the effects of stress on the sympathetic nervous system. According to a report on the effects of cigarette smoking from the U.S. Surgeon General's office, nicotine (the active and addictive ingredient in cigarettes) promotes the release of epinephrine from the adrenal glands, producing the "fight-or flight" reaction classically associated with stress. The smoker's heart rate increases, fatty acids are released into the bloodstream, and blood pressure rises. (For more on the harmful effects of cigarette smoking to your health, and for tips on how to quit, see Chapter 7.)

According to the National Institute on Alcohol Abuse and Alcoholism, you're likely to feel stronger effects from a given amount of alcohol when you're emotionally upset or under stress than you would when drinking the same amount while relaxed. And research has shown that, drink for drink, the hangover you experience during a time of stress is worse than that suffered during normal periods.

When It's More Than Stress

It's not unusual for stress to make you feel depressed, anxious, or even a little panicky at times. If these feelings can't be dispelled by a healthy diet, exercise, and/or the use of relaxation techniques, if they persist even after the stressful episode has passed, or if they cause serious disruption in your life, this could be a sign of a more serious problem that may require professional help.

Depression

An estimated 5 million women suffer from major depression at any given time—a rate twice as high as that of men. Depression is *not* a passing blue mood, nor is it a sign of personal weakness or a condition that can be willed away. Rather, it is a serious mental illness with biochemical, genetic, and environmental roots and can be treated with appropriate drugs and/or psychotherapy.

Experts now recognize two main types of depression: *major depression* (also known as *unipolar* depression) and *manic-depressive illness* (or *bipolar* depression).

Major depression: Symptoms of major depression include incapacitating feelings of despair and worthlessness, fatigue, lack of interest in activities that usually bring pleasure, inability to get to sleep and/or early-morning awakenings, agitation, inability to concentrate, diminished interest in sex, social withdrawal, and possibly suicidal thoughts. Often, symptoms are worse in the morning and improve as the day goes on. A person suffering from major depression may either lose interest in food altogether or overindulge in food. Some people with major depression experience persistent physical symptoms that do not respond to treatment, such as headaches, digestive disorders, and chronic pain.

How long the depression lasts is also a clue to its seriousness. Generally speaking, if five or more of these symptoms persist for more than two weeks or recur on a regular basis, they are considered to be symptoms of major depression.

Major depression generally doesn't make an appearance until the middle years, and can occur once, twice, or several times in a lifetime.

Manic-depressive illness: Bipolar depression is not nearly so prevalent as major depression, but it is just as incapacitating. People with manic-depressive illness may experience cycles of depression and elation or mania. Sometimes the mood switches are dramatic and rapid, but more often they are gradual. When in the depressed cycle, you may experience all of the symptoms of a depressive disorder. When in the manic cycle, you may experience inappropriate elation, irritability, severe insomnia, grandiose notions, increased talking, disconnected and racing thoughts, increased sexual desire, a burst of energy, poor judgment, or inappropriate or embarrassing social behavior.

134

Generally, the onset of manic-depressive illness occurs in a person's twenties, and affected people have more episodes of illness than people with major depression.

The first episodes of a depressive disorder may be triggered by stressful life events, such as the breakup of a relationship or the loss of a job. But, as we pointed out earlier, genetic, biochemical, and environmental influences play a part, as well. If one of your parents or a sister or brother has suffered serious depression, you have a 15 percent chance of experiencing a major depressive episode yourself. If a close family member has manic-depressive illness, you are at a greater risk of developing either manic-depressive illness *or* major depression.

There's ample evidence that both major depression and manic-depressive illness are frequently caused by an imbalance in certain *neurotransmitters* (brain chemicals that relay messages between nerve cells), notably *norepinephrine, serotonin,* and *dopamine.* Indeed, antidepressant drugs are believed to help lift depression by remedying neurotransmitter imbalances.

The environment you were raised in also factors into the equation. Children whose parents were overly critical, exploitative, or emotionally unresponsive tend to be more prone to suffer depressive episodes as adults. Children living in such an environment often grow up with low self-esteem and consequently have trouble effectively coping with stress in adulthood.

Symptoms of depression can also be caused by physical illness, such as diabetes, a vitamin deficiency, a hormonal imbalance, or a thyroid disorder. Dozens of prescription and over-the-counter drugs, including birth-control pills, blood-pressure medication, antibiotics, and cold preparations, can cause symptoms of depression. The depression usually lifts once the illness is cured or the drug is discontinued.

If left untreated, a major depressive episode may last from seven to fourteen months, and some 20 percent of untreated cases may drag on for up to two years. However, thanks to the advent of antidepressant drugs and psychotherapies, depression is the most treatable of any mental disorder. More than 80 percent of those who suffer from depression can be helped with appropriate treatment.

To make a diagnosis of depression, your doctor will consider your medical and family history, perform a physical exam, and administer a few psychological tests.

Once depression is diagnosed, a variety of antidepressant medications and psychotherapies can be used to treat it. Some people do well with psychotherapy, others with antidepressants. Some may benefit most from combined treatment: medication for relatively fast relief of symptoms and psychotherapy to learn more effective ways of dealing with life's problems.

Anxiety

Feelings of anxiety can be useful: They alert you to impending trouble and signal the need for change or adaptation. When anxiety is present most or all of the time, however, it becomes destructive. A hallmark of generalized anxiety disorder is excessive anxiety or apprehension about two or more of life's circumstances, such as worrying about possible harm to a child, even when the child is in no danger, or being overly concerned about finances for no apparent reason. Physical symptoms include a rapid or pounding heartbeat, difficulty in breathing, shakiness, sweating, dry mouth, tightness in the chest, sweaty palms, and dizziness. If these kinds of concerns occupy your thoughts for more days than not and persist for a period of six months or longer, you are probably suffering from generalized anxiety disorder.

Diagnosing anxiety is a process of elimination, since numerous physical ailments (including premenstrual syndrome, menopause, iron-deficiency anemia, hypoglycemia, hyperthyroidism, and mitral-valve prolapse), can produce many of the same physical symptoms. Certain over-the-counter and prescription drugs, caffeine, and alcohol abuse can mimic symptoms, as well. Moreover, people with generalized anxiety disorder are more likely to suffer from panic attacks and panic disorder (see below) and may suffer from depression at the same time. Your doctor will review your family and medical history and perform a physical examination, including urinalysis, complete blood count, other blood tests, and an electrocardiogram, before making a diagnosis.

Treatment involves behavioral therapies, such as biofeedback and relaxation techniques (see page 132). A program of mild to moderate exercise (such as brisk walking) early in the day may also help you relax. You will probably be advised to limit or totally eliminate your consumption of caffeine and other stimulants to the central nervous system.

Drugs used in the treatment of anxiety disorder include a class of sedative drugs known as *benzodiazepines* (Ativan, Centrax, Librium, Lipoxide, Mitran, Valium, Xanax), which are generally prescribed for six weeks. Because it's fairly easy to become dependent on these drugs, they are given intermittently for the six-week treatment period, then gradually withdrawn. Some patients may be helped by taking antidepressants, and still others, particularly those with severe physical symptoms, such as hand tremors and heart palpitations, may benefit from beta blockers, drugs normally used in the treatment of hypertension and heart disease.

Panic Attacks and Panic Disorder

In some people, anxiety can become so severe that they begin to experience sudden and intense feelings of fear and apprehension for no apparent reason. Panic attacks, as these episodes are called, are accompanied by such physical symptoms as shortness of breath, dizziness, heart palpitations, trembling, or sweating. People in the throes of a panic attack often fear they are dying or going crazy. If you suffer more than three unprovoked panic attacks in a three-week period, you are said to have panic disorder. But many people who have even one panic attack per month should be considered for treatment.

The condition can be confused with various physical ailments, such as hypoglycemia, mitral-valve prolapse, and thyroid disease. Many people who experience chest pains during a panic attack end up in the emergency room, thinking they're having a heart attack.

Panic attacks usually last only a minute or two. But repeated attacks can leave deep psychological scars, making it impossible for those affected to lead normal lives. Sufferers often develop a fear of the location where a panic attack occurred. Many shun closed-in places such as elevators, automobiles, and tunnels. Others refuse even to leave the house.

No one's sure what causes panic attacks, although they tend to run in families and appear to have biological or genetic roots. Attacks may be triggered by carbon dioxide, caffeine, and a chemical called sodium lactate. Some illicit drugs, such as marijuana and cocaine, can also induce panic attacks. Cocaine triggers attacks in susceptible people not only while they're using the stimulant but also after drug use stops.

How to Find a Counselor

Sometimes stress becomes so severe that it's wise to get help. Left untreated, it may keep you from functioning normally.

If you decide to undergo counseling, choose a counselor carefully. This person will be very important in your life and should be someone with whom you feel comfortable enough to share your innermost thoughts and feelings. Most therapists fall into one of the following categories:

Psychiatrists have completed four years of medical school in addition to three years of training in a psychiatric residency program. They are the only therapists who can prescribe drugs. In general, psychiatrists tend to be medically oriented and deal more with severe mental illness than other therapists. The psychiatrist should be licensed to practice in your state and may be certified by the American Board of Psychiatry and Neurology. If you have medical insurance, the fees of a psychiatrist are likely to be reimbursed.

Clinical psychologists have Ph.D. degrees in psychology and at least one year of supervised clinical training. They must have passed a state licensing examination to practice. Often their services are covered by medical insurance. They may also be certified by the American Board of Examiners in Professional Psychology.

Social Workers generally hold master's degrees, although some have Ph.D. degrees, as well. They have completed at least two years of graduate study and two years of clinical internship. Many social workers are employed by hospitals and clinics, but some have private practices. They may or may not be eligible for insurance payments. Social workers may be listed in the National Registry of Health Care Providers in Clinical Social Work.

Counseling degrees may be held by other health-care professionals. Some counselors hold master's degrees or Ed.S. degrees from graduate programs in education. They are usually called *mental-health counselors*. Others hold degrees in psychiatric nursing and are also trained to counsel.

While it's important that any counselor you choose have graduate education in counseling and supervised training, the expertise and skill of the individual counselor is often more critical than a specific degree. This is why it's so important to choose a person you trust and with whom you feel compatible.

Your first step in seeking counseling should be to interview one or more counselors before making a decision. At the initial visit, ask about the counselor's theories of counseling and whether short- or long-term counseling is used. Ask about fees and insurance coverage, too.

Certain psychological traumas—especially separation anxiety or the loss of a loved one at an early age—can make people more susceptible to panic attacks later in life. Extreme shyness in childhood may also predispose you to panic attacks later in life. And for reasons that aren't known, twice as many women as men suffer from such attacks.

About 80 percent of patients with panic disorder can be cured. Because the symptoms associated with panic attacks overlap with those of physical illnesses, you should first see a doctor to rule out heart disease or other physical problems. If no obvious physical condition can be found to explain the symptoms, your doctor may refer you to a specialist in treating panic symptoms.

A number of drugs have recently been found to be effective in treating panic disorder. The most commonly used are tricyclic antidepressants and MAO inhibitors. Benzodiazepines may also be helpful.

A number of psychotherapy approaches are also being developed. Cognitive and behavioral therapies, in which the patient is desensitized by exposure to fearful situations and to the symptoms themselves, can reduce the frequency of attacks. Deep breathing and relaxation techniques also appear to help.

A Final Word

You can learn to control the stress in your life before it controls you. First, understand why your body reacts as it does. Second, identify the people and events that throw you off balance. Finally, make some simple changes in the way you handle the situations that undermine your peace of mind and well-being.

Resources and Support

National Institute of Mental Health, Public Inquiries, Room 15C-05, 5600 Fishers Lane, Rockville, MD 20857. This government office provides information on depression, anxiety, and other mental illnesses. Write for a publication list.

National Self-Help Clearinghouse, 25 West 43rd Street, New York, NY 10036. This organization maintains a list of thousands of self-help groups nationwide for individuals and their families coping with special physical and/ or psychological problems. Enclose a stamped self-addressed business envelope with your request for information about groups in your area.

Anxiety Disorders Association of America, 6000 Executive Blvd., Rockville, MD 20852. This national nonprofit organization provides referrals to clinicians who treat phobias, panic attacks, and related anxiety disorders. Write or call for a list of publications, catalogs, and cassettes with the latest information on phobias and panic disorder.

Suggested Reading

Benson, Herbert. *The Relaxation Response.* New York: Avon Books, 1976.

Gold Mark S., and Lois B. Morris, *The Good News About Depression: Cures and Treatments in the New Age of Psychiatry,* New York: Bantam Books, 1988.

Gold, Mark S., M.D., *The Good News About Panic, Anxiety and Phobias.* New York: Bantam Books, 1990.

Chapter 7

*Alcohol, Tobacco,
and Drugs:
Why Now Is the
Time to Break
the Habit*

The physical differences between men and women are precisely why chemical substances such as alcohol and tobacco take a harsher toll on a woman's health—including her reproductive health. Overreliance on over-the-counter and prescription medications can pose health problems, too. Older women are particularly vulnerable.

Take a few moments now to learn how substance use (yes, even social drinking), misuse, and abuse may be undermining your efforts at keeping healthy in the middle and later years and what you can do about it.

Alcohol

It's not your imagination. Women *do* respond differently from men to alcohol. You're probably aware that alcohol's intoxicating effects are measured in a rough way by your blood-alcohol level (BAL). A BAL of .10—the legal definition of intoxication in most states—means that there is one part ethanol for every one thousand parts blood in your body. But your BAL doesn't depend just on how much alcohol you consume. How quickly it is absorbed into the bloodstream and how fast it is eliminated from the body also factor into the equation—an equation in which women are on the losing end.

When you have a drink, alcohol—or, more accurately, *ethanol,* its active ingredient—first passes through the stomach, where it is partially broken down by an enzyme called *gastric alcohol dehydrogenase* before being absorbed into the bloodstream. Research now shows that women have lower levels of this enzyme than men. As a result, alcohol passes more quickly through a woman's stomach and into the bloodstream, raising blood-alcohol levels at a much faster rate than in men.

As it circulates in the bloodstream, alcohol is distributed throughout your body's fluids and tissues. But because a woman's body is generally smaller than a man's and has less total body water, a woman drinking the same amount as a man ends up with a higher concentration of alcohol in her bloodstream.

Fluctuations in hormones during the menstrual cycle may also affect the way in which you metabolize alcohol. The highest peaks in blood-alcohol levels appear to occur just before your period.

Alcohol's most significant effects are on the central nervous system and the brain. Ethanol depresses higher brain functions such as conscience, making you feel less inhibited, even after as little as one or two cocktails in an hour. As you continue to drink, it depresses other functions, such as memory, reflexes, and coordination. The effects last until the alcohol is metabolized (broken down) by the liver and eliminated from the body.

How Alcohol Affects Your Health

We've known for some time that chronic heavy drinking can lead to such complications as permanent liver damage, high blood pressure, dangerous enlargement of the heart muscle, low bone mass, impaired brain function, and menstrual problems. We now know that it takes less alcohol over a shorter period of time for women to sustain this kind of serious, sometimes irreversible damage. Indeed, heavy drinking for men is considered more than four drinks per day. For women, it is in the range of two or more drinks per day.

More recently, research has shown that even light to moderate drinking—what's known as social drinking—may adversely affect a woman's health.

• **Osteoporosis:** Having three drinks per day on a regular basis may contribute to low bone mass, although no one is sure how. Heavy drinkers typically are poorly nourished and simply may not get the calcium and vitamin D they need to keep their bones healthy. Alcohol appears to impair the liver's ability to activate vitamin D, which boosts calcium absorption. Alcohol inhibits calcium absorption, as well.

Even more disturbing are reports that women under age sixty-five who drink moderately (two to six drinks per week) are at a significantly increased risk of suffering a hip fracture.

If you are at a higher risk of developing osteoporosis—that is, if you are small-boned, fair-skinned, have a family history of osteoporosis, or have low bone mass—you should limit your consumption of alcohol to no more than two drinks per day—preferably fewer. If you already have osteoporosis, having even one drink can impair your balance, predisposing you to a fall that could lead to a debilitating fracture. For this reason, you should probably abstain from drinking altogether.

• **Breast cancer:** Still controversial is the link between moderate drinking and breast cancer. Studies conducted in the late 1980s reported that having as few as three drinks per week could increase the risk for breast cancer by 40 to 50 percent. Most of those studies were criticized for being poorly designed. But one well-designed study by Walter C. Willett, M.D., and his colleagues at Harvard Medical School found that women who had one drink or more per day were 60 percent more likely to develop breast cancer than nondrinkers.

More research needs to be conducted before we can say for certain just what role alcohol consumption plays in raising your risk of breast cancer. Until we know more, experts now recommend that you avoid drinking altogether if you are at greater risk of developing breast cancer (that is, if you are overweight, have had few children, had your first pregnancy after age thirty, or if your mother or a sister had breast cancer).

•   **Obesity:** There's some evidence that women who drink are more likely to be overweight than male drinkers, even though the women in the studies drank less than the men. Other researchers have found no association between alcohol consumption and increased body fat in women. Nevertheless, alcohol contains seven calories per gram, compared to four calories per gram of carbohydrate or protein, and each of those seven calories is an "empty" calorie with virtually no nutritional value. At a time in your life when your metabolism is slowing, your need for calories is declining, and your need for certain nutrients is rising, there's simply not much room in your diet for empty calories.

•   **Pregnancy-related concerns:** Of concern to women of childbearing age who may have postponed starting a family is fetal alcohol syndrome (FAS), a cluster of symptoms including low birth weight, mental retardation, and deformities of the heart, face, and limbs, caused by alcohol crossing the placenta to the fetus. Most babies with FAS are born to mothers who drink heavily during pregnancy—an average of six drinks per day. But some studies suggest that even moderate drinking (two drinks per day) can increase a woman's odds of having a miscarriage or giving birth to an underweight baby. For this reason, most experts, including the U.S. Surgeon General, recommend that you have no alcohol if you're pregnant or planning to get pregnant in the near future.

•   **Heart disease:** Confounding the issue of *adverse* effects on a woman's health are reports that for both men *and* women, moderate drinking (no more than two drinks per day) can *reduce* your risk of developing heart disease, which affects many times more women than breast cancer or osteoporosis. Alcohol raises levels of HDL_3, one of two types of high-density lipoprotein (HDL) cholesterol, which is thought to protect against heart disease. Alcohol also affects certain blood-clotting mechanisms (see page 319), which may reduce the likelihood of developing a blood clot that could trigger a heart attack or stroke.

The studies showing that alcohol has a protective effect are by no means conclusive, however. One Harvard University study involving women showed that moderate drinkers had an increased risk of suffering a cerebral hemorrhage (a type of stroke caused by excessive bleeding in the brain).

For the time being, the American Heart Association and other national health organizations recommend that you limit your consumption of alcohol to no more than two drinks per day, especially since heavy drinking has been associated with high blood pressure, damage to the heart muscle, and high triglycerides, all of which can raise your risk of heart disease.

•   **Alcohol use among older women:** Older women may be seriously affected by even moderate amounts of alcohol. For instance, older women are more likely to have heart disease, and the chest pain caused by *angina* (an important warning sign of developing heart disease) may be deadened by alcohol. Chronic alcohol use may also lead to nutritional deficiencies, peptic ulcer, gastritis, and diarrhea.

142

Since older women tend to take a larger number of medications, the chances of experiencing dangerous drug interactions with alcohol are substantially higher.

....
Sensible Social Drinking
....

Remember, you can control alcohol only on its way into your body; once it's in your system, only time can undo its effects. If you do drink, there are some ways in which you can do so more sensibly.

• **Be aware that a drink is not a drink is not a drink.** One drink is equivalent to twelve ounces of beer, four ounces of wine, or one ounce of hard liquor. The alcohol in beer and wine is more diluted than in hard liquor, but if you drink enough beer or wine, the effects are the same.

• **Don't drink on an empty stomach.** Instead, drink during or after eating. Food helps slow alcohol's entry into the bloodstream.

• **Dilute drinks with plenty of ice and water or juice.** If you are drinking white wine, add sparkling water for a refreshing wine spritzer.

• **Drink slowly—no more than one drink per hour.** This is the *average* time it takes for alcohol to reach peak blood levels. (See Blood-Alcohol Levels and Behavior on page 144.) Remember, though, that most studies on peak blood levels of alcohol were conducted on men; it will likely take even less time for alcohol to enter your bloodstream, depending on your size, the time of the month (if you're still menstruating), how much stress you're under, and when you last ate. Slow down—or, better yet, *stop* drinking—the moment you start to feel a little tipsy.

• **If you want to appear social but don't want to imbibe, order sparkling water with a twist of lime, or your favorite soft drink.** If you're in a restaurant, try to be the first to place your drink order so that you don't feel pressured into having what others are having. You may also want to try one of the sparkling juices that look like champagne but contain no alcohol. Several brands of nonalcoholic beer are now on the market, as well.

• **Avoid mixing alcohol with over-the-counter or prescription drugs.** Antihistamines, decongestants, and sedatives may increase the sedative effect of alcohol on the central nervous system. Oral contraceptives may slow down the metabolism of alcohol. Certain drugs, including aspirin and the ulcer medications *cimetidine* (Tagamet) and *ranitidine* (Zantac), may reduce the activity of gastric alcohol dehydrogenase, raising blood-alcohol levels even more rapidly. Mixing alcohol with certain antibiotics (notably Flagyl) can make you violently ill.

• **Designate a driver who agrees not to drink at all.** One overlooked health hazard of drinking is fatal car accidents. The National Highway Traffic Safety Administration estimates that half of all automobile fatalities are alcohol-related. If you have no designated driver, call a cab.

Blood-Alcohol Levels and Behavior

BAL (150-lb. person)	Number of drinks (in two hours)	Effect on Behavior and Judgment
0.05	2	Relaxed, judgment not as sharp
0.10	4	Legal limit for driving intoxicated in most states; movement and speech clumsy, judgment impaired
0.15	6	Reflexes poor, speech slurred, judgment severely impaired
0.20	8	Very drunk; loud and difficult to understand; emotions unstable
0.40	16	Difficult to wake up; incapable of voluntary action
0.50	20	Dead drunk; coma and/or death

Recognizing an Alcohol Dependency

While men are more likely than women to develop chronic drinking problems, women who drink heavily have as many or more alcohol-related health problems as men. Alcoholism progresses faster and more severely in women, and such physical complications as cirrhosis of the liver develop more rapidly and at lower intakes of alcohol in women than in men. Alcoholic women have a mortality rate 4.5 times what is expected and lose an average of fifteen years from their life expectancy.

During the middle and later years, the most vulnerable women appear to be those who are either divorced or separated, those who are living with an alcoholic partner, or married women who aren't employed outside the home and whose children no longer live at home. Women with a family history of alcoholism are also at greater risk, as are women who suffer from depression or anxiety. Various surveys now show that a significant number of older woman may be susceptible to developing an alcohol dependency, even if they've never had a drinking problem in the past.

In addition, it may be more difficult to recognize an alcohol dependency in a woman than in a man. Experts often diagnose alcoholism based on how much a person drinks, but women generally drink less than men. One survey of women entering federally funded treatment programs found that the women reported drinking only slightly more than half as much as men. In addition, women are more likely than men to drink alone and to hide their drinking more effectively. "If there is any one trait that characterizes the woman alcoholic, it is the solitary, hidden nature of her drinking," says Sheila Blume, M.D., a psychiatrist at the State University of New York at Stony Brook and an expert on women and alcoholism. "She drinks in the bedroom or in the kitchen and, since she is likely to be divorced or separated, the only people who may know about her drinking may be minor children who are not in a position to intervene." Finally, women are twice as likely to combine their alcohol dependence with a dependence on a sedative drug. "We tend to think of an alcoholic as someone who takes a morning drink," says Dr. Blume. "For a woman, it is often a morning Valium, a morning tranquilizer, or a morning sedative. She may not use any alcohol until evening."

Women who develop an alcohol dependency late in life may be even more difficult to diagnose, since they often live alone and they don't fit the stereotype of the skid-row bum. Because they are often retired, they don't have work-related problems that could call attention to their alcoholism. When older women do develop behavioral problems related to alcohol consumption, other causes, such as senile dementia or depression, are often considered first.

Getting Help

Admitting that you have a problem may be the hardest step you take toward recovery. But the sooner you accept your problem, the sooner you can get the help you need to put your health—and your life—back on track. When an alcohol dependency is treated early, many of the adverse effects on your health can be reversed.

The ultimate goal of treatment is to break your dependence on alcohol altogether. This is usually achieved by entering a detoxification program (either as an inpatient or an outpatient) or by taking the drug disulfiram (Antabuse), which causes violent vomiting when alcohol is consumed. Therapy should also include individual or group counseling and regular attendance at meetings of Alcoholics Anonymous or another support group for recovering alcoholics (see page 155 for a listing of self-help groups). Some women may prefer women-only support groups, such as Women for Sobriety, or working with a female therapist. It's often worthwhile for family members to attend Al-Anon meetings. This support group can help family members break old habits that may have enabled the drinking problem to continue.

Tobacco

The U.S. Surgeon General has pronounced cigarette smoking the number-one hazard to a woman's health today. The average thirty-year-old who smokes fifteen cigarettes a day will lose at least five years off her life, usually from an increased risk of lung or heart disease. Some experts even predict that cigarette smoking alone will soon wipe out the seven-year longevity edge that women now enjoy over men.

Fortunately, cigarette smoking is also the most important *preventable* cause of disease and death. From the moment you quit, your body begins to repair much of the damage that smoking has wrought. Even if you've smoked cigarettes for twenty-five years, in just a few years you can have a healthier heart and cleaner lungs by quitting now.

Quitting isn't easy. In fact, it may be one of the hardest things you do in your life. Nicotine is a powerful addictive substance—as addictive as cocaine or heroine. Quitters today, however, will find more support than ever before—from stop-smoking groups to help break the psychological addiction, to nicotine-laced chewing gum and skin patches to ease you out of the physical addiction.

How Smoking Affects Your Health

You probably know that cigarette smoking raises your risk of lung cancer. Indeed, the increase in cigarette smoking among women after World War II has been largely responsible for making lung cancer the most common cause of cancer death in women today. However, you may not be aware of some of the *other* health risks associated with smoking.

• **Heart disease:** Although most people associate tobacco use with lung cancer, cigarette smoking contributes to three times more deaths from heart disease, the leading cause of death in women over age forty. Women who smoke more than twenty-five cigarettes per day (a little over a pack) are nearly six hundred times more likely to suffer a heart attack than nonsmokers. Women who smoke and take oral contraceptives are thirty-nine times more likely to develop heart disease than oral contraceptive users who don't smoke. In fact, we now know that cigarette smoking, not birth-control pills, is largely responsible for the increased risk of cardiovascular disease once associated with oral contraceptive use (see page 186).

• **Chronic lung disease:** Cigarette smoking accounts for some 85 percent of chronic obstructive lung disease, which includes chronic bronchitis and emphysema. Emphysema, a condition in which the tiny air sacs in the lungs become distended, is a leading cause of disability. One-fourth of the estimated 2 million people affected are so handicapped by the illness that they can't work or run a household.

• **Cervical cancer:** Women who smoke are more likely to develop cervical cancer than nonsmokers. The more cigarettes you smoke and/or the longer you smoke, the greater the risk.

- **Peptic ulcer:** Smokers are more likely to develop peptic ulcers and suffer more sickness and death from them than nonsmokers. Some studies suggest that ulcers heal more rapidly in patients who stop smoking than in those who continue to do so.

- **Reduced fertility:** It may take smokers longer to conceive a child, since the chances of conception may be reduced by nearly 30 percent. This could become a major problem for women over thirty-five who want to have children, since fertility naturally declines as you grow older (see page 200). Smokers also have about a 46 percent higher infertility rate than nonsmokers.

  Researchers believe this reduced fertility may be related to cigarette smoking's antiestrogen effect; that is, cigarette smoking somehow interferes with your body's production and/or use of the hormone estrogen, resulting in lower estrogen levels. Infertility appears to be the result of damage to the delicate Fallopian tubes (where conception takes place), possibly caused by some of the more than four thousand compounds in cigarette smoke.

- **Pregnancy-related complications:** Smokers are at increased risk of suffering a miscarriage or stillbirth. They also risk developing some potentially serious complications of pregnancy, including bleeding during pregnancy and premature rupture of the membranes (the sac of amniotic fluid that surrounds and protects the baby in the womb) Smokers are more likely to deliver babies with low birth weights, the leading cause of death in the first year of life. Babies born to women who smoke during pregnancy are also more likely to succumb to sudden infant death syndrome (SIDS). Moreover, a mother's smoking during pregnancy may have long-term effects on a child's physical and emotional development. Follow-up studies on infants and children born to women who smoked during pregnancy show deficits in growth, intellectual and emotional development, and behavior.

- **Early menopause:** Women who smoke experience menopause and all of its attendant health risks (including an increased risk of heart disease and osteoporosis) an average of one or two years earlier than do nonsmokers. Again, the antiestrogen effect of cigarette smoking may be to blame.

- **Osteoporosis:** There's some evidence that women who smoke are at an increased risk of developing osteoporosis, possibly as a result of lower estrogen levels and a negative effect of cigarette smoking on the bone-remodeling cycle.

- **Incontinence:** Cigarette smokers are more likely to suffer from incontinence (loss of bladder control) than nonsmokers.

- **Premature aging of the skin:** Studies have shown that cigarette smoking causes earlier and more severe skin wrinkles.

Cigarette smoke is also capable of harming the health of those around you. Reports by the Surgeon General and the National Academy of Sciences now show that healthy nonsmokers who inadvertently breathe in cigarette smoke of nearby smokers are at a greater risk of developing lung cancer and heart disease than people who are not exposed to secondhand smoke. Passive smoking can also worsen the symptoms of asthma, chronic bronchitis, and allergies in nonsmokers. And children of parents who smoke experience more respiratory infections and other respiratory problems than children of nonsmoking parents.

When you quit, however, you can substantially reduce your smoking-related risk of heart disease and lung cancer. Two years after you quit, your elevated risk of heart disease is cut in half. Some fifteen years after kicking the habit, your risk of lung cancer declines to the level of nonsmokers. Many of the other health risks associated with cigarette smoking will be reduced after you've quit, as well.

Calling It Quits

If you're like most smokers, you probably *want* to quit. The key to success is to develop a plan to quit that is designed to help you over the biggest hurdles. For women, the major obstacles appear to be the physical addiction, the psychological addiction, and worries about weight.

The physical addiction: Nicotine, the addictive substance in cigarettes, appears to be much more addictive than previously believed. As we mentioned earlier, the Surgeon General has declared nicotine a substance as addictive as heroin. Moreover, women may be more vulnerable to the physical addiction of cigarettes than men are. The reason is that men metabolize nicotine faster than women, so it takes fewer cigarettes for a woman to achieve the same blood levels of nicotine as a man. This may be one reason why women purportedly have a harder time kicking the habit than men.

If you are determined to quit, however, you can. Just remember that withdrawal symptoms—cigarette cravings, irritability, difficulty concentrating, sleep disturbances, drowsiness, headache, and stomach upsets—are strongest during the first two or three days after you quit, then gradually subside over the next couple of weeks. *Physical withdrawal symptoms for even the heaviest smokers disappear altogether after a month.*

You'll find it easier to manage withdrawal symptoms as each day goes by. One way to deal with withdrawal symptoms is to occupy yourself with activities that preclude smoking during the first few days after you quit. Go to the movies, take long walks, go for a bike ride. Be sure to get plenty of rest, too.

If you are a heavy smoker (that is, you have your first cigarette within thirty minutes after waking up in the morning, or you smoke more than a pack a day), you may want to ask your doctor about using nicotine chewing gum (Nicorette) or the more recently FDA-approved nicotine skin patch (Nicoderm, Habitrol). Both the gum and the twenty-four hour skin patch (which are available only with a doctor's prescription) help ease physical withdrawal symptoms by keeping some nicotine in your bloodstream for several weeks after you quit.

The psychological addiction: When you smoke, you develop not just a physical addiction to cigarettes but also a psychological one. You may use cigarettes to relax or to deal with anger, stress, boredom, or frustration. Many women report that smoking helps them cope with stress or handle difficult situations or emotions.

The psychological addiction may be harder to break than the physical one. It may take months before you begin to feel comfortable without a cigarette in your hand. That's why it's important to find substitute behaviors. Here are some suggestions:

• Keep your hands busy. Fiddle with a paper clip. Take up knitting. Play cards.

• Find something else to put in your mouth: Chew sugarless gum; eat carrot or celery sticks.

• Stay busy with activities that discourage you from smoking. For example, it's hard to enjoy a cigarette while washing the car, riding a bicycle, or taking a shower.

• Brush your teeth often. Enjoy that fresh, clean taste. Go to your dentist for a professional cleaning as soon as you've stopped smoking.

• Spend time in places that don't allow smoking, such as movie theaters and libraries.

• Ask your friends for support. If you must, avoid smokers for a while.

• Limit your alcohol intake. Drinking is often associated with smoking, and alcohol can weaken your resolve.

• Learn relaxation techniques such as deep breathing (see page 132) to reduce tension when the urge to light up strikes.

• Avoid eating too much sugar. Maintaining a stable blood-sugar level helps prevent fatigue and depression.

• Exercise regularly. This is an ideal way to relieve stress and anxiety.

Worries about weight: Fear of gaining weight is another major stumbling block for women who smoke. But don't let it keep you from quitting. According to the American Cancer Society, only one-third of smokers who quit gain weight. Another one-third actually lose pounds as they substitute exercise for smoking.

As for the argument that gaining weight may be more hazardous to your health than cigarette smoking, by some estimates you'd have to put on an additional seventy-five pounds to offset the health benefits gained by quitting. On the average, ex-smokers who do gain weight put on only about five or six pounds.

There are several possible reasons for the weight gain. Some studies have found that smoking speeds up your metabolism. When you quit, your metabolism may slow down a little, causing you to gain weight in the weeks after you quit. Weight gain may also be more likely if you feel a need to put something in your mouth to replace cigarettes, you indulge in extra food as a reward for stopping smoking, you enjoy eating more because your sense of taste has improved, or you develop a better appetite because your overall health has improved.

Whatever the cause of the weight gain, it can often be easily managed. A few tips:

• Get regular exercise. Exercise burns calories and may help rev up a sluggish metabolism. Walking is especially helpful because it is an aerobic activity that is not too strenuous.

• Drink a lot of water—six to eight glasses per day.

• Substitute low-calorie foods for cigarettes. Munch on raw vegetables, plain crackers, bread sticks, cinnamon sticks, unbuttered popcorn, and sugarless hard candies or chewing gum.

Developing a Plan to Quit

When you're ready to quit smoking, develop a clear plan. Start by writing down all the reasons why you want to quit. Next, choose a method. By far the most successful way to quit is to go it alone. In one of the largest surveys to date on smokers who quit, more than 90 percent did so on their own, without any help from organized smoking-cessation programs. Smokers who quit cold turkey were more likely to succeed than those who gradually decreased their daily consumption of cigarettes, switched to cigarettes lower in tar and nicotine, or used special filters or holders. (If you decide to go it alone, check out the numerous books, pamphlets, videotapes, and other materials available to help you. See Resources and Support on page 155 for a list of organizations that provide free information on how to quit.)

If you are a heavier smoker who hasn't been able to quit on your own, you may benefit from joining a stop-smoking group. These groups meet at least once a week for about ten weeks, providing support and helping you find constructive alternatives to smoking. Local chapters of the American Heart Association, the American Cancer Society and the American Lung Association offer stop-smoking clinics. You might also check with hospitals in your area.

As we mentioned earlier, heavy smokers may also benefit by using Nicorette gum or the Nicoderm or Habitrol skin patches (available from your doctor), along with individual counseling or group support to help ease the psychological addiction.

Once you've decided on a method, set a quit date about two weeks away and circle the date on your calendar. Some smokers find it helpful during this time to switch to a brand of cigarettes that's low in tar and nicotine and start to taper down. You might also keep a record of when, where, and under what circumstances you light up. This smoker's diary will help familiarize you with your habit and help you find substitutes to smoking after you quit. You should also write down some alternatives to smoking, such as the ones discussed earlier.

On the day you quit, throw away all cigarettes and matches. Hide all lighters and ashtrays and follow the suggestions in your quit plan for coping with any withdrawal symptoms you may experience.

Even if you don't succeed the first time, keep trying. Many smokers attempt to quit at least twice before finally quitting for good. As you learn new strategies for quitting, each attempt will be a little easier than the last and will bring you closer to success.

Drug Misuse and Abuse:
The Hidden Addiction

Although much ado has been made in the press about addiction to illicit drugs, a much more pervasive problem for women in the middle and later years is misuse or abuse of prescription and over-the-counter drugs.

Older women may be particularly at risk for several reasons. To begin with, there are simply more older women than there are men. Second, older women tend to have more chronic health problems that require medication. Older women also make significantly greater use of potentially addictive prescription drugs, such as tranquilizers, sedatives, antidepressants, and antipsychotics.

Compounding the problem is the fact that since women have more body fat than men, drugs that are deposited in body fat, such as tranquilizers and barbiturates, may be broken down and cleared from the body more slowly in women than in men. And because women have less body fluid and a lower body weight than men, these drugs tend to act more quickly on a woman's central nervous system. These differences in metabolism increase after menopause, when a woman's relative proportion of body fat rises. As a result, women—particularly older women—are at a greater risk of experiencing toxic side effects from these drugs, as well as dangerous drug and alcohol interactions.

The Effects on Your Health

We tend to think of prescription and over-the-counter medications as safe—and most *are* fairly safe when used properly. However, misusing or abusing these drugs can result in serious health consequences.

• **Drug addiction:** Using psychotropic drugs such as tranquilizers may lead to such complications as chronic dependency and addiction, emotional disturbances, insomnia, or overdose. These drugs may also cloud your thinking and interfere with your ability to perform even simple motor tasks. Sometimes, the effects of the drugs are so severe that they may lead to institutionalization. Women who take psychotropic drugs are at a greater risk of falling and, if they have osteoporosis, of suffering a hip fracture. Women who abuse these drugs are at a greater risk of committing suicide, as well.

• **Adverse drug reactions:** Older women are more likely than younger women to experience adverse drug reactions—usually from taking a combination of medications—and to be hospitalized as a result. The drugs most commonly associated with adverse reactions in older women are analgesics, antibiotics, anticoagulants, antidepressants, antihypertensives, antiparkinsonian drugs, antipsychotics, bronchodilators, the heart medication digitalis, diuretics, nonsteroidal anti-inflammatory agents, oral hypoglycemics (prescribed for diabetics), and sedatives. Common symptoms and signs of adverse drug reactions include restlessness, falls, depression, confusion, loss of memory, constipation, and incontinence. More serious complications include upper GI bleeding with nonsteroidal anti-inflammatory drug use and hip fracture with psychotropic drug use.

• **Noncompliance:** If you take a lot of different pills during the day, there's a greater chance you will forget to take something that is essential or that you'll take something in the wrong amount.

Even such seemingly harmless over-the-counter medications as laxatives, analgesics, diuretics, and diet pills may become problematic, and some may be potentially addictive.

• **Laxatives:** Laxatives are often advertised as a "safe and gentle" way to relieve constipation, a common problem among women in the middle and later years. However, long-term use of certain types of laxatives, known as *stimulant laxatives* (see Common Over-the-Counter Laxatives) can actually aggravate the problem. Chronic use of stimulant laxatives may cause inflammation of the mucous lining of the colon and weaken the muscles in the colon wall, a potentially severe and irreversible condition known as *cathartic colon*. Over-reliance on stimulant laxatives may also cause electrolyte imbalances and fluid loss, possibly triggering dizzy spells, light-headedness, irregular heart rhythms, dehydration, and weakness. Chronic use of these drugs could also cause gastrointestinal bleeding, which could lead to anemia, allergic reactions, and reduced nutrient absorption. Moreover, prolonged laxative use may actually cause you to become *more* constipated, creating a vicious cycle of laxative-dependence.

• **Analgesics:** Analgesics are among the most frequently used drugs in women age sixty-five and older, particularly since arthritis and other painful conditions increase with age and since a wide variety of analgesic drugs is available without a prescription. Aspirin, however, may irritate the stomach. It also has an anticoagulant effect and can promote bleeding. For this reason, people with blood-clotting disorders, a vitamin K deficiency, and those with a history of peptic ulcer or gastrointestinal bleeding may be advised to use the nonaspirin substitute acetaminophen instead.

Common Over-the-Counter Laxatives

BULK-FIBER LAXATIVES
Fiberall
Metamucil
Serutan

STIMULANT LAXATIVES

Correctol	Ex-Lax
Carter's Little Pills	Feen-a-Mint
Colace	Fletcher's Castoria
Dialose	Milk of Magnesia
Dialose-Plus	LaxCaps
DOSS	Perdiem
Doxidan	Peri-Colace
Dulcolax	Senokot

Ibuprofen (Motrin IB, Advil), an antiinflammatory analgesic, may cause indigestion, nausea, stomach pains, and diarrhea. The drug may also decrease kidney function and cause you to retain sodium and water. This may be a problem for women with congestive heart failure. Older women, those with hypertension, diabetes, or atherosclerosis may also be at an increased risk of developing renal (kidney) toxicity when they take these drugs; they should take acetaminophen instead.

As "safe" as acetaminophen is, even this over-the-counter analgesic can cause problems, particularly when taken for long periods of time. Chronic excessive use of acetaminophen (more than 5 grams per day for several weeks) can produce liver toxicity.

And it may be easier than you think to take an overdose. Many over-the-counter multisymptom cold and flu preparations contain a decongestant *and* an analgesic (usually aspirin or acetaminophen). Often, however, cold sufferers use these products *along with* an analgesic, inadvertently taking a double dose. Check the labels of these products before using them to ensure you don't make this mistake.

• **Diuretics:** Many over-the-counter and prescription diuretics, usually used by women to relieve premenstrual bloating and water retention, may produce a rebound effect; that is, after you stop taking them, you gain even more water weight than before you started using them.

• **Diet pills:** While over-the-counter diet pills, such as Acutrim, Dex-a-Diet, and Dexatrim, may initially suppress your appetite and cause you to lose weight, the effects last only for as long as you take them. The U.S. Food and Drug Administration is currently investigating the safety and effectiveness of phenylpropanolamine, the "active" ingredient in many over-the-counter diet pills. Phenylpropanolamine, also found in more than one hundred over-the-counter and prescription nasal decongestants, psychostimulants, and treatments for premenstrual syndrome, can cause severe hypertension, seizures, strokes, and even death when it is unknowingly ingested by someone who is sensitive to it or who may consume more than the recommended dosage.

Some Tips for Safe Drug Use

• **Keep a list of drugs you are taking, including over-the-counter preparations, and share it with your physician and your pharmacist.** As a service to their clients, some pharmacies now keep track of your prescription medications for you. This will help prevent adverse drug interactions and duplication of medications.

• **Don't mix alcohol with over-the-counter or prescription medications.** Of the one hundred most frequently prescribed drugs, fifty interact with alcohol; of the ten most prescribed drugs, all do.

• **Ask your physician if there are nondrug alternatives that may help your condition.** For instance:

If you regularly use laxatives: Constipation is more likely a result of poor bowel and dietary habits and chronic laxative use than "normal" aging. Instead of using laxatives, get into the habit of having a bowel movement at a set time each day (in the morning, for example), drink plenty of fluids, eat foods high in fiber (try eating three or four prunes just before bedtime), and exercise regularly. (For more tips on how to avoid constipation, see page 69.)

There are times when a laxative may be appropriate. For example, many drugs, including aluminum-containing antacids, calcium, iron, codeine, certain antihypertensive drugs, antidepressants, antihistamines, and nonsteroidal anti-inflammatory agents, are potentially constipating. However, you should take laxatives *only* on your doctor's advice.

If you use an over-the-counter diuretic: Instead of taking diuretics for bloating and water retention, try reducing the salt in your diet. Cutting back on salt can be as effective as a mild diuretic without any of the side effects. (For advice on how to reduce the salt in your diet, see page 74.)

If you use nonprescription diet pills: Try a more sensible weight-loss diet and exercise regimen (see Chapter 15). It may take longer for you to measure the results, but your efforts will more likely be long-lasting.

Even such serious chronic health conditions as hypertension and high cholesterol are often *best* managed with nondrug therapies (see Chapter 16).

A Final Word

When it comes to substance use, misuse, or abuse, it's almost never too late to make a change for the better. And as difficult as it may be to change your ways, the returns to your health are enormous. So why not make a fresh, clean start today?

Al-Anon Family Group Headquarters, P.O. Box 862, Midtown Station, New York, NY 10018-0862. Office phone: (212)302-7240; for free pamphlets: (800)356-9996; for meeting information in New York: (800) 245-4656; in the United States: (800)344-2666; in Canada: (800)443-4525. Al-Anon provides support for friends or relatives of problem drinkers. Look in the phone directory under Al-Anon for a chapter near you.

Alcoholics Anonymous, General Service Office, Box 459, Grand Central Station, New York, NY 10163. Look in the phone book under Alcoholics Anonymous or write to this address for information on AA's 12-step program for recovery from alcoholism.

American Lung Association, 1740 Broadway, New York, NY 10019. The ALA is dedicated to the fight against lung disease (including asthma, tuberculosis, emphysema, and lung cancer) and its causes, such as cigarette smoking, air pollution, and hazards of the workplace. For literature and more information, contact your Lung Association, listed in the white pages.

For more information on kicking the smoking habit, check with the *American Cancer Society,* the *National Cancer Institute* (see page 405 for addresses), or the *American Heart Association* (see page 337 for address).

National Clearinghouse for Alcohol and Drug Information, P.O. Box 2345, Rockville, MD 20852. Phone: (800) 729-6686 or (301) 468-2600. This branch of the National Institutes of Health contains the largest body of information about alcohol and other drugs in the nation. The NCADI provides referrals to alcohol and drug-treatment centers around the country and publishes the *National Directory of Drug Abuse and Alcoholism Treatment and Prevention Programs.* The NCADI also publishes free fact sheets on a variety of topics, including *Women and Alcohol, Aging and Alcohol Abuse, The Fact Is . . . It's Dangerous to Drink Alcohol While Taking Certain Medications,* and *Using Your Medicines Wisely: A Guide for the Elderly.* Write or call for a publications catalog.

Women for Sobriety, P.O. Box 618, Quakertown, PA 18951. Phone: (800) 333-1606. This organization, founded in 1975, is geared specifically toward helping women alcoholics overcome their addiction. Send a business-size stamped self-addressed envelope for a referral to a support group near you.

Chapter 8

Looking Your Best at Any Age: New Options and Proven Techniques

When you feel your best on the inside, it's only natural to want to look your best on the outside. Here is a look at some of the cosmetic concerns you may have in the middle and later years.

Skin Wrinkles

Your skin, your body's largest organ, consists of three layers: the *epidermis* (outermost layer), *dermis* (inner layer), and *subdermis* (a layer of fat just under the skin—see Figure 8.1). How well your skin ages depends on a variety of factors. Some skin changes are written in your genes at birth: Generally speaking, dark-skinned people have thicker skin with more oil, so lines and wrinkles come later in life. Dark-skinned people are also better protected against skin cancer because they have more protective melanin in their skin. You can determine your skin type, based on how readily your skin burns or tans when exposed to sunlight, by consulting What's Your Skin Type on page 157.

Natural aging plays a part, too. The connective tissues in skin, *collagen* and *elastin*, which normally maintain skin tone, lose their elasticity (ability to stretch and flex) as you grow older. Production of collagen in the dermis declines, too. What's more, both of these fibers tend to deteriorate with age. As a result, the dermis begins to bunch and fold underneath the epidermis, which retains its original size. Those folds are wrinkles. Sebaceous glands produce less lubricating sebum, as well, causing the skin to become more dry. The number of melanocytes in the skin diminishes, too, somewhat reducing your body's natural protection against the sun.

Even your menopause appears to affect the quality of your skin. Low estrogen levels have long been suspected of contributing to the wrinkles of postmenopausal women. The exact role that estrogen plays in skin wrinkling and dryness still isn't clear, but studies have shown that estrogen receptors

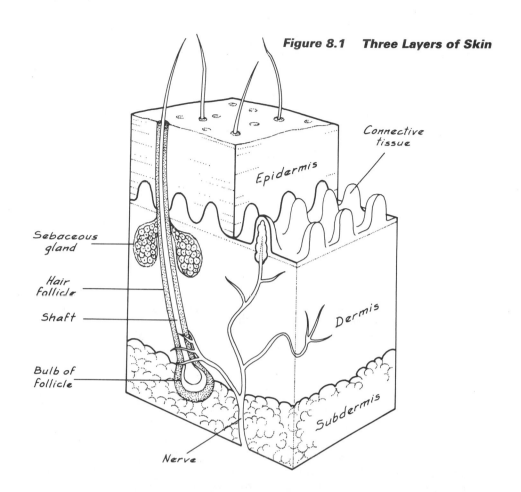

Figure 8.1   Three Layers of Skin

Connective tissue

Epidermis

Sebaceous gland

Hair Follicle

Shaft

Bulb of Follicle

Dermis

Subdermis

Nerve

....
What's Your Skin Type?
....

Skin type	History of sunburning or tanning*
I	Always burns easily, never tans
II	Always burns easily, tans minimally
III	Burns moderately, tans gradually and uniformly (light brown)
IV	Burns minimally, always tans well (moderate brown)
V	Rarely burns, tans profusely (dark brown)
VI	Never burns, deeply pigmented (black)

*Based on first forty-five to sixty minutes of sun exposure after winter or no sun exposure.

Note: Reprinted with permission from "Harmful Effects of Ultraviolet Radiation," The Council on Scientific Affairs, American Medical Association, in the *Journal of the American Medical Association* (July 21, 1989) 262, no. 3: 380–384. Copyright © 1989 by the American Medical Association.

exist in the skin (particularly in the face) and that estrogen levels affect the condition of your skin. Premenopausal women who have had their ovaries removed and who don't take estrogen experience thinning of the epidermis— the longer the time elapsed from surgery, the thinner the skin becomes. When the women begin taking estrogens, however, the epidermis plumps up again and continues to thicken during the first six months of estrogen therapy. It's not known yet how much of this thickening is a result of fluid retention. Estrogen has also been shown to affect the amount of collagen in the skin. In one study, collagen production in the skin of postmenopausal women who didn't take estrogen fell by two percent a year for up to fifteen years. On the other hand, women who were given estrogen implants experienced a significant increase in collagen after three to six months of receiving the implant.

Of course, as anyone with laugh lines or frown lines knows, facial expressions can influence the development of wrinkles, too.

Preventing Skin Wrinkles

A majority of skin changes over the years are a result of sun exposure, cigarette smoking, and other environmental assaults over the course of a lifetime. This means there is a lot you can do to slow down or stop skin wrinkling and other skin changes.

• **Protect yourself from excessive or chronic sun exposure.** Up to 90 percent of the skin changes we once associated with normal aging, including wrinkling, sagging, and a leathery appearance, may actually be a result of damage from the sun's ultraviolet radiation. Ultraviolet radiation damages the skin's elastic fibers, causing them to thicken and tangle, a condition known as *elastosis*. The amount of collagen in photodamaged skin also decreases, as does the skin's ability to hold water. The sun causes skin inflammation and damages the microscopic blood vessels that nurture the skin.

In addition to wrinkles, broken capillaries (facial telangiectasias), freckles, age spots and pigmentation on the upper lip, cheeks, and forehead (called *chloasma*) may become more visible with increased sun exposure.

More serious to your overall health is the increased risk of skin cancer that accompanies excessive sun exposure (for more on skin cancer, see Chapter 18).

To protect yourself from photoaging, wear protective clothing when you go out in the sun, avoid sun exposure during peak daylight hours (10:00 A.M. to 3:00 P.M.), and *use a sunscreen any time you are outdoors for more than twenty to thirty minutes a day.* Get into the habit of using sunscreen in your daily makeup routine. Apply an ounce of sunscreen (about a palmful) to all exposed areas not well covered by clothing *at least thirty minutes before going outdoors or before applying makeup.* Most screens take between ten to thirty minutes to bond to the outer layer of skin. If you apply makeup before the screen has had a chance to bond, some of the sunscreen may be removed and your foundation will not go on smoothly.

What kind of sunscreen is best? Most sunscreens state on the package label their ability to protect against UVB, the part of the sunlight spectrum most responsible for causing sunburns as well as skin cancer. The sun protection factor (SPF) rating tells you approximately how many times longer you can expect to stay out in the sun before suffering a sunburn than if you were unprotected.

We now know that ultraviolet A (UVA) radiation, long considered to consist of relatively harmless tanning rays, can also cause skin damage, including premature aging and the promotion of skin cancer. So for the best protection, you should use one of the newer broad-spectrum sunscreens that also protect against UVA radiation. The U.S. Food and Drug Administration is in the process of revising regulations for sunscreen labeling to reflect how much protection is provided by the new sunscreens. Until the new regulations go into effect, you should look for products with one or more of the following ingredients, which protect against UVB *and* UVA radiation:

oxybenzone	dioxybenzone
Eusolex 6300 and 8020	Parasol 1789
lawsone with dihydroxyacetone	sulisobenzone
2-ethylehexyl	titanium dioxide
2-cyano-3, 3-diphenylacrylate	red petrolatum

An SPF rating of 15 or greater is adequate protection for most people. These products filter more than 90 percent of the UVB responsible for sunburn. (If your skin tans easily and you choose a lower SPF rating with the intent of getting a tan, keep in mind that there's no such thing as a "safe" tan. In fact, a suntan is a sign of sun damage.)

If you have dry skin, look for a sunscreen with a cream or creamy lotion base, such as Presun Creamy, Total Eclipse, Piz Buin, or Estee Lauder's Sun Waterworld. Be sure to protect your lips with a lip protectant, as well. And don't forget to wear sunglasses, which not only protect your eyes from the sun's harmful rays but also help keep you from squinting, which could contribute to wrinkles.

A precaution about sunscreens: Sunscreens block the UVB rays that trigger the skin's manufacture of vitamin D, which aids in calcium absorption and bone formation. Some experts worry that liberal use of sunscreens may cause a vitamin D deficiency in postmenopausal women. At least one preliminary study has shown that users of sunscreens at midday in summer (when seasonal vitamin D levels are at their peak) had 50 percent lower blood levels of vitamin D compared to nonusers. More research needs to be conducted before we know whether sunscreens actually do make you more susceptible to a vitamin D deficiency. Until we know more, postmenopausal women may want to take a dietary supplement (200 I.U., or half of the recommended dietary allowance of 400 I.U.). (For more on vitamin D, see Chapter 4.)

Strong winds, high altitudes, humidity, and temperature extremes can exacerbate sun damage. Remember, too, that a thin cloud cover filters out just 20 to 40 percent of the sun's harmful rays, so, in effect, you can get a sunburn even when the sky is overcast. Wearing a hat or sitting in the shade isn't enough protection from the sun, either, since you can still receive reflected light. Be sure to cover up and use a suncreen under these conditions, as well.

• **Quit smoking.** Smoking cigarettes also prematurely wrinkles your skin. The more heavily you smoke, the more quickly and severely your skin will age. Smokers in their forties often have facial wrinkles equivalent to those of nonsmokers in their sixties. Particularly prominent are tiny wrinkles spreading from the upper and lower lips and crow's-feet around the eyes.

No one is sure exactly how cigarette smoking increases skin wrinkling. Some researchers suggest that the toxins in cigarette smoke damage the tiny blood vessels that nourish the skin. Others speculate that the lower estrogen levels associated with cigarette smoking in women may contribute to premature aging. Still others suggest that squinting to keep cigarette smoke out of the eyes plays a part. For advice on quitting smoking, see Chapter 7.

• **Vary your sleep pattern.** If you always sleep on your side, you may develop diagonal wrinkles on your cheek or forehead. Many models learn to sleep on their backs to prevent such wrinkles. To avoid these wrinkles, try to rotate your sleep position every night. (Placing a pillow under your knees may make sleeping on your back more comfortable.)

If You Already Have Wrinkles

While photoaging of the skin was once considered permanent, a variety of treatment regimens are available that can minimize—and sometimes erase— some of the damage wrought by the sun. For most of the treatments or proce-dures here, you'll want to find a dermatologist or a *qualified* plastic surgeon. Some of the procedures can be quite risky when performed by untrained or inexperienced practitioners.

Nonsurgical Treatments

• **Retin-A:** Not long ago, Retin-A (*topical tretinoin*) made headlines as a revolutionary new antiaging cream that could take years off your looks. The prescription cream, a vitamin A derivative that's been used for more than eighteen years to treat acne, *does* appear to have an antiaging effect. But it has not yet been approved by the U.S. Food and Drug Administration for use as an antiaging cream (although it is frequently prescribed for this reason). And it's not for everyone. The best candidates are women between fifty to seventy years old who have fine to moderate wrinkles, particularly crow's-feet around the eyes. You should consult with a dermatologist to determine whether you're a good candidate for Retin-A and to get a prescription.

• **Dermabrasion:** This treatment, usually conducted by a dermatologist or a plastic surgeon on an outpatient basis, involves mechanically removing super-ficial wrinkles and scars with high-speed rotating brushes. The brushes scrape away the top layer of skin (epidermis) and a small portion of the dermis, allowing new, smooth skin to form. The best candidates are women with acne scars or fine wrinkles, especially around the mouth. The results are permanent.

• **Chemical peels:** If you have fair, thin skin with fine wrinkling on your face, you may want to consider having a chemical peel. This involves the use of chemicals to remove the top layer of skin, permanently erasing or fading fine facial wrinkles. The procedure is usually done by a qualified physician on an outpatient basis (unless you have a full face peel, which may require a one-night hospital stay).

- **Collagen injections:** Collagen injections can be used to fill out deep facial wrinkles, add fullness to lips, and smooth out the backs of your hands. The injections work particularly well on wrinkles between the nose and mouth (laugh lines), crow's-feet around the eyes, or frown lines at the top of the nose. This outpatient procedure takes fifteen to twenty minutes, and a local anesthetic is included in the collagen mixture. Your physician will probably want to pretest you to determine whether you are allergic to collagen.

  The biggest drawback to collagen injections is that they don't last. You may have to have repeated injections every six to nine months.

- **Moisturizers:** One class of products that *won't* cure (or prevent) wrinkles includes moisturizing creams and lotions, so don't be taken in by the antiaging claims made by many of these products. (Moisturizers *can* help temporarily relieve dry skin associated with aging. But their use is limited. See "Dry Skin.")

- **Estrogen therapy:** While it's true that estrogen therapy plumps up your skin and increases collagen production in skin, estrogen is a drug and, like any drug, it has side effects. (See Chapter 20.) There are more effective ways to retain a more youthful-looking appearance than to take postmenopausal estrogen.

Surgical Options

For more severe wrinkles and sagging skin (as well as other cosmetic problems associated with middle age, such as sagging breasts), you may want to consider plastic surgery. New surgical techniques, a trend toward money-saving outpatient surgery, and financing offered by plastic surgeons have all helped make cosmetic surgery more accessible and affordable. As the population grows older, attitudes about cosmetic surgery have changed, too. There's simply no reason to be embarrassed about wanting to look as young as you feel. Remember, though, that cosmetic surgery is just that—surgery. Like any type of surgical procedure, cosmetic surgery is not without risks. While complications are rare, they can be fairly serious, including anesthesia-related reactions and post-operative infection.

If you are considering cosmetic surgery, you should learn as much as you can about the procedure(s) before making a decision (see Suggested Reading on page 176). Two excellent resources are the American Society of Plastic and Reconstructive Surgeons and its affiliate, the American Society for Aesthetic Plastic Surgery (see Resources and Support on page 177 for their addresses and toll-free phone number).

Keep in mind that finding a qualified surgeon is a key to successful and safe results. Unfortunately, as the number of people seeking aesthetic surgery has risen, so has the number of unqualified surgeons performing the procedures. To find a qualified plastic surgeon, you should

- Ask your regular physician for a referral.

- Get referrals from friends who have had successful operations.

- Call the toll-free number of the American Society of Plastic and Reconstructive Surgeons for a referral (see page 177). All members are certified to perform plastic surgery by the American Board of Plastic Surgery.

- Call the American Board of Plastic Surgery (215-586-4000) to confirm that a doctor is *board-certified in plastic surgery.*

- Call local hospitals to find out whether the doctors on your list have hospital privileges for the same procedures they perform in their office. Even if the procedure will be done in the doctor's office, hospital affiliation means a doctor has the respect of his or her peers.

- Interview several surgeons. Ask how frequently and for how long the physician has been performing the procedure you want. A plastic surgeon who specializes in liposuction (removal of excess fat deposits) may not be the best choice if you want an eyelid lift.

- Ask if the surgeon has voluntarily had his or her clinic accredited by the American Association for Accreditation of Ambulatory Plastic Surgery Facilities (AAAAPSF), which provides added insurance that the clinic is properly staffed and equipped to handle medical emergencies.

- Look for a physician who asks about your motivation for wanting the surgery, and your expectations.

- Avoid physicians who try to talk you into undergoing additional procedures. They may be more interested in your money than your looks.

Dry Skin

Dry skin may become more of a problem as you get older and the sebaceous glands in your skin produce less lubricating sebum. To help prevent dry, scaly, itchy skin, follow our head-to-toe guidelines below.

- **For your face:** Use a cleansing cream or lotion to remove your makeup. Mineral oil is a cheap and effective makeup remover, but cleansing creams are more aesthetically pleasing because they don't leave a greasy residue.

  Use a superfatted soap or soapless lotion to wash your face. Many soaps can dry your skin—even those that claim a reputation for gentleness. Ivory soap, for example, is actually too harsh to use on your face. Better choices are Dove, Basis, Eucerin, Cetaphil, Aquanil, SC Lotion, or Moisturil. Lever 2000 is the one deodorant soap that's not harsh. Avoid deep-cleaning skin-care products, such as abrasive sponges, granules, and cleansing machines, which are harsh and may strip away your skin's natural oils. Stay away from astringents containing alcohol, which can dry your skin.

  Wash your face once a day; this is usually sufficient. Washing your face too frequently can rob your skin of moisture and protective oils. After washing, pat your skin dry (don't rub) with a clean towel.

  Use a moisturizer. Generally speaking, moisturizing creams are more effective than lotions, but some women find that creams clog their pores. If this is the case, choose products labeled *noncomedogenic,* which have been laboratory tested and are less likely to clog pores. Good choices are Neutraderma, Moisturel, Aquaflor, and Eucerin. If your skin is still acne-prone, stay away from lanolin, heavy oils, and cocoa butter. Don't waste your money on expensive creams and lotions in attractive containers with exotic-sounding ingredients.

Contrary to claims made by some manufacturers, ingredients such as avocado, collagen, and aloe can't replace collagen lost in the aging process. These products can't penetrate the outer layer of skin to the dermis, where most of the skin's collagen fibers are. Nor can these products repair the broken or damaged elastic fibers that cause wrinkles.

If you use a moisturizer in the morning, first rinse your face with water and pat dry. Wait fifteen to twenty minutes before applying your makeup so that the moisturizer has a chance to soak into your skin. (This also ensures that your makeup will go on more smoothly.)

• **For your body:** When bathing, use a mild soap, and use it only on the areas of your body that need washing. Soaking in a warm (not hot) tub will help hydrate the skin. (Avoid using bath oils; they have limited effectiveness and can make your tub slippery, which can increase your risk of falling.) If your skin is scaly, lightly rub it with a washcloth or an abrasive sponge (such as Buff-Puff) to remove the scales. Apply a moisturizing cream or lotion immediately after your shower or bath to help lock moisture into your skin. If your skin is extremely dry, you may need to apply a moisturizer in the morning and again at night.

• **For your hands:** You may need a thicker moisturizer for your hands than for the rest of your body, and you may need to apply it several times a day. Try Shepherd's hand cream, Purpose dry skin cream, or Neutrogena hand cream.

• **For your heels:** Heels, which have a tendency to become dry and cracked, may require a thicker moisturizing cream, such as Carmol cream or Aquacare HP cream. Use a pumice stone to help remove and smooth roughened skin. Then apply the cream to soften the skin.

Age Spots, Pigmentation, Moles, and Other Skin Lesions

Most of us have a number of moles and blemishes on our skin. For the most part, these pose more of a cosmetic problem than a health problem. Some of the more common harmless blemishes include the following:

• **Skin tags (acrochordons):** These soft brownish-colored growths commonly arise on the neck, upper eyelids, armpits, and groin. Skin tags are benign and are usually asymptomatic; however, they may become irritated from rubbing against clothing, or they simply may be cosmetically unacceptable.

Your doctor can easily remove skin tags with a pair of surgical scissors. Since the lesions are raised off the skin, local anesthesia is usually unnecessary. Tiny lesions may be treated by electrodesiccation, in which a low-level electrical current is used to remove the growths.

• **Cherry angiomas:** These smooth, bright red, dome-shaped lesions, arising from dilated capillaries, vary in size from a pinpoint to a quarter inch or more in diameter. They begin to appear at about age forty, and some 75 percent of people over age seventy have them. The lesions may be removed by electrodessication or cryosurgery (freezing the growth).

- **Seborrheic keratoses:** These growths begin to appear after age thirty, usually on the face, trunk, and extremities. They start out as oval, waxy, flat-topped bumps that are beige-colored or tan, eventually growing to between a third of an inch to several inches in diameter.

If the growths become inflamed or take on an unusual appearance, a dermatologist may recommend a biopsy to rule out malignant melanoma or pigmented basal-cell carcinoma. Otherwise, flat seborrheic keratoses that appear early can be treated with topical acids or with cryosurgery. More raised lesions may need to be surgically removed.

- **Hyperpigmentation:** Age spots (also known as liver spots) are tan to dark brown flat, pigmented areas up to an inch in diameter that typically appear on the face and the backs of the hands. Contrary to popular belief, age spots are *not* so much a part of natural aging. Rather, they are the result of overactivity of melanin, due to overexposure to the sun. Increased pigmentation on the upper lip, cheeks, and forehead, called *chloasma,* may appear both during and after pregnancy, use of birth-control pills, or other hormonal changes.

Since these types of irregular pigmentation darken after even minimal sun exposure, you'll need to regularly use a sunscreen with an SPF of 15 or greater to help prevent further darkening.

Often the pigmented areas on your face can be lightened with bleach creams. For age spots, fading creams may help, but it may take months of therapy before a noticeable improvement occurs. Treatment with cryosurgery is the most effective treatment. However, the surgery sometimes leaves a residual ring of pigmentation. If you're concerned about this, your physician can treat one or two lesions initially as test areas.

- **Potentially harmful skin changes:** Some skin changes may be early signs of skin cancer and warrant a close watch. For this reason, you should perform a skin self-examination (see page 165) at least once every six months (once a month if you are at a greater risk of developing skin cancer). Report to your doctor any of the following changes:

  - a persistent scaly red patch with irregular borders that sometimes crusts or bleeds
  - an open sore that bleeds, oozes, or crusts and remains open for three or more weeks.
  - an elevated growth with a central depression that occasionally bleeds
  - a shiny bump or nodule that's pearly, translucent, pink, red, white, tan, brown, or black in color.
  - a white, yellow, or waxy scarlike area that often has poorly defined borders.
  - a wartlike growth that crusts and occasionally bleeds
  - any change in the size, color, or shape of a mole or pigmented area of the skin.

How to Perform a Skin Self-Examination

You will need a good light, a chair or stool, two mirrors (one full-length and one hand-held), and a blow-dryer. For skin areas that are difficult for you to see yourself, you may need the assistance of a family member or friend. You are looking for any of the skin conditions described on pages 163–164. You might find it helpful to use Figure A.1 on page 484 to record the location and size of moles or other spots that are not a problem now but that might change in appearance or size over time, possibly signifying a skin cancer.

Begin by examining your hands, including the palms, backs, fingernails, and between the fingers. Examine the front and back of your wrists and forearms. Standing in front of the full-length mirror, hold your arms up and examine your inner arms and armpits (see Figure 8.2).

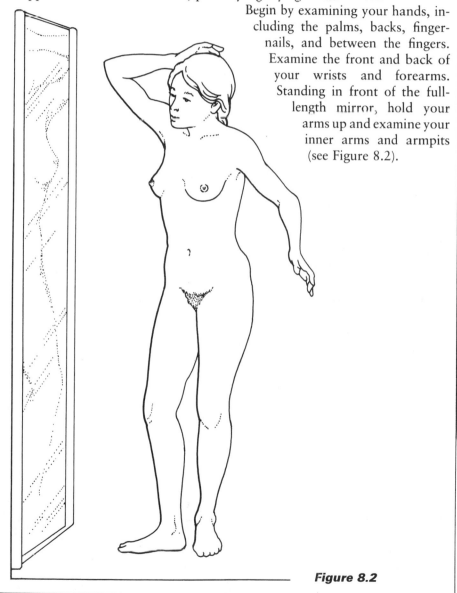

Figure 8.2

165

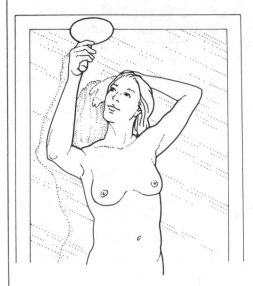

Figure 8.3

Next, with your back to the full-length mirror, use the hand mirror to examine your upper back and the backs of your upper arms. Now examine your neck and chest area. Examine your breasts carefully, including areas that may be subjected to pressure from straps or elastic bands.

Examine your face, particularly the rims and lobes of your ears, and your nose, lips, and mouth. Remember, 80 percent of skin cancers appear on the head and neck. Use the blow-dryer to part your hair section by section and examine your entire scalp (see Figure 8.3).

Figure 8.4

While seated, check the soles of your feet, your toenails, between the toes, your heels, ankles, shins, calves, and thighs (see Figure 8.4).

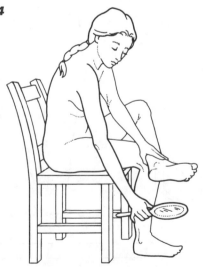

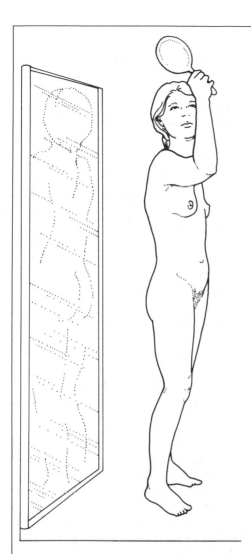

With the aid of both mirrors, examine your lower back, buttocks, and genital areas (see Figure 8.5). (For more information on skin cancer, see Chapter 18.)

Figure 8.5

Note: Instructions for skin self-examination excerpted from Perry Robins, M.D., *Sun Sense*. New York: The Skin Cancer Foundation, 1990. Reprinted with permission from the publisher. Copyright © 1990 by Perry Robins, M.D.

Hair

Most women in the middle and later years will eventually have to come to terms with graying hair, one of the earliest and most inevitable signs of aging. Hair turns gray when the melanocytes that give hair its color produce less pigmentation as you age. Tiny bubbles in the hair shaft may also contribute to gray hair. Occasionally, a medical condition, such as hypothyroidism (an underactive thyroid gland), can cause prematurely gray hair. But when you go gray is largely determined by heredity. And what you do about it (color it or let nature take its course) is really your own personal preference.

Two other problems may be far more emotionally devastating than graying hair for some women in the middle and later years. These women suffer from either excessive hair growth, medically known as *hirsutism,* or excessive hair loss, known as *alopecia.* For most women, medical help is available to help remedy the problem.

• **Hirsutism:** Excessive hair growth typically occurs on the face, chest, lower back, and lower abdomen of women, and often becomes more apparent after menopause.

Some women are simply born with more body hair than others. This is because the type of hair, its rate of growth, and its distribution over the body differ among different racial groups. Generally speaking, Orientals and American Indians have less body hair. Women whose ancestors came from the southern parts of Europe have more body hair and are more likely to experience excessive hair growth on the upper lip and the lower part of the face, on the chest, around the nipples of the breasts, and on the lower abdomen.

Certain drugs may increase the growth of body hair, particularly hormonal medications, such as anabolic steroids, used by some athletes to build muscle and improve performance, and testosterone, used to treat certain menopausal symptoms. Drugs such as *diazoxide* (Proglycem), used to treat hypoglycemia (low blood sugar); the anticonvulsant *phenytoin* (Dilantin); the immunosuppressive drug *cyclosporin* (Sandimmune); and the blood-pressure medication *minoxidil* (Loniten) cause excess hair to grow anywhere on the body in both men and women. (In fact, the ability of minoxidil to stimulate hair growth has made it a promising new treatment for baldness.)

More often than not, however, the problem is tied to the "male" hormone testosterone, which is produced in small amounts by the adrenal glands and ovaries in women. Testosterone can convert the short, fine, colorless *vellus* hairs on your body into *terminal* hairs, which are long, coarse, pigmented, and, in certain areas of the body, responsive to hormonal fluctuations. Changes in testosterone levels or in the way your body metabolizes testosterone often play a role in the development of hirsutism. For instance, menopause is associated with lower levels of a liver protein known as *sex hormone–binding globulin,* which binds to and decreases the biological effectiveness of the reproductive hormones estrogen, progesterone, and testosterone. And while the ovaries' production of estrogen and progesterone declines after menopause, both the ovaries and the adrenal glands continue to secrete testosterone. As a result, many menopausal women have an increase in levels of the more biologically active *free testosterone,* which may stimulate hair growth.

Increased testosterone production by either the adrenal glands or ovaries may also trigger excessive hair growth. Possible causes include benign or malignant tumors of the adrenal glands (which are fairly uncommon) and Cushing's syndrome, in which the adrenal glands produce excessive amounts of the hormone *cortisol*. Women with polycystic ovarian disease, in which numerous small cysts develop within and enlarge the ovaries, and those with certain benign or malignant ovarian tumors may also have elevated testosterone levels. High insulin levels caused by insulin resistance are also associated with excessive testosterone production, as is obesity. Hair growth associated with elevated testosterone often comes on rather suddenly and is often accompanied by other signs of masculinization, such as deepening of the voice and enlargement of the clitoris.

Often, hirsutism can't be traced to any apparent medical cause, and levels of testosterone are normal or only slightly elevated. This is what's known as *simple*, or *idiopathic, hirsutism*. It may be that your body has slightly increased its production and metabolism of testosterone, or that your hair follicles have become more sensitive to normal levels of testosterone. Most women with idiopathic hirsutism have had the problem since puberty, but they may notice that it worsens with age.

Since hirsutism is a possible sign of an underlying medical problem, your physician will first review your medical history (including any drugs you may have taken) and perform a physical examination to rule out serious illness. He or she may also administer blood and urine tests to check for elevated levels of testosterone and cortisol.

If your doctor finds an underlying cause of elevated testosterone levels, the problem will be corrected. If you're taking a medication associated with excessive hair growth, your physician may recommend that you switch to another medication (if possible). Any tumors will be surgically removed, and women with Cushing's syndrome will be appropriately treated.

If your doctor finds no hormonal imbalances or tumors and you have mild hirsutism, you may consider bleaching the hair, electrolysis, using a depilatory, or shaving the excess hair. Shaving is the safest and easiest method of removing excess hair and doesn't make the hair grow back faster.

Several drug therapies are available for more severe cases of hirsutism. Glucocorticoids reduce hair growth in up to 50 percent of women who use them. The drugs work by reducing testosterone secretion from the adrenal glands and, to a lesser extent, from the ovaries. However, side effects include a possible drug-induced case of Cushing's syndrome and, if treatment is abruptly discontinued, adrenal insufficiency.

Since the most common cause of hirsutism is excessive testosterone production by the ovaries, low-dose oral contraceptives may be prescribed for premenopausal women. Birth-control pills essentially shut down the ovaries by suppressing the pituitary gland's release of follicle-stimulating hormone and luteinizing hormone. This also reduces the ovaries' secretion of testosterone. The estrogens in oral contraceptives stimulate the liver's manufacture of sex hormone–binding globulin, as well, resulting in lower blood levels of free testosterone. Postmenopausal estrogen may help, too.

Some women have found that the progestogen *medroxyprogesterone acetate* (Amen, Curretab, Cycrin, and Provera) works, too.

The diuretic *spironolactone* (Aldactone), which has antiandrogenic properties, may also be prescribed. However, spironolactone may cause such side effects as nausea, fatigue, irregular menstrual periods, and headaches, particularly at higher dosages. Spironolactone has also been known to induce ovulation in previously infertile women with polycystic ovarian syndrome, so if you are premenopausal and have polycystic ovarian syndrome, be sure to use a reliable form of contraception when taking this drug.

You should be aware, too, that it may take weeks or months before you see a noticeable improvement with most drug therapies. For faster results, you may want to consider combining drug therapy with electrolysis, which removes the actively growing hairs.

• **Alopecia:** Generally speaking, the hairs you find on your pillowcase, in your hairbrush, and around the bathroom drain after a shower are part of your hair's natural growth cycle. This includes an actively growing (*anagen*) phase, lasting from two to six years, and a resting (*telogen*) phase, lasting about two to three months. Hair in the resting phase, comprising about 15 percent of the hair on your head at any given time, sheds when a newly developing hair forms in its place. Then the cycle begins again. On an average, both men and women lose from 50 to 75 hairs a day—and up to 250 hairs after shampooing.

It's perfectly normal for your hair to begin progressively thinning out after age fifty. Most women won't notice any difference in the thickness of their hair for years. But a sudden or greater-than-average hair loss may indicate a more serious problem. If you notice obvious bald patches or increasing numbers of hair in your comb, or bathtub drain, you should notify your doctor, who can often diagnose the condition simply by gently pulling a few hairs from your scalp and examining them under a microscope. Rest assured that for most women a certain degree of hair regrowth can be expected within one year of medical intervention.

The most common type of hair loss is a condition known as *telogen effluvium*, or loss of resting hair. A variety of conditions can trigger a change in the normal hair cycle, resulting in an increased transition from anagen (growing) hair to telogen (resting) hair, which in turn causes increased shedding. These include:

- acutely stressful events, which may have occurred as long as six to eight months earlier
- prolonged surgery or anesthesia
- sudden weight loss from crash dieting or from gastric-bypass surgery for obesity
- high fever
- exposure to a variety of drugs, including amphetamines, anticonvulsants, antidepressants, and lithium
- a recent pregnancy or use of oral contraceptives
- poor nutrition, especially iron deficiency
- thyroid or pituitary-gland problems

170

- chronic illnesses such as diabetes or Hodgkin's disease, kidney or liver failure, cancer, or systemic lupus erythematosus.

Fortunately, the condition rarely results in a loss of more than 40 percent of the scalp hair, and regrowth often occurs after the underlying cause is corrected.

Another type of hair loss, *anagen effluvium,* occurs when the hairs in the growing phase die suddenly. Prolonged fasting, cancer treatments (radiation and chemotherapy), and occupational exposure to such toxins as arsenic, bismuth, gold, borax, or thallium may be the culprit. Extensive hair loss may occur within several days to a week. Again, once the cause is determined and treated, the hair usually regrows.

When the cause of hair loss cannot be determined, it is often referred to as *alopecia areata.* There's some evidence that the condition is somehow linked to an autoimmune mechanism. Generally, people with alopecia areata develop patches of baldness caused by a combination of hair loss and breakage of existing hairs. These patches develop over a period of three to six months. In rare instances, the condition progresses to total loss of scalp hair (*alopecia totalis*) or loss of all body and scalp hair, including eyelashes and eyebrows (*alopecia universalis*).

The less severe the hair loss, the better are the chances that it will regrow. Indeed, 90 percent of women with mild hair loss experience a gradual regrowth of hair in another three to six months.

Some women may inherit a genetic predisposition to hair loss that can be triggered by high levels of the "male" hormone androgen, a condition called *androgenetic alopecia* (also known as male-female pattern baldness). Unlike men, who develop an M-shaped hairline with thinning in the temporal areas, thinning of hair in women occurs in a more diffuse pattern. Some women with this condition may also suffer from hirsutism, deepening of the voice, increased muscle mass, and other signs of masculinization.

For women with androgenetic alopecia, medications to counter the action of the androgens may be effective in preventing further hair loss, but usually don't promote regrowth of hair. However, a topical form of the blood-pressure medication minoxidil (Rogaine), the drug that has brought hope to bald men, may also stimulate hair growth in some women.

Sometimes, hair loss occurs because the hair shaft becomes weakened and breaks off too easily. Tints, bleaches, straighteners, and permanents can cause this kind of damage. Using a cream rinse and protein conditioner after shampooing helps reduce friction and strengthen individual hair fibers.

Repeated use of certain hairstyles, such as braiding and ponytails, wearing elastic hair bands, curling your hair with rollers, and excessive teasing can also lead to hair loss. You can avoid this kind of hair loss simply by varying your hairstyle.

Teeth and Gums

Contrary to popular belief, tooth loss is *not* a normal part of aging. With proper care, your teeth should last a lifetime. But certain dental problems do become more prevalent in the middle and later years. Among them: gum disease (which can lead to tooth loss), cosmetic changes, and dry mouth.

Gum Disease

You tend to become more prone to periodontal, or gum, disease as you age. In its earliest and mildest stage, gum disease is an inflammation of the gums called *gingivitis*. At this point, it is reversible and has yet to cause serious damage. But as gum disease progresses, it develops into *periodontitis*, an infection that affects the bony socket of the tooth and can eventually lead to tooth loss.

Gum disease is caused by the bacteria in plaque, a sticky, nearly invisible film that constantly forms on teeth and gums. Plaque needs to be removed every twenty-four hours; otherwise, the bacteria begin producing toxins that destroy the bones anchoring your teeth. The severity of the disease can often be measured by the loss of the gum attachment to the tooth, creating what are called pockets.

About three out of four adults are believed to suffer from gingivitis. And while studies have shown that gingivitis doesn't always progress to periodontal disease, no one knows which cases will and which won't. Good news for women with low bone mass (osteopenia) and osteoporosis: Although early studies suggested that periodontis may be made worse by low bone mass, our research and that of others has failed to show a correlation between osteoporosis and the progression of gum disease. On the other hand, the hormonal and vascular changes of pregnancy may increase the risk for gingivitis and often cause inflammed, swollen gums. Oral contraceptives can have the same effect.

Gum disease may or may not cause pain and can easily go unnoticed. Be sure to tell your dentist if you notice any of the symptoms of gum disease: bleeding gums when you brush or floss, a bad taste in your mouth, or swollen gums. Your dentist can look for signs of periodontal disease during regular checkups. X rays can help diagnose bone loss, and a tool called a *periodontal probe* can be used to measure the depth of gum pockets: less than 3 to 5 millimeters indicates moderate disease; more than 5 millimeters often requires corrective surgery.

Regular dental checkups and professional cleanings (every six months) can help prevent the progression of gum disease. There's a lot you can do at home, too. The most important: Brush and floss. Use a soft-bristled brush and replace it every three months (sooner if the bristles mat or splay). Only flossing can remove plaque that collects between your teeth, where the brush can't reach, and at the gumline.

If you find flossing difficult, your dentist or hygienist can recommend other methods of cleaning between the teeth, such as Stim-u-dents, triangular-shaped toothpicks of soft wood, and interproximal brushes, which look like miniature bottle brushes.

A host of products has entered the marketplace purporting to remove plaque and fight gingivitis. What's the truth behind their claims?

Tartar-control toothpastes: These products help prevent the formation of tartar (hardened plaque) above the gumline. The problem: Tartar above the gumline plays little role in gum disease and is actually more of a cosmetic problem.

Antiplaque toothpastes: These share the same problem as brushing—they don't reach between the teeth.

Mouth rinses and mouthwashes: Only two, Listerine and the prescription mouth rinse Peridex, have met the American Dental Association's guidelines to receive its Seal of Acceptance. Listerine contains essential oils, such as eucalyptol, menthol, thymol, and methyl salicylate, that penetrate the cell walls of bacteria and disrupt the organisms' chemistry. However, Listerine can burn the mouth, and many people complain about its taste.

Peridex, approved by the U.S. Food and Drug Administration in 1986, contains chlorhexidine (the same chemical used in surgical scrub rooms), which binds to bacteria and kills them. But Peridex can stain your teeth and alter your sense of taste, so it is most commonly prescribed after periodontal surgery, when brushing and flossing are difficult.

The controversy still rages over Plax, a prebrushing rinse that claims to remove plaque. Independent research studies have failed to substantiate the manufacturer's claims.

Dental devices: Some high-tech dental tools also claim to help fight plaque. You can probably get just as good results with a manual toothbrush, but you may find an electric toothbrush, such as WaterPik's PlaqueControl 2000, the Interplak, or Braun's Oral-B Plaque Remover, easier to use. Oral irrigators, such as Teledyne's WaterPik, remove plaque at the gumline with a stream of water. Many dentists believe these devices do more harm than good, however, because the force of the water can push plaque below the gumline, where it can cause abscesses and infection. Your dentist or hygienist can show you how to use the device properly without injuring your gums.

Cosmetic Changes

Your smile ages as you age. Stains accumulate and enamel thins, darkening the color of your teeth. Gums recede, giving you a "long in the tooth" look. Teeth wear, changing the smile line. The contour of your lips may even change. Many people are now turning to cosmetic dentistry to give their smile a face-lift. What are your options?

• **Bleaching:** This is one of the simplest ways to lighten the color of teeth. It is usually harmless to the teeth (although it may increase their sensitivity to heat and cold) and does not require an anesthetic. Your dentist applies an oxidizing agent (hydrogen peroxide) to your teeth and exposes them to heat or light for about half an hour. Results are cumulative and may take up to six visits. However, stains can return and you may need to have the procedure repeated.

Also popular are do-it-yourself bleaching kits to use at home, but their safety and effectiveness have been questioned. A milder version of the peroxide solution is put into a mouthpiece that you wear for several hours a day or even overnight for several weeks. But peroxide can irritate the gums, and some of the solution could be swallowed.

• **Bonding:** If stains are too dark to respond to bleaching, bonding may be the answer. The technique can also be used to fill in chipped or broken teeth or gaps between teeth. During the procedure, a bonding material (a paste made up of plastic resins containing microscopic ground glass) is painted on your teeth and hardened under a special light. Then the bonding material is shaped and polished. Bonding can often be done in a single visit without an anesthetic. The only drawback is that bonding can chip, break, or stain and requires special care. It may need touching up or replacing in several years.

• **Porcelain veneers:** These false fronts, resembling artificial fingernails, are laminated to the front surface of teeth after a small amount of enamel is removed. Veneers cost more than bonding and require several visits, but they are stronger, last longer, and can cover darker stains.

• **Crowns:** Also called caps, these were once the only option for people with stained, chipped, or broken teeth. New all-porcelain or ceramic crowns look more natural but require the removal of much more of the tooth. They're not reversible and may have to be replaced within fifteen years.

• **Contouring:** Years of use can wear down the edges of your teeth, changing the line of your smile. A technique called cosmetic contouring, which is nothing more than grinding down the edges of your teeth, can revamp your look.

Sometimes a combination of techniques may be necessary to get the look you want. Computer imaging—using a computer to show how a particular procedure will change your appearance—may help you make a decision.

Because cosmetic dentistry is not a recognized specialty, it's important to find a qualified dentist. Start with your family dentist; about 80 percent of them now do cosmetic work. Ask friends for recommendations. Periodontists (specialists in gum disease) are good sources for recommendations, too. Or call the restorative or operative dentistry department of the nearest dental school.

Dry Mouth

Also known as *xerostomia,* this condition becomes more common with age. It's also a side effect of more than four hundred different medications, including antidepressants, antihypertensives, and antihistamines. The lower estrogen levels associated with menopause may exacerbate the problem in some women. Besides causing discomfort, the reduced salivary flow associated with dry mouth can increase the risk of gum disease and cavities.

If you suffer from dry mouth, try chewing sugarless gum or sucking on sugarless mints to help stimulate your saliva flow. Take frequent sips of water to keep your mouth moist.

Varicose Veins and Spider Veins

Another concern for women in midlife are varicose veins and spider veins, unsightly distended blood vessels that usually appear on the legs. Both varicose veins and spider veins tend to worsen as your veins and skin lose elasticity with age.

Until recently, treatment of varicose veins usually meant surgery—sometimes multiple surgeries—leading to scarring that was often as cosmetically unacceptable as the varicose veins themselves. Today, the treatment of both varicose veins and spider veins is much more effective, allowing many women to once again bare their legs.

Varicose Veins

The veins in your legs help carry blood back to the heart for oxygenation. Since the blood has to work against gravity, these veins contain one-way valves to prevent blood from flowing in the opposite direction. When the valves fail, blood flows backward and accumulates in one spot, causing the vein to balloon outward.

For reasons that aren't clear, women are four times more likely than men to develop varicose veins. The condition tends to run in families, especially among people of Irish or German descent. Reproductive hormones play a role, as well: During pregnancy, higher hormone levels may dilate and weaken the walls of the veins, leading to valve failure. Women with a genetic predisposition who take oral contraceptives appear to be particularly susceptible, as are women with thrombophlebitis (blood clots in the superficial veins of the legs) and deep vein thrombosis (blood clots in the deep veins of the legs).

Wearing tight-fitting clothing (particularly girdles) and having a job that requires you to stand rather than walk or sit have been associated with an increased incidence of varicose veins. Sitting with your legs crossed may also impede venous blood flow back to the heart, thus increasing the risk of developing varicose veins, but there's no scientific evidence to substantiate this. A sedentary lifestyle plays a part, too. Your calf muscles are so important in helping push blood back to the heart that they are sometimes called the "calf pump" or "peripheral heart." Inactivity stifles the pumping action of the calf muscles and may allow blood to pool in the veins, causing them to swell.

Varicose veins aren't usually a major threat to your health, although they can cause problems in some women. For instance, poor blood circulation may cause swelling of the calf and ankle (especially after standing for long periods of time), itching, and skin ulcers. In rare instances, phlebitis (inflammation of the vein), often associated with a blood clot, may occur. These clots cause local pain but rarely travel to the heart or lungs.

Surgery involves stripping or tying off parts of the varicose vein, forcing blood to flow through veins with good valves. Four weeks after surgery, what is left of the superficial varicose veins can often be treated with sclerotherapy, in which a chemical solution is injected into the vein, killing the cells lining the vein, and making it incapable of carrying blood. Blood that was once circulated through the vein is rerouted through other veins with working valves.

Spider Veins

These are spindly red or blue spiderlike veins that typically appear on the legs and ankles. They most commonly develop among women ages thirty to fifty, although no one is sure why. Somehow the capillaries (the tiniest blood vessels in your body) near the surface of the skin become dilated, resulting in a visible network of red or blue veins. As with varicose veins, the condition seems to be partly hereditary. Physical trauma, such as a fall or a blow, standing or sitting for long periods of time, and hormonal changes, particularly during pregnancy, factor into the development of spider veins, as well. Often spider veins develop as a result of varicose veins.

Most spider veins pose no threat to your health whatsoever, and treatment is purely for cosmetic reasons. The most common treatment is sclerotherapy.

• Avoid sitting with your legs crossed or standing for long periods of time.

• **Put your feet up above hip level periodically during the day.** This helps encourage blood flow back to the heart.

• **Maintain proper weight.** Added weight puts additional strain on the veins in your legs.

• **Avoid heavy lifting or straining.**

• **Don't smoke.** Cigarette smoking has been associated with varicose veins.

• **Don't wear tight shoes, garters, belts, or other restrictive clothing.** An exception is support hose, which may help prevent both spider veins and varicose veins by discouraging blood from pooling in the legs.

• **Exercise.** Physical activity helps your calf muscles push blood back to your heart; regular exercise also helps keep your weight in check.

If for some reason sclerotherapy doesn't work, electrodesiccation, in which a small electrical current is applied to the blood vessels using microscopic needles, may be used. For stubborn spider veins, surgery is an option.

A Final Word

Many of the most common cosmetic problems that arise during the middle years—skin wrinkles, dry skin, age spots, varicose veins, tooth loss—can be prevented by taking a few simple precautions in your premenopausal years. Moreover, most of these and other cosmetic problems in midlife, such as excessive hair growth or loss of hair, can be treated with the help of a qualified physician, so don't be afraid to ask for help. You have every right to look as good as you feel in the middle and later years.

Suggested Reading

Schoen, Linda Allen, and Paul Lazar, M.D. (sponsored by the American Academy of Dermatology). *The Look You Like: Medical Answers to 400 Questions on Skin and Hair Care*, New York: Marcel Dekker, Inc., 1989.
Wilson, Josleen. *The American Society for Plastic and Reconstructive Surgery's Guide to Cosmetic Surgery*. New York: Simon & Schuster, 1992.

The American Society of Plastic and Reconstructive Surgeons and The American Society for Aesthetic Plastic Surgery, 444 East Algonquin Road, Arlington Heights, Illinois 60005, (800) 635-0635.

With a membership of about 3,600 board-certified plastic and reconstructive surgeons, many of whom specialize in aesthetic plastic surgery, these affiliated professional organizations seek to educate the public on the specialty of plastic surgery (both aesthetic and reconstructive), and to help individuals in selecting a properly trained and experienced physician. Both organizations offer a toll-free referral and information service (callers interested in aesthetic plastic surgery should specify "The Aesthetic Society"), as well as pamphlets and brochures describing numerous aesthetic and reconstructive procedures.

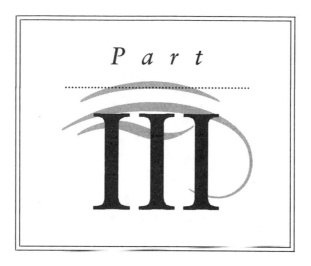

Part

III

*Special
Reproductive-Health
Concerns of
the Middle Years*

Chapter 9

....

Midlife
Contraception:
You Have More
Choices
Than You Think

While your patterns of ovulation become more erratic in the years preceding menopause, it's still possible to get pregnant—for as long as you're menstruating. Indeed, the abortion ratio (the number of abortions to live births) in women ages forty to forty-four is second only to that of teens under age fifteen. Clearly, one essential but often overlooked concern for women in midlife is finding and *using* a reliable form of contraception. Contraception is important during the middle years for another reason: The risks associated with pregnancy rise with the mother's age.

Contrary to what you may think, your contraceptive options in the middle years are every bit as broad as they were when you were younger. Even birth-control pills—once believed to be too risky for women over thirty-five—have now broken the age barrier and are considered safe even for women over forty. Most women are limited only by their personal preferences.

Sterilization

This is the best method once you and your partner have made a permanent decision regarding future pregnancies.

• **Vasectomy:** We personally prefer this form of sterilization because the operation is easy to perform, can be done on an outpatient basis under a local anesthetic, and has no long-term side effects. During the procedure, the physician makes a small incision in the man's *scrotum* (the pouch of skin containing the testes, where sperm is produced), then severs and ties off the *vas deferens*, the tubes through which sperm travel to the urethra (see Figure 9.1). The procedure has no effect on a man's sex drive or his ability to ejaculate, since most of the fluids in a man's ejaculate are released from the *seminal vesicles* (which contain no sperm) and the prostate gland. But because the vas deferens has been tied off, the ejaculate no longer contains active sperm.

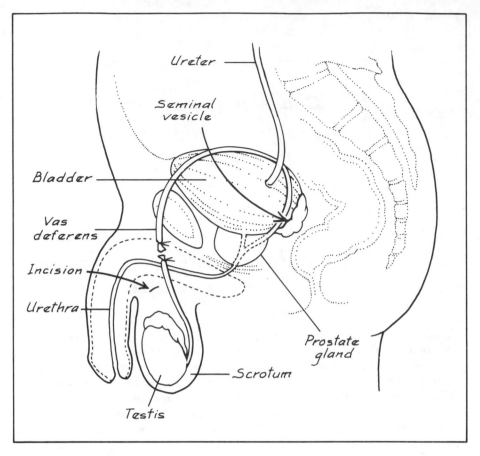

Figure 9.1   Vasectomy

While some studies have raised concerns about a link between vasectomy and an increased risk of prostate cancer later in life, the results have been called into question because of the way the studies were designed and carried out. Several other studies have found no association between vasectomy and prostate cancer. And no study has shown an increase in deaths from prostate cancer among vasectomized men. At this time, the American Urological Association says that the relationship between vasectomy and prostate cancer is "unproven." Nevertheless, until more research is done, the organization recommends that men who had a vasectomy more than twenty years ago, or who were at least forty years old when vasectomized, should have an annual digital exam of the rectum and a blood test for prostate-specific antigen (PSA), two screening tests for prostate cancer.

As for an increased risk of cardiovascular disease, thought by some to be a complication of vasectomy, several large studies have not found any increase in heart disease among men who have undergone a vasectomy.

After the procedure, couples should wait at least four weeks before having unprotected intercourse, since the male organs will still contain active sperm for a while.

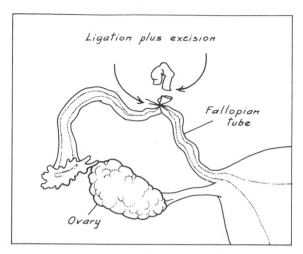

Figure 9.2   Tubal Sterilization Using Ligation Plus Excision

• **Tubal sterilization/interruption:** Tubal interruption, or having your tubes tied, is a good contraceptive alternative to vasectomy, although the operation is a little more involved. Essentially, the procedure involves surgically blocking a woman's Fallopian tubes to prevent conception. The tubes may be blocked in several ways:

Ligation: During the operation, each Fallopian tube is pulled up into a loop and tied across with a suture.

Ligation plus excision: In addition to being tied, the top part of the loop is cut (See Figure 9.2).

Clips or bands: The tubes are interrupted by placing a small plastic or metal clip over the tubes, which blocks the tubes completely without crushing the surrounding tissue (see Figure 9.3). Alternatively, silicon bands have been

Figure 9.3   Tubal Sterilization Using Clips or Bands

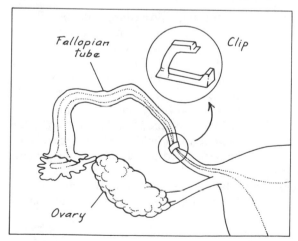

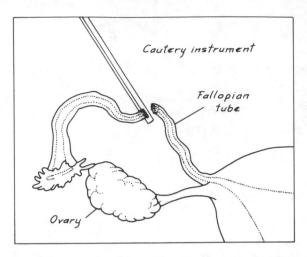

Figure 9.4   Tubal Sterilization Using Cautery

used to block the tubes. However, the bands have been associated with a relatively high incidence of postoperative pain.

Cautery: A heated probe is used to destroy a limited area of the tubes (see Figure 9.4). The main drawback is possible damage from heat extending to the blood vessels that supply the ovaries. For this reason, care needs to be taken when using cautery.

Sterilization of women can usually be performed on an outpatient basis using laparoscopy. This procedure, also known as "belly button" surgery because it requires a small incision just inside or below the navel, may be performed under local or general anesthesia. Carbon dioxide is pumped through the incision into the abdomen to separate the organs. A laparoscope (a thin lighted tube) is then inserted through the incision to provide a clear view of the uterus, ovaries, and Fallopian tubes. The tubes are then interrupted using one of the methods discussed earlier.

Tubal ligation may also be performed using a procedure called *minilaparotomy* (sometimes called "bikini" surgery because the remaining scar can be concealed by most bikini bathing suits). This operation involves making a small incision just above the pubic hairline, gently lifting the Fallopian tubes through the incision, and dividing and excising a small portion of the tubes between sutures placed precisely around the tubes only (see Figure 9.5). With this method, there is very little chance that the vital blood supply to the ovaries will be compromised. Because this procedure is so precise, there's also a greater likelihood of successfully *reversing* the operation should you have a change of heart later on. Minilaparotomy may be performed under regional or general anesthesia.

Complications arising from tubal ligation are rare and recovery time is short. You can usually resume your normal activities within forty-eight hours of the procedure.

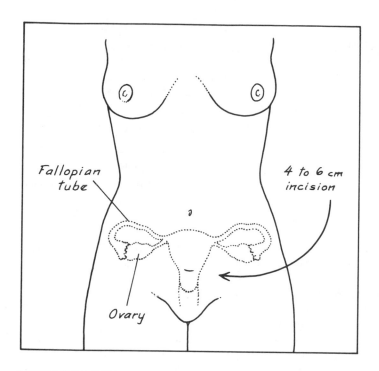

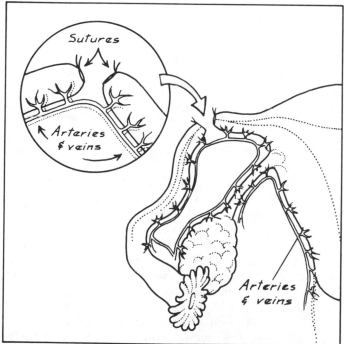

Figure 9.5 Tubal Sterilization Using the Minilaparotomy Technique

Sterilization is probably the most effective form of contraception available, preventing pregnancy 99.8 percent of the time. However, the procedures are not 100 percent fail-proof. From two to four out of one thousand women who have their tubes interrupted with either clips or bands subsequently get pregnant, usually because the devices were not properly placed on the Fallopian tubes and failed to block the tubes entirely.

Remember, too, that all sterilization procedures should be considered *permanent*. While it is sometimes possible to reverse the procedures, the surgery can be tricky. Success rates for reversal of vasectomy are somewhat lower than that for tubal sterilization: the pregnancy rate for women whose partners have had reverse vasectomies ranges from 31 to 47 percent. However, the rate drops to only 9 percent if the reverse operation is performed ten years or more after vasectomy. The outlook for tubal ligation is more optimistic, thanks to new microsurgery techniques. Depending on which procedure is used to interrupt the tubes, between 44 to 90 percent of women who undergo surgery for reverse sterilization subsequently manage to conceive a child.

Oral Contraception

Today's birth-control pills are a far cry from the ones introduced in 1960. Overall, the new pills prevent pregnancy in the same way: When taken on a daily basis, the estrogen and progestogen in combination birth-control pills suppress the monthly release of an egg. Oral contraceptives also thicken a woman's cervical mucus, making it difficult for sperm to penetrate. As a final measure of protection, oral contraceptives make the uterine lining unfavorable for implantation of a fertilized egg.

But today's oral contraceptives contain drastically lower doses of hormones. The pills of thirty years ago contained 10 milligrams of progestogen and up to 150 micrograms of estrogen, compared with just 1 milligram of progestogen and 30 to 35 micrograms of estrogen in today's. The result is oral contraceptives that are highly effective in preventing pregnancy, with a much improved safety record. In fact, oral contraceptives may well be the best type of *reversible* contraception for women in midlife—in terms of both safety and efficacy.

Yet only about 5 percent of women over thirty-five use birth-control pills. This is largely because of concerns that oral contraceptives raise the risk of a heart attack among older women. We now know that early studies showing an increased risk of heart attacks among older oral-contraceptive users failed to take into account the effects of cigarette smoking on a woman's risk of heart disease. Indeed, when cigarette smokers were removed from those studies, there was *no pill-related increase in heart attacks at any age*—in spite of the high levels of estrogen and progestogen in the pills. Several other studies have now confirmed that cigarette smoking, not birth-control pills, is the main culprit.

Still, while the increased cardiovascular risk associated with birth-control pills is due *largely* to cigarette smoking, oral contraceptives themselves have been found to aggravate certain risk factors for heart disease. Past studies have associated the progestogen in birth-control pills with higher levels of detrimental LDL cholesterol and lower levels of protective HDL cholesterol, decreased glucose tolerance, and elevated insulin levels, all of which raise the risk of heart disease. So questions have remained about the safety of oral contraceptives in women over age thirty-five, whose risk of heart disease naturally increases with age.

Again, most of these studies were conducted with older oral contraceptives containing larger doses of hormones (particularly progestogen) than today's pills. We are among a number of researchers now conducting studies investigating the newer, low-dose oral contraceptives and their impact on various heart-disease risks. So far, the results are extremely encouraging. Among our findings:

• While triglyceride levels rise and protective HDL levels fall among users of low-dose oral contraceptives who are ages thirty-four and older, the altered levels are still within "safe" ranges that *are not associated with an increased risk of heart disease*. Moreover, a month after study participants stopped taking birth-control pills, triglyceride and HDL levels returned to their prepill levels.

• Glucose tolerance fell and insulin levels rose among users of the new, low-dose triphasic oral contraceptives, but again the changes were not serious enough to raise the risk of heart disease.

New types of progestogens, including *gestodene, desogestrel,* and *norgestimate* will probably make oral contraceptives safer still. Most of the progestogens being used today can produce side effects similar to those associated with the "male" hormone androgen, including acne, weight gain, and negative changes in blood-cholesterol levels. However, the new progestogens have few androgenlike properties, so these side effects are unlikely to occur.

What about blood clots? As the doses of estrogen in oral contraceptives have decreased, so has the incidence of blood clots that develop in the veins (*venous* blood clots). In a recent study, we looked at the effects of low-dose oral contraceptives on certain coagulants and anticoagulants in the blood that govern the development of these blood clots. We found that the changes hormones had on blood coagulants were balanced by changes in anticoagulants. Essentially, the new, low-dose oral contraceptives appear to have a minimal effect on the development of blood clots in the veins—usually in the legs (deep-vein thrombosis).

While the risk of developing arterial blood clots (the kind that can precipitate a heart attack or stroke) is very low, these types of blood clots do occasionally occur among women taking oral contraceptives. We don't fully understand how or why these blood clots develop. We suspect that *platelets* (substances in the blood that help form a blood clot) may be somehow affected by hormones (specifically estrogen), making them more likely to stick together.

One way to counteract this effect is to take a junior aspirin (60 milligrams) every three days. Aspirin stimulates the anticoagulant prostacyclin in the blood-vessel wall and suppresses the blood coagulant thromboxane produced by the platelets. In this way, aspirin prevents spasms of the arteries and makes platelets less likely to stick together and form a clot. (For more on aspirin and heart-disease protection, see page 319.)

Overall, oral contraceptives are safe for women over thirty-five—and even over forty. The evidence was so convincing that, in 1990, the FDA broke the age barrier for oral contraceptives by deleting the package labeling suggesting the increased risk of heart attack among healthy nonsmoking women age forty

TABLE 9.1 *Effectiveness of Oral Contraceptives*

Conscientious use means taking your pill at about the same time *every day*. If you miss a pill, take it as soon as you realize that you have forgotten it and resume your tablet-a-day schedule for the remainder of the cycle. If you miss two pills, take them as soon as you realize that you have forgotten them, continue your regular tablet-a-day schedule, *and use a back-up method of contraception for the remainder of the cycle.* If you miss three or more pills in a row, notify your doctor, who will give you further instructions.

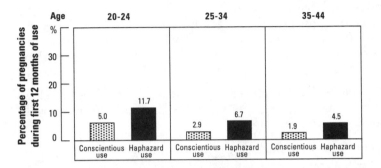

Note: Table reprinted with permission of The Alan Guttmacher Institute from Susan Harlop, Kathryn Kost, and Jacqueline Darroch Forrest, *Preventing Pregnancy, Protecting Health: A New Look at Birth Control Choices in the United States.* New York: The Alan Guttmacher Institute, 1991.

and older. (If you smoke more than fifteen cigarettes a day, however, you should choose another form of contraception. Cigarette smoking appears to act synergistically with birth-control pills to increase your risk of a heart attack.)

What about the risk of breast cancer? The weight of evidence still suggests there's no overall increased risk of breast cancer associated with the use of oral contraceptives. Several major studies involving thousands of women have found no statistically significant link between breast cancer and birth-control pills. There doesn't appear to be any increased risk among oral-contraceptive users with a family history of breast cancer or existing benign breast disease, either. The only group of women who may be at a slightly increased risk of developing breast cancer are young, childless women who take birth-control pills for more than eight years. Even given this, researchers are quick to point out that the association is weak and study results have been conflicting.

Oral contraceptives are still the most effective form of reversible contraception available (see Table 9.1). This is especially important in the middle years, when pregnancy-related risks rise, as do the number of unintended pregnancies. In theory, birth-control pills are 99.5 percent effective in preventing pregnancy. In practice, only about two of every one hundred users will get pregnant each year. Still, when compared to other methods of birth control, oral contraceptives have one of the best track records.

Plus, oral contraceptives offer a number of other health benefits that are particularly important to women in midlife, including:

•   **Protection from ovarian cysts and ovarian cancer.** Oral contraceptive users are 70 percent less likely to develop benign ovarian cysts than nonusers and 40 percent less likely to develop ovarian cancer than nonusers. Protection from ovarian cancer begins in as little as three to six months of oral-contraceptive use and continues for up to fifteen years after you stop taking birth-control pills.

•   **Protection against endometrial cancer.** Birth-control pills provide 50 percent increased protection from endometrial cancer after just one year of use. Effects last for at least fifteen years after you stop using birth-control pills.

•   **Protection from benign cysts of the breast.** Users of oral contraceptives enjoy a 65 to 85 percent decrease in fibroadenoma, a 35 to 50 percent decrease in chronic fibrocystic breast disease, and a 50 percent decrease in breast biopsies compared with nonusers.

•   **Increased bone mass.** Columbia University's Robert Lindsay, M.D., found that premenopausal women taking oral contraceptives experienced an increase in vertebral bone mass of about 1 percent per year. Other researchers have reported increases in bone mass of the wrist among oral-contraceptive users.

•   **Protection from iron-deficiency anemia.** Women who take birth-control pills are 50 percent less likely to develop iron-deficiency anemia than nonusers.

•   **Protection from pelvic inflammatory disease.** Oral contraceptive users have a 20 to 50 percent lower risk of pelvic inflammatory disease (PID), a bacterial infection of the reproductive tract, than women using no contraception. This is possibly because of a thickening of the cervical mucus, which may block bacterial invasion. Decreased menstrual flow among birth-control pill users may also be protective. If you do develop PID while taking oral contraceptives, it's often less severe and less likely to cause infertility.

Birth-control pills also help to maintain regular bleeding cycles and a consistent hormonal pattern right up to menopause. They help relieve PMS symptoms 30 percent of the time.

It's possible that oral contraceptives may even protect against heart disease. Animal studies suggest that oral contraceptives, in particular, may have a protective effect *in spite of changes in blood-cholesterol levels that would appear to raise the risk of developing heart disease.* In one study, two groups of monkeys were fed a high-fat, high-cholesterol diet—the kind of diet that promotes narrowing of the coronary arteries (*atherosclerosis*) and often leads to a heart attack. One group of monkeys was given oral contraceptives. The other group received a vaginal ring (a small rubber ring inserted into the vagina like a diaphragm) that secretes contraceptive hormones. As expected, the monkeys in both groups experienced a drop in protective HDL cholesterol, a drop that is associated with a greater risk of heart disease. However, when the two-year study was over, the monkeys taking oral contraceptives were found to have fewer and smaller artery-clogging plaques than those who had received the vaginal ring. In a later study, the researchers expected to find a twofold increase in the extent of atherosclerosis among monkeys taking oral contraceptives who ate a high-fat diet. Instead, they found a *50 to 75 percent decrease in the extent of atherosclerosis—in spite of reduced HDL–cholesterol levels caused by the oral contraceptives.* The findings suggest that oral contraceptives—specifically the estrogen in them—protect against atherosclerosis in ways we don't yet fully understand.

Moreover, a large population study has found no increased risk of cardiovascular disease among former users of oral contraceptives—including women who took birth control pills with higher doses of hormones than today's. Meir Stampfer, M.D., and his colleagues at Harvard University's School of Public Health compared the number of heart attacks and strokes suffered by women who had used oral contraceptives in the past with that of women who had never used birth-control pills. In the eight-year study involving over 100,000 women, there was little difference in the incidence of heart attack and stroke between users and nonusers.

Today's new, low-dose contraceptives are associated with far fewer minor side effects, as well. When side effects such as headaches, breast tenderness, or breakthrough bleeding do occur, they usually go away after the first three months of using birth-control pills.

Which type of oral contraceptive is best for older women? Obviously, you want to choose the preparation with the lowest combination of estrogen and progestogen. (See Some Commonly Prescribed Oral Contraceptives on page 191.) One way to bridge the gap between your peak reproductive years and menopause is by using one of the new multiphasic brands of birth-control pills, such as Ortho-Novum 7-7-7, Tridesogen, or Triphasil. These pills contain varying levels of hormones that fluctuate as needed throughout the cycle to provide adequate protection with the minimum dosage of hormones. Another appropriate oral contraceptive is Loestrin 1 + 20.

Keep in mind, however, that every woman responds differently to the same type of oral contraceptive, so no one type of pill is right for everybody. If one brand of birth-control pills gives you problems for more than three months, try switching to another.

Generally speaking, most healthy women over age thirty-five can take oral contraceptives right up until menopause *as long as they do not smoke.* However, women over forty should be screened by their physicians to ensure they don't have any underlying health conditions that may be exacerbated by the use of birth-control pills. If you're over forty and otherwise healthy, you should have your blood cholesterol checked by undergoing a lipid profile (see page 311). You should also have a test for fasting blood-sugar levels. If you have a family history of diabetes or have developed gestational diabetes during a past pregnancy, you should undergo a two-hour postglucose screen, in which your blood-glucose levels are measured two hours after ingesting a glucose solution. If results of the screening test are positive, you should also have a glucose-tolerance test. Women who previously had thrombophlebitis (blood clots in the legs) should undergo tests for *prothrombin time* (which helps determine how quickly your blood clots), *fibrinogen* (a blood coagulant), and *antithrombin III* (an anticoagulant in the blood that helps prevent clots).

For added protection against possible increased cardiovascular risks, we recommend that you take a junior aspirin every three days (under your doctor's supervision, of course) and that you remain physically active. Regular physical

There are four basic types of oral contraceptives from which to choose. Each has its advantages and disadvantages.

1. **Monophasic** pills are the easiest to use, since all pills for each cycle contain the same amount of estrogen and progestogen. However, the pills have a higher total hormonal content than other formulations, and higher doses mean a greater potential for side effects and complications. Some brand names include Brevicon, Demulen, Desogen, Genora, Levlen, Loestrin, Lo-Ovral, ModiCon, Nelova, Nordette, Norethin, Norinyl, Norlestrin, Ortho-Novum, Ovcon 35, and Ovral.

2. **Biphasic** pills (which are not frequently prescribed) have a lower total hormone content than monophasic pills and more closely mimic the hormonal changes in the menstrual cycle, but they are associated with a greater incidence of breakthrough bleeding. Brand names include Nelova 10/11 and Ortho Novum 10/11.

3. **Triphasic** pills have the lowest total hormone content of all combination oral contraceptives, but these pills contain up to four different doses of hormones per cycle; if you miss a pill or experience other problems, it's more difficult for your doctor to tell where you are in the pill cycle and what precautions you should take to protect yourself from unwanted pregnancy. Brand names include Ortho-Novum 7–7–7, Tridesogen, Tri-Levlen, Tri-Norinyl, and Triphasil.

4. **Progestogen-only** pills have the advantage of sparing you from such estrogen-related side effects as headaches and nausea. But "minipills" are not as effective in preventing pregnancy as combination pills. In addition, your menstrual patterns may be less predictable and you may experience irregular bleeding problems. Brand names include Micronor, Nor QD, and Ovrette.

activity is especially important, since it has been shown to confer protection against heart disease and since, for reasons that aren't clear yet, oral contraceptives can have a negative impact on a woman's fitness level. In one study of ours, women who started taking oral contraceptives experienced an 8 percent decline in physical fitness.

How will you know when to *stop* taking birth-control pills? In your late forties and early fifties, your physician may want to check periodically to see whether you are menopausal. This involves taking a blood test during the pill-free week to check for levels of follicle-stimulating hormone (see page 36). Levels over 40 mIU/ml mean that you are menopausal and don't have to worry about contraception anymore.

Why not continue taking birth-control pills even after menopause to relieve such menopausal symptoms as hot flashes? Low-dose oral contraceptives contain approximately four to seven times the amount of estrogen that's effective for relieving menopausal symptoms. If you have a problem with hot flashes and other menopausal symptoms, it's better to switch to the lower (and even safer) doses of hormones prescribed in postmenopausal hormone therapy. (For more on postmenopausal hormone therapy, see Chapters 20 and 21.)

Norplant

This recently approved contraceptive device consists of six tiny silicone rubber tubes containing the progestogen *levonorgestrel*. The device is surgically inserted under the skin of the arm by a trained medical practitioner, where the tubes slowly release the drug into the bloodstream. The implant, which lasts at least five years, is a highly effective reversible method of contraception. The implant frequently causes menstrual irregularities, however; and it *should not* be used by women with dysfunctional bleeding.

Intrauterine Devices (IUDs)

When inserted into the uterus by a physician, the IUD prevents pregnancy by somehow altering the delicate chemical balance of the uterus, making it either inhospitable to sperm or impossible for a fertilized egg to implant. Although the safety of the IUD was called into question in the 1970s and 1980s, most of the problems stemmed from a design flaw in the A. H. Robins Company's Dalkon Shield. The Dalkon Shield's multifilament tail (the part of the IUD that passes through the cervix and into the vagina) acted as a wick to allow bacteria to enter the uterus, resulting in hundreds of cases of pelvic inflammatory disease (PID), infertility, and a number of deaths among its users. The FDA banned further sales of the Dalkon Shield in 1983, but the government agency considers all other IUDs (which have monofilament tails) to be safe and effective birth-

TABLE 9.2 *Effectiveness of Intrauterine Device*
Conscientious use involves checking for the tail of the IUD in your vagina at least once a month, and having the IUD replaced every four to six years, as necessary.

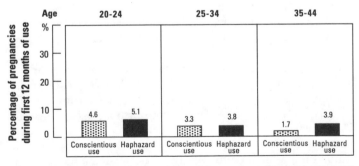

Note: Table reprinted with permission of The Alan Guttmacher Institute from Susan Harlop, Kathryn Kost, and Jacqueline Darroch Forrest, *Preventing Pregnancy, Protecting Health: A New Look at Birth Control Choices in the United States.* New York: The Alan Guttmacher Institute, 1991.

control methods *provided you are in a mutually monogamous relationship.* (Women with multiple sex partners and those who are not in a mutually monogamous relationship are at a greater risk of contracting a sexually transmitted disease, and sexually transmitted diseases are more likely to develop into PID [pelvic inflammatory disease] among IUD users.)

Two types of IUDs are now available in the United States, the Copper T and the Progestasert.

•   **Copper T:** This small plastic T-shaped device that's coated with copper has a pregnancy rate of less than 1 percent in the first year of use. The Copper T can be worn for up to six years.

•   **Progestasert:** This IUD releases a small amount of progestogen into the uterus. The Progestasert is very good for premenopausal women, particularly if they are obese, because the IUD protects the endometrium from unopposed estrogen and potential overgrowth (*hyperplasia*) of endometrial cells. (In fact, this may be an ideal method of protecting the endometrium in women taking postmenopausal estrogens.) The Progestasert also has been shown to reduce heavy bleeding, which can be a problem among women approaching menopause. A large number of studies show that the Progestasert reduces average menstrual-blood loss by 40 percent compared with other IUDs.

The principle advantage of using an IUD in your middle years is that it doesn't interfere with your hormonal cycle. This makes it easier to recognize the onset of menopause. The main disadvantage of the IUD (including the Progestasert) is that it may be associated with some irregular bleeding. Since the risk of endometrial cancer rises with age, your physician may want to ensure that the irregular bleeding is associated with the IUD and *not* an early sign of endometrial cancer. This may involve endometrial sampling—in which cells from the endometrial lining are removed and examined for possible precancerous changes—or ultrasound (see page 393).

Progestogen Injections (Depo Provera)

In 1992, the U.S. Food and Drug Administration approved yet another form of birth control, a long-acting synthetic hormone known as *depot medroxyprogesterone acetate* (Depo Provera). Depo Provera, which has been used for contraception in other countries for many years, is administered as an injection by your physician every three months. The injections are more than 99 percent effective in preventing pregnancy. However, Depo Provera may cause irregular menstrual bleeding, weight gain, fatigue, dizziness, and headaches. Moreover, some women may have trouble conceiving for up to nine months after they stop taking the injections. The drug doesn't have any long-term effects on a woman's fertility, however.

Barrier Methods

Barrier methods of birth control—the diaphragm, sponge, cervical cap, condom, and spermicides—can be highly effective when used correctly and consistently (see tables 9.3, 9.4, 9.5, and 9.6). Condoms have another advantage for

TABLE 9.3 *Effectiveness of Diaphragm/Cervical Cap*

Conscientious use means using the diaphragm or cap *along with a spermicide* every time you have intercourse; periodically inspecting the diaphragm or cap for leaks (hold the device up to a bright light and visually check for holes or tears in the rubber, or pour a small amount of tap water into the diaphragm or cap and check for signs of leakage); inserting the diaphragm or cap properly (your doctor can show you how); leaving the diaphragm in place *at least eight hours after intercourse*; periodically checking to ensure that the diaphragm or cap is in place while you wear it; and re-applying spermicide every time you have intercourse.

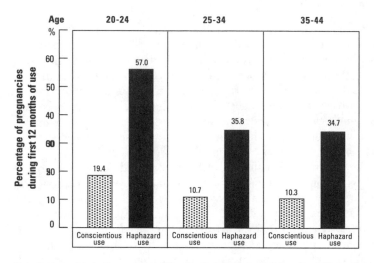

Note: Table reprinted with permission of The Alan Guttmacher Institute from Susan Harlop, Kathryn Kost, and Jacqueline Darroch Forrest, *Preventing Pregnancy, Protecting Health: A New Look at Birth Control Choices in the United States.* New York: The Alan Guttmacher Institute, 1991.

women who *aren't* in a monogamous relationship: They help prevent the spread of sexually transmitted diseases, including the HIV virus that causes AIDS.

Barrier methods have several other advantages, as well. Except for the diaphragm and the cervical cap, barrier methods can be purchased over the counter. They need to be used only at the time of intercourse, so they are particularly suitable for couples who have intercourse only occasionally. Barrier methods are relatively inexpensive, easy to use, and don't require periods of abstinence. Cervical caps, sponges, and the new female condom may be inserted at some point before lovemaking, thus increasing spontaneity. Latex condoms are particularly useful as protection against the spread of sexually transmitted diseases (see page 280). As some of the oldest forms of birth control around, barrier methods have a good safety record, too.

On the other hand, barrier methods are only as effective as the people who use them. While they can be as high as 97 to 99 percent effective in preventing pregnancy when used properly and consistently, in practice, barrier methods have an efficacy rate ranging from 40 to 95 percent.

TABLE 9.4 *Effectiveness of Contraceptive Sponge*

Conscientious use involves inserting the sponge properly (follow the directions in the package insert), keeping the sponge in place for at least 8 hours after intercourse, and changing the sponge at least once every 24 hours.

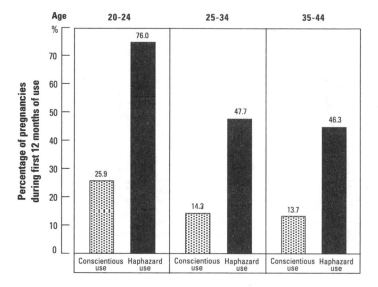

Note: Table reprinted with permission of The Alan Guttmacher Institute from Susan Harlop, Kathryn Kost, and Jacqueline Darroch Forrest, *Preventing Pregnancy, Protecting Health: A New Look at Birth Control Choices in the United States.* New York: The Alan Guttmacher Institute, 1991.

TABLE 9.5 *Effectiveness of Condoms*

Conscientious use means using a fresh condom with every act of intercourse. Using spermicides along with condoms (or using spermicidally treated condoms) improves their effectiveness.

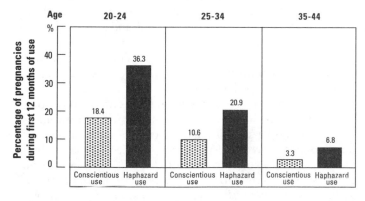

Note: Table reprinted with permission of The Alan Guttmacher Institute from Susan Harlop, Kathryn Kost, and Jacqueline Darroch Forrest, *Preventing Pregnancy, Protecting Health: A New Look at Birth Control Choices in the United States.* New York: The Alan Guttmacher Institute, 1991.

TABLE 9.6   *Effectiveness of Spermicides*

Conscientious use means re-applying spermicides with every act of intercourse. Spermicides alone aren't terribly effective in preventing pregnancy, but when used together with a barrier method of birth control, such as the diaphragm, cervical cap, or condoms, these agents can be highly effective.

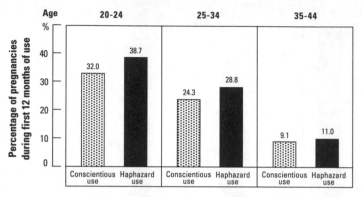

Note: Table reprinted with permission of The Alan Guttmacher Institute from Susan Harlop, Kathryn Kost, and Jacqueline Darroch Forrest, *Preventing Pregnancy, Protecting Health: A New Look at Birth Control Choices in the United States.* New York: The Alan Guttmacher Institute, 1991.

Some of the main drawbacks to barrier methods are also some of the major reasons why compliance is so low: Many couples find the spermicides messy. Some users find that interrupting lovemaking or preparing in advance detracts from spontaneity and sexual enjoyment. Condoms may cause a partial loss of sensation in the man or discomfort in the woman. And, as we stressed earlier, these methods must be used *with every act of intercourse* to obtain maximum protection against unwanted pregnancy and sexually transmitted diseases.

While side effects are minor, they may keep some couples from using barrier methods. About 2 to 4 percent of men and women become sensitive to spermicides. An even smaller percentage are allergic to latex and rubber. The diaphragm has been associated with an increased rate of urinary-tract infections, and the cervical cap sometimes produces cervical and vaginal trauma. However, most couples can use barrier methods without a problem.

Barrier methods are a good choice for women who can't use other methods of contraception or who have reservations about them. And while the effectiveness of barrier methods is lower than that of birth-control pills or IUDs, they may actually be somewhat more effective for women in midlife than for other age groups, simply because ovulation patterns become more erratic in the middle years. If you have multiple sexual partners or are not in a mutually monogamous relationship, barrier contraception may be the method of choice to help protect yourself against sexually transmitted diseases. Indeed, if you are sexually active with a new partner or with more than one partner, *you should use a barrier method (particularly latex condoms) in addition to your regular birth-control method* in order to protect specifically against sexually transmitted diseases.

196

TABLE 9.7   *Effectiveness of Periodic Abstinence*

Conscientious use involves taking your basal body temperature every day, checking your cervical mucus daily for characteristic changes associated with ovulation (ask your physician for details), and abstaining from intercourse or using a barrier method of contraception during your fertile period.

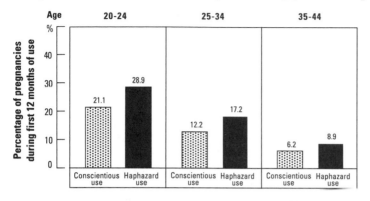

Note: Table reprinted with permission of The Alan Guttmacher Institute from Susan Harlop, Kathryn Kost, and Jacqueline Darroch Forrest, *Preventing Pregnancy, Protecting Health: A New Look at Birth Control Choices in the United States.* New York: The Alan Guttmacher Institute, 1991.

Periodic Abstinence

The contraceptive methods known collectively as periodic abstinence or natural family planning are simply too unpredictable for climacteric women. These methods work best among women with predictable menstrual cycles, and even then the methods are only 70 to 80 percent effective in preventing pregnancy. (see Table 9.7) The irregular periods and ovulation patterns characteristic of the middle years make periodic abstinence too chancy. Also, one of the methods used to predict ovulation requires that you monitor changes in cervical mucus over the course of the menstrual cycle. However, the climacteric itself alters the quality of cervical mucus, making this barometer of ovulation unreliable.

If you use periodic abstinence or natural family planning and your period *does* come late, you may find yourself constantly wondering whether or not you are pregnant. Why not take the worry out of midlife contraception by choosing a more reliable birth-control method than this one.

The Morning-After Pill

This method is better described as an "interceptive" rather than a contraceptive, since the goal is to prevent implantation of a fertilized egg. The morning-after pill is only for women who've had unprotected intercourse around the time of ovulation and suspect they may have conceived.

There are several different morning-after regimens, but all must be started within seventy-two hours of ovulation, which again is a problem for women in midlife, since ovulation becomes more unpredictable as you approach menopause.

Probably the most reliable regimen involves taking two tablets of Ovral (containing 50 micrograms of estrogen) within seventy-two hours of unprotected intercourse. The regimen is repeated twelve hours later. This method has a success rate of 98 to 99.8 percent.

Another regimen is to give high doses of conjugated estrogen (Premarin) three times a day for five days. Among 359 women we treated in this way, only one woman got pregnant—a success rate of 99.7 percent.

Nausea, vomiting, and breast tenderness are common side effects associated with all morning-after regimens. Your physician may prescribe an antiemetic to curb nausea and vomiting.

If your period doesn't start within two to three weeks from the time you take the morning-after pill, your doctor will want you to undergo a pregnancy test.

RU-486

You've undoubtedly heard rumblings about RU-486, the synthetic progestogen being used in France to prevent unwanted pregnancy after conception. The drug works by blocking the ovaries' production of progesterone, which prevents the implantation of a fertilized egg in the uterus, or the growth of an egg that has already become implanted. RU-486 has been used in France since January 1989, with more than two thousand patients per month. In a French study involving 2,115 women who took RU-486 within forty-nine days of their last menstrual period, the drug induced abortion in 96 percent of the women, with no serious side effects. The authors of the study concluded that RU-486 was as safe and effective as suction abortion, the most common method of abortion used in the first three months of pregnancy.

As of this writing, the drug is not available in the United States. However, the FDA has cleared the way for quick approval of RU-486 in this country by stating that clinical trials conducted in Europe may be sufficient for the agency to review the safety and effectiveness of the drug.

A Final Word

When deciding on the most suitable form of birth control for your middle years, be sure to take into account not just the safety and efficacy of the various methods but also your personal preferences. Are you likely to remember to take a birth-control pill every day? (Taking your pill at the same time every day helps get you into the habit.) If you're thinking about one of the barrier methods of birth control, will you (and your partner) be motivated enough to use it correctly *every time you have intercourse*? (Some couples find that inserting a diaphragm or putting on a condom can be a part of sexual foreplay, thus adding to the spontaneity and enjoyment of sex.)

Once you've made a decision, make sure you are well versed in the proper use of your method of choice. This way, you can enjoy freedom from unwanted pregnancy straight through to menopause.

....
Suggested Reading
....

Winikoff, Beverly, and Suzanne Wymelenberg, eds. *The Contraceptive Handbook: A Guide to Safe and Effective Choices for Men and Women*. Mount Vernon, NY: Consumers Union, 1992.

....
Resources and Support
....

American College of Obstetricians and Gynecologists, Resource Center, 409 12th St., SW, Washington, D.C. 20024. The college provides free brochures on contraception and a wide range of other subjects, including pregnancy after thirty-five, menopause, and hysterectomy. Send a stamped self-addressed business envelope along with your request.

Planned Parenthood Federation of America, 810 Seventh Avenue, New York, NY 10019. Planned Parenthood publishes pamphlets and produces videos on contraception, pregnancy, and a variety of other topics. Contact your local affiliate of Planned Parenthood or write to the national office for a publication list.

Chapter 10

....

Midlife Fertility and Pregnancy: New Discoveries and New Hope

There *are* some advantages to postponing pregnancy. Older mothers tend to be better educated, established in professional occupations, and financially better off than younger mothers. And while delaying pregnancy until later in life does carry certain risks, overall the chances of having a healthy baby in the middle years far outweigh the slightly increased risks to mother and baby from midlife pregnancy (see Table 10.1). What's more, most of these risks can be managed by preparing yourself well in advance of pregnancy (a new trend in obstetrics called *preconception care*), having regular medical checkups throughout your pregnancy, and taking good care of yourself from the moment of conception until the baby's birth. Let's look at some of the more common risks associated with pregnancy after age thirty-five and what you can do to increase your odds of having a healthy baby—even in midlife.

Declining Fertility

Women in the middle years tend to raise two common questions about their fertility: Those who *don't* want to get pregnant ask, "Will I?" Those who *do* wish to conceive ask, "Can I?" The answer to *both* questions is yes. Although fertility does decline somewhat as you grow older, your ovaries will continue to release eggs until you experience menopause. This means that if you *don't* want to get pregnant, you will still need to diligently use some form of contraception. If you do want to conceive a child, however, you should realize that it may take a little longer now than when you were younger. Studies have shown that the percentage of women age twenty-five who conceive after twelve months of unprotected intercourse is 73 percent. The number drops to 53 percent for women over thirty-five.

The reasons for this decline in fertility are many. To begin with, your ovaries have already started producing less progesterone and estrogen, and

TABLE 10.1 *Putting Midlife Pregnancy Risks Into Perspective*

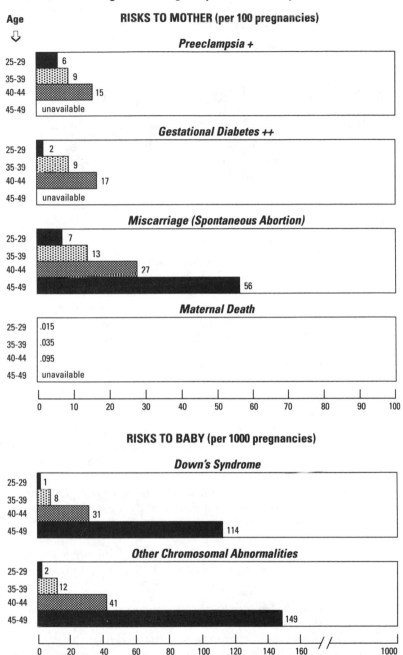

Age ⇩   **RISKS TO MOTHER (per 100 pregnancies)**

Preeclampsia +

Age	
25-29	6
35-39	9
40-44	15
45-49	unavailable

Gestational Diabetes ++

Age	
25-29	2
35-39	9
40-44	17
45-49	unavailable

Miscarriage (Spontaneous Abortion)

Age	
25-29	7
35-39	13
40-44	27
45-49	56

Maternal Death

Age	
25-29	.015
35-39	.035
40-44	.095
45-49	unavailable

0   10   20   30   40   50   60   70   80   90   100

RISKS TO BABY (per 1000 pregnancies)

Down's Syndrome

Age	
25-29	1
35-39	8
40-44	31
45-49	114

Other Chromosomal Abnormalities

Age	
25-29	2
35-39	12
40-44	41
45-49	149

0   20   40   60   80   100   120   140   160 // 1000

† Shown here are risks to first-time mothers. Risks may be lower for women who have already given birth to at least one child without developing the condition.

†† Shown here are risks for first-time mothers of normal weight who have no family history of gestational diabetes. Risks are slightly greater for women who are overweight or who have a family history of gestational diabetes. At greatest risk are obese women over 40 with a family history of the condition. About 34 percent of these women will develop gestational diabetes.

201

TABLE 10.2 *Percentage of Women with Menstrual Irregularities*
Menstrual cycles that have become more irregular indicate a decline in ovulation—and in fertility.

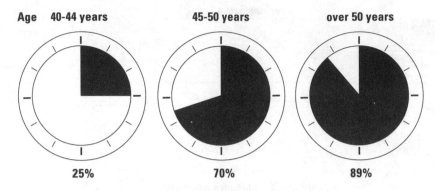

Age	40-44 years	45-50 years	over 50 years
	25%	70%	89%

your pattern of ovulation is gradually becoming more erratic (see Table 10.2). Also, your reproductive system has had more time to be exposed to such insults as infection and illness, which can cause fertility to decline. For instance, women with *endometriosis* (a condition in which the uterine lining grows outside of the uterus) may suffer damage to the delicate Fallopian tubes, where conception takes place. Women who have had pelvic inflammatory disease (PID), a severe infection of the Fallopian tubes that's often caused by an untreated or inadequately treated sexually transmitted disease, also may have more difficulty conceiving. Apparently, changes in the uterus as you grow older make implantation of a fertilized egg more difficult, too.

Remember also that there are only about two days out of every month that you can actually conceive—right around the time of ovulation. If you're determined to get pregnant and don't want to leave conception to chance, you may want to try one of these methods of pinpointing your time of ovulation:

• **Basal body temperature:** This method involves taking your basal (or resting) temperature every morning before you get up and charting any changes during the course of your menstrual cycle. (Note: You'll want to use a basal thermometer, which has larger numbers and easier-to-read temperature increments.) A change in body temperature from 0.5 to 1 degree Fahrenheit indicates approximately when you are ovulating (see Figure 10.1). (You'll find a basal body temperature chart on page 482.)

• **Ovulation predictor tests:** Several home tests are available to help predict your time of ovulation (Clearplan, First Response, Fortel, OvuKit, OvuQuick). These tests, which involve taking a urine sample for several days in the middle of your menstrual cycle, can detect the surge of luteinizing hormone (LH) at midcycle that is associated with ovulation. Release of an egg by your ovaries usually occurs within about thirty hours of the surge in LH. You are most likely to become pregnant if you have sexual intercourse within the first twenty-four hours after detecting the surge in LH. (Note: These tests are not reliable

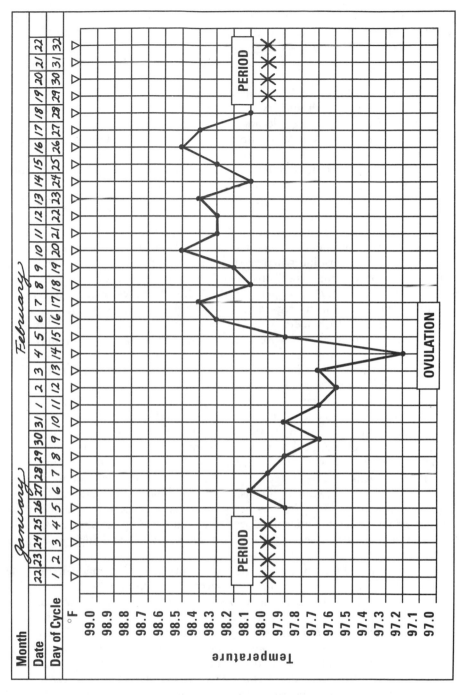

Figure 10.1   Sample Basal Body Temperature Chart

enough to be used for contraception.) The test kits, which contain enough chemicals to perform six to nine tests, cost around twenty-five dollars, which can get expensive if you use them for several months in a row. On the other hand, they're more accurate than measuring daily basal body temperature.

Because fertility declines rapidly after age forty-five, it's best not to wait *too* long. Ideally, you should try for pregnancy between ages thirty-five and forty-five—the "last chance" decade.

If you still haven't conceived after a year of unprotected intercourse—the technical definition of infertility—you may want to consider having an infertility work-up. (If you undergo infertility testing, it's essential that *both* you and your partner participate in the examination; although we typically tend to think that most infertility problems reside with the woman, up to 40 percent can be traced to the male.)

A typical infertility work-up includes a medical history and physical examination for both partners. The woman will undergo blood-hormone tests, as well as tests to determine whether she is ovulating, her Fallopian tubes are open, her uterine lining is receptive to a fertilized egg, and her cervical mucus is normal (to help transport sperm to the Fallopian tubes, where conception occurs). The man will undergo a sperm analysis to determine whether he is producing sufficient numbers of motile sperm to penetrate the cervical mucus and reach the Fallopian tubes. Keep in mind that the entire work-up may take a month or two to complete. And some of the tests (such as the *hysterosalpingogram,* in which a dye is injected into the woman's uterus and Fallopian tubes to ensure that the tubes are open) can be somewhat uncomfortable.

The outlook for infertile couples today is better than ever, thanks to such treatment advances as microsurgery and in vitro fertilization. According to the American Fertility Society, up to two-thirds of infertile couples today do go on to conceive and deliver healthy babies. One of the most common problems for women—failure to ovulate, or *anovulation*—is fairly easy to treat. Sometimes, a minor problem in each partner—low sperm motility in the man and hostile cervical mucus in the woman, for instance—combined can result in infertility, and treating one or both partners brings success. To find out more about the causes of and cures for infertility, see Suggested Reading on page 214. For a referral to an infertility specialist near you, see Resources and Support on page 215.

The new technology for treating infertility has even made it possible for some postmenopausal women to become pregnant. In one instance, a postmenopausal woman gave birth to her own grandchild. The woman was first treated with hormones to thicken the uterine lining in preparation for pregnancy. At the same time, her daughter underwent in-vitro fertilization, in which several ripe eggs were taken from her ovaries and fertilized with her husband's sperm in a laboratory dish. The resulting embryo was placed in the older woman's uterus, and the child was successfully carried to term. Still, while pregnancy may be possible after menopause, it is an option that should be reserved for only the most desperate couples, especially since the health risks to the mother rise with age.

Miscarriage

The loss of a pregnancy in the first twenty-eights weeks of pregnancy (*miscarriage*, or *spontaneous abortion*) can happen to a woman of any age. But for women forty and older, the risk is somewhat greater. No one's sure why this is so. There are numerous possible causes for miscarriage, including fibroid tumors of the uterus, hormonal imbalances, and chronic illness, such as hypertension. But the most likely cause is a genetic abnormality of the fetus that keeps it from developing properly.

What signs should you look for? A *threatened abortion* occurs whenever you have a bloody discharge or bleeding from the uterus in the first half of pregnancy. You may or may not experience mild cramping (resembling that of a menstrual period) or low backache. Keep in mind, however, that *as many as 30 to 40 percent of all women experience some spotting during the early weeks of pregnancy, and most go on to deliver healthy babies.*

If you notice any spotting or light bleeding early in your pregnancy, you should notify your practitioner as soon as possible during regular office hours (you needn't rush to the hospital emergency room unless you are bleeding heavily, are in severe pain, or are passing blood clots). Your practitioner may perform a blood test to measure levels of the hormone *human chorionic gonadotropin*, which is present in predictable levels during early pregnancy. You may also be advised to have an ultrasound test, which can determine whether the fetus's heart is beating (after the fifth or sixth week), whether the fetus is active, and whether it is growing and developing as expected for its age. If tests reveal that the pregnancy is not viable, your physician may recommend that you undergo a dilatation and curettage (D&C), in which the contents of the uterus are removed.

If You Suffer a Miscarriage

Whatever the reasons for a miscarriage, experts are just beginning to recognize that early pregnancy loss can have serious emotional ramifications. Although we typically think of the first trimester as too early for a mother to form an emotional bond with her baby, research now shows that bonding may begin at the moment you start planning a pregnancy. And grief reactions can be as deep as if the baby had been stillborn or died during childbirth.

Women who have an ectopic pregnancy (in which the embryo implants in a Fallopian tube rather than in the uterus), and even those who have an elective abortion, may experience similar emotions. This is particularly true if the pregnancy was planned and you chose an abortion to avoid giving birth to a child with birth defects.

If you do experience a miscarriage, you may take little comfort in knowing that at least you can get pregnant, or that it was a blessing in disguise because the child probably could not have survived outside the womb. Mourning over the loss is more complicated because there's no baby, no funeral, and none of the other channels through which we normally process grief.

It helps to know that strong feelings of grief and sorrow are normal after a miscarriage, and you should allow yourself to grieve. It's also not unusual to feel anger, guilt, sadness, fear, and a sense of failure. Your partner and children may also be deeply affected by the loss. To help resolve some of these feelings, you may want to seek comfort from other women who have had a miscarriage. Several good books have been written on the subject (see Suggested Reading on page 214). Some communities have support groups specifically for couples who have suffered a miscarriage. These groups can be enormously helpful. Ask your practitioner or local hospital whether there's a group in your area.

Try not to compound your grief with guilt about what you could have done differently during your pregnancy. While it's not always possible to pinpoint the exact causes of a miscarriage, the chances that you did something to cause it are low. We know, for example, that emotional upsets (resulting from an argument, stress at work, or family problems), a fall or other *minor* accidental injury, normal physical activity (such as housework, lifting children, and moderate exercise), and sexual intercourse (unless you have a history of miscarriage) *don't* cause miscarriages.

On the other hand, some factors within your control *do* increase your risk of having a miscarriage, and it's useful to know what they are so you can prepare for the next time. If you smoke cigarettes, you are twice as likely to suffer a miscarriage as a nonsmoker. Heavy drinking is associated with an increased risk of miscarriage, too. So is exposure to rubella (German measles) or other diseases that can harm the fetus, radiation exposure, or exposure to drugs harmful to the fetus.

When should you try to conceive again? Most physicians generally recommend that you wait at least two or three months before trying to get pregnant again. This allows your body to return to a normal pattern of menstruation. However, it may take longer than this for you to come to terms with your feelings about the miscarriage. Let your feelings be your guide in determining when you're ready to try again.

Pregnancy-Related Risks to the Mother

While your chances of experiencing certain medical complications during your pregnancy rise as you grow older, most problems can be monitored effectively with regular visits to your physician and usually pose no long-term threat to your health or your baby's.

Diabetes

Women over forty are at a somewhat greater risk of developing *diabetes mellitus*, which may be why women in midlife are also more likely to develop *gestational diabetes*, a form of diabetes that occurs only during pregnancy.

Indeed, it's not always clear how many women diagnosed with gestational diabetes actually had diabetes *before* they got pregnant. At any rate, with proper treatment, including a controlled diet, exercise, and regular glucose (blood-sugar) monitoring, a woman with diabetes or gestational diabetes has just about as good a chance of having a healthy baby as a nondiabetic mother.

How does gestational diabetes develop? Even a normal pregnancy puts added strain on your body's ability to process carbohydrates. Your growing fetus relies on sugar (glucose) as a major source of energy, so glucose is constantly being drained from your bloodstream. This leads to much lower blood-sugar levels in the mother after fasting. In addition, blood-sugar levels remain high for several hours after eating a meal, probably because your gastrointestinal tract takes longer to digest food during pregnancy. To help your body's tissues absorb blood sugars, your pancreas produces roughly two to three times more insulin during the second half of your pregnancy.

Women who develop gestational diabetes either don't produce enough insulin to clear glucose from the bloodstream or become "resistant" to the effects of insulin on blood sugars. As a result, these women have elevated blood sugar levels until the baby is delivered.

If left untreated, gestational diabetes can cause the fetus to absorb excess sugar, stimulating the baby to grow unusually large. Sometimes the baby grows too large to pass through the birth canal, necessitating a cesarean delivery. Women with diabetes mellitus that isn't well controlled during pregnancy are at a greater risk of developing preeclampsia, a form of high blood pressure that occurs in pregnancy (see page 208), infections, and cardiorespiratory problems. Their babies also are at a greater risk of developing birth defects and respiratory problems.

Since diabetes can be a serious problem for the older mother-to-be, you should have a glucose tolerance test *before* you conceive. If you do have diabetes, you can take steps to control blood sugar levels before you get pregnant. Even if you don't have diabetes when you conceive, your doctor will recommend that you undergo another blood glucose test between 24 to 28 weeks after conception to screen for gestational diabetes.

Treatment includes a diet high in complex carbohydrates (beans, rice, whole-grain bread), moderate in protein, and low in cholesterol and fat. Sugary sweets should be cut out of your diet altogether. Whether you have diabetes mellitus or gestational diabetes, it is imperative that you stick strictly to your diet. Most cases of gestational diabetes are mild and can be managed through dietary measures alone. Your physician may also recommend that you participate in a moderate exercise program and undergo regular glucose testing. Only women with more severe cases of diabetes will need insulin injections.

You will be monitored more closely than other expectant mothers if you have diabetes or develop gestational diabetes. This is simply to ensure that the diabetes is kept under control and ultimately to ensure the health of you and your baby.

If you develop gestational diabetes, your body should return to normal after you deliver the baby. However, many women who develop gestational diabetes are at a greater risk of developing overt diabetes later in life. By keeping up the good eating and exercise habits you learned during your pregnancy, you will substantially reduce your odds of developing diabetes in the years to come.

Pregnancy-Induced Hypertension

The number of women who develop high blood pressure during pregnancy also rises with age, which is why routine monitoring of your blood pressure by your physician throughout your pregnancy is essential. Again, it's not clear how many women suffer from chronic, or *essential* hypertension (which increases with age, too) that's compounded by pregnancy. Keep in mind that only 5 to 15 percent of *all* women develop pregnancy-induced hypertension. And there's some evidence that taking one junior aspirin a day during pregnancy (under your doctor's supervision, of course) may actually help prevent pregnancy-induced hypertension.

Actually, there are three forms of pregnancy-induced hypertension: If your blood pressure rises above 140/90 during your pregnancy, you have hypertension. *Preeclampsia* is a term used to describe high blood pressure combined with protein in the urine, water retention(*edema*), or both. *Eclampsia* is preeclampsia plus convulsions. Eclampsia is the most severe form of pregnancy-induced hypertension, and the most dangerous to mother and baby.

No one's sure why some women develop pregnancy-induced hypertension. We do know that you are more likely to develop pregnancy-induced hypertension if:

- this is your first pregnancy
- your grandmother, mother, or sister developed preeclampsia
- you already have hypertension
- you have diabetes or kidney disease
- you are carrying twins

Black women are also more prone than white women to develop preeclampsia, possibly because black women are at a greater risk of developing hypertension than white women.

Most cases of hypertension occur after the twentieth week of pregnancy. Preeclampsia doesn't appear until the late stages of pregnancy—usually not until the last trimester.

If you develop preeclampsia, you may experience swelling of your hands and face and gain weight rapidly. Your blood pressure will rise and there may be protein in your urine. Women with severe cases may experience blurred vision, headaches, irritability, a decrease in urine production, confusion, and severe stomach pains.

Your doctor will need to take your blood pressure on at least two separate occasions (at least six hours apart) before making a diagnosis. Generally, a blood pressure reading of 140/90 or greater that remains elevated at least six hours later indicates that you have high blood pressure. Your urine will also be checked for elevated protein levels, which indicate preeclampsia. (Most women with high blood pressure go on to develop preeclampsia.)

If left untreated, preeclampsia can lead to damage of the mother's nervous system, blood vessels, or kidneys and can cause growth retardation or oxygen deprivation in the baby. If you are receiving regular medical care, your physician should spot the problem in time to provide the necessary intervention and prevent most of the serious complications.

Treatment varies according to the severity of the problem, but most experts agree that the best cure for pregnancy-induced hypertension is delivery of the baby. If you are close to your due date, your physician often will induce labor (or in some cases perform a cesarean section) to avoid any harm to you or the baby. If you have mild preeclampsia and it is too early for a safe delivery, your practitioner may recommend bed rest at home or (more likely) in the hospital with close medical supervision, and possibly antihypertensive medications (with the exception of ACE inhibiters, which have been associated with an increased risk of fetal injury and death when used in the last two trimesters of pregnancy).

In severe cases, you may be treated with *magnesium sulfate,* a medication that controls one of the most serious complications of the disease—convulsions. Your physician will want to deliver the baby *immediately*—even if the baby is premature. Sometimes steroids are given to help a premature baby's lungs mature faster.

For most women with preeclampsia, blood pressure returns to normal within twenty-four hours after delivery. (If your blood pressure remains elevated even after you deliver the baby, it's a good indication that you probably had high blood pressure even before you got pregnant. See page 303 for more on how high blood pressure can be managed after pregnancy.)

Several studies now suggest that preeclampsia may be prevented by taking a low dose of aspirin (60 to 150 milligrams) during the second and third trimesters. Since aspirin may also prolong labor and increase the likelihood of bleeding for both the mother and the baby, especially when taken during the last three months of pregnancy, it should be used only under your doctor's supervision.

Cesarean Birth

For reasons that aren't clear, your chances of having your baby delivered by cesarean section (in which the baby is surgically removed from the uterus via an incision in your abdomen) go up as you grow older. One 1991 study from the University of Washington in St. Louis found that 33 percent of first-time mothers over thirty-five had cesarean deliveries, compared with 24 percent of younger women.

Some experts speculate that the higher rate of cesarean deliveries among older women is a result of the increased medical complications (including pregnancy-induced hypertension and gestational diabetes) associated with mid-life pregnancy, which often require a C-section. Others argue that the high rate isn't explained even when those complications are taken into account. For example, in the University of Washington study, first-time mothers with no complications of pregnancy, labor, and delivery that would require a cesarean section *still had more than twice the rate of cesarean births as younger women (14 percent versus 6 percent).*

A cesarean section can save your life and your baby's if you have such pregnancy-related complications as preeclampsia or gestational diabetes or if certain problems arise during labor and delivery that endanger either your health or that of your baby. However, cesarean deliveries as a whole have risen dramatically in the last twenty years. Indeed, *C-sections are the most commonly performed surgery in the United States today.*

Remember, cesarean delivery is *major surgery* and, as such, carries risks of its own for both the mother and baby, including anesthesia-related risks to mother and baby and a much longer recovery time for the mother. What's more, some of the most common indications for a C-section—a single previous cesarean delivery and breech birth (in which the baby comes out feet-, knees-, or buttocks-first, rather than headfirst)—are also some of the most controversial.

Some C-sections are unavoidable, and it certainly wouldn't be in your best interest to put your life (or your baby's) on the line simply because you'd prefer a vaginal birth. On the other hand, most experts now agree that the old saw, "Once a C-section always a C-section," no longer holds true. We now know that many women who gave birth to their first baby by cesarean section can safely deliver subsequent babies vaginally. Breech babies can often be turned around prior to labor if your practitioner is willing to work with you, and, in many instances, can be safely delivered vaginally as a breech. The experience and judgment of the obstetrician is critical, however.

What you can do to protect yourself from possible unnecessary C-sections is to become informed. Read as much as you can about cesarean sections and the circumstances under which they are necessary. Discuss with your physician his or her philosophy and practices and share your feelings. If you strongly disagree with your physician's practices, you may want to consider switching to a practitioner whose philosophy is more in line with your own. (You should try to have this discussion in the early part of your pregnancy—or even before you conceive—to ensure that you'll receive continuous care throughout your pregnancy.)

Remember, however, that when all is said and done, what matters most is not *how* you delivered the baby but the fact that you and your baby are healthy.

Risks to the Baby

Another concern to women considering midlife pregnancy are the increased risks to the baby. The good news is that older women are not at significantly greater risk of delivering a low-birth-weight baby (weighting less than five pounds at birth) or of having a preterm delivery. Nor is a higher fetal death rate associated with midlife pregnancy.

That's not to say, however, that certain risks to your baby don't rise with maternal age. As you are probably aware, the risk of having a child with Down's syndrome—the most common chromosomal abnormality—increases significantly with age. This genetic defect, caused by an extra copy of the twenty-first chromosome, is characterized by mild to severe mental retardation and certain physical abnormalities, including slanted eyes, a small head flattened at the back, short stature, and heart defects. One in 365 infants born to women age thirty-five will have the syndrome, while 1 in 32 babies born to women age forty-five have Down's syndrome.

The incidence of neural-tube defects (NTDs)—the second-most-common birth defect in the United States—also increases with age. NTDs are abnormalities of the brain or spinal cord of the fetus. The neural tube (the brain and spinal-cord tissues) may fail to close as the fetus develops, leaving the brain and spinal cord exposed. In other cases, the neural tube may close improperly and be covered by skin or bone.

Two common NTDs are *anencephaly* and *spina bifida*. Babies with anencephaly are born with small or missing brain hemispheres and die soon after birth. Spina bifida babies are born with an improperly fused spinal column. In its mild form, the infant may suffer only a slight physical disability. In more severe forms, the lower half of the body may be paralyzed and the child may suffer from chronic illness and mental retardation.

Chromosomal abnormalities as a whole also rise with maternal age. Fortunately, a number of excellent prenatal tests are available now that can alert you to problems early in your pregnancy.

- **Ultrasound:** Your physician may recommend that you have an *ultrasound* test, in which sound waves are used to create an image of your baby on a video screen, for several different reasons. In the first trimester, ultrasound can be used to rule out a possible *ectopic* pregnancy (in which the fetus implants in a Fallopian tube instead of the uterus) by establishing the location of the pregnancy in your uterus. Ultrasound is also used to determine the age of the fetus and its heartbeat (as early as five and a half weeks into your pregnancy). In the second trimester, ultrasound can gauge the size of your baby as well as alert you to certain physical deformities, including neural-tube and heart defects, cleft palate, and possible problems with the abdominal wall, stomach, kidneys, and bladder. (The baby's sex can sometimes be determined, too, if the genitals are in clear view. Tell your doctor or the ultrasound technician if you'd rather not know your baby's sex.)

Third trimester ultrasound is used mainly to determine the size and position of the baby and whether it is growing as expected.

Ultrasound is a painless procedure that takes about five to ten minutes. The examination can be conducted abdominally or vaginally. During an abdominal exam, you lie on your back on an examining table and an oil gel is spread over your abdomen. The practitioner moves a hand-held ultrasound transmitter slowly across your abdomen.

A vaginal exam differs only in that a probe is placed in your vagina instead of on your abdomen. (Some women prefer vaginal ultrasound in early pregnancy; unlike the abdominal exam, it does not require that you have a full bladder.)

- **Maternal serum alpha-fetoprotein screening:** Alpha-fetoprotein (AFP) is a protein produced by the fetus. High levels in the mother's blood may indicate the presence of a neural-tube defect or other congenital abnormality. Extremely low levels of AFP in the mother's blood suggest there may be a chromosomal abnormality, such as Down's syndrome.

The AFP screening test involves taking a small sample of blood from your arm and measuring the levels of alpha-fetoprotein. The test is generally performed between the fifteenth and eighteenth weeks of pregnancy.

Remember, though, this is just a screening test. It will not tell you definitively whether your baby has an NTD. If your baby's age has been miscalculated, the test may be conducted too early or too late, which can skew the results. Carrying twins also can result in a higher reading.

Essentially, a positive test result means further testing is in order. Generally, your physician will probably perform another blood test to confirm the results. If the results come back positive a second time, an ultrasound test will be performed to determine the baby's age, to see whether you are carrying twins, or to check for any visible NTDs or abnormalities.

If ultrasound fails to reveal the source of the problem, an amniocentesis is performed (see below) to check AFP levels in the amniotic fluid surrounding the fetus. Amniocentesis is 90 percent accurate.

• **Amniocentesis:** Women over thirty-five are routinely offered amniocentesis to check for a number of birth defects, including Down's syndrome. During the test, a long needle is inserted into the amniotic sac (the "bag of waters") surrounding the fetus. The removed amniotic cells are cultured, or grown in a laboratory dish, and examined under a microscope for numerous genetic abnormalities.

The test can yield other valuable information as well, including the baby's sex, which may be important if you are a carrier of a sex-linked disorder, such as hemophilia or muscular dystrophy; the maturity of the baby's lungs, which is important if your baby is at risk of premature delivery; and the presence of neural-tube defects.

There are a number of birth defects that amniocentesis *cannot* detect. These include cleft lip and cleft palate, most heart defects, and clubfoot.

The procedure itself is relatively painless. You lie on your back on an examining table, with your abdomen exposed. Your physician will use ultrasound to locate the fetus and placenta so that when the needle is inserted neither are injured. Your abdomen is swabbed with an antiseptic. If you prefer, the injection site can be numbed with a local anesthetic. However, the anesthetic injection hurts as much as the needle used for the procedure, so some physicians omit this step. Next, a long, hollow needle is guided into the uterus, where a small amount of amniotic fluid is taken. Your vital signs are checked before and after the procedure, as well as your baby's heart tones. In all, amniocentesis takes about thirty minutes.

After the procedure, you may experience some vaginal cramping, a slight leakage of fluid, or vaginal bleeding. Be sure to discuss any leakage or bleeding with your physician.

The risk of miscarriage is increased slightly with amniocentesis. As you may recall, miscarriage occurs spontaneously in 15 to 20 percent of pregnancies, and usually happens in the first trimester. With amniocentesis, the risk of miscarriage for the remainder of your pregnancy increases by less than 1 percent.

One of the biggest drawbacks to amniocentesis is that it takes three to four weeks to get the test results back. Should you decide to terminate your pregnancy at this time, the procedure is a little more risky and traumatic than having an abortion in the early part of your pregnancy.

• **Chorionic villus sampling** (CVS): This is a relatively new procedure for testing for chromosomal abnormalities and can be performed between the ninth and twelfth weeks of your pregnancy. Results are available within one to seven days, giving you plenty of time to have a safe abortion, should you choose that option.

The procedure involves taking a sample of cells from tiny fingerlike projections of the placenta, called chorionic villi. Since these cells have the same genetic makeup as the fetus, the cell samples can be used to detect essentially all of the same chromosomal abnormalities as amniocentesis, including Down's syndrome. However, CVS cannot diagnose neural-tube defects. NTDs diagnosis requires a sample of amniotic fluid.

The procedure can be performed both vaginally or abdominally. During the vaginal procedure, your cervix is numbed with a local anesthetic as you lie on an examining table. Then, a long, thin tube is inserted through the vagina and cervix and into the uterus. Using ultrasound as a guide, the practitioner places the tube between the uterine lining and the placenta. A sample of chorionic villi is then snipped or suctioned off for study.

During the abdominal procedure, the practitioner first numbs your abdomen with a local anesthetic. Then, with the help of ultrasound, a long, hollow guide needle is inserted through the abdomen and uterine wall to the placenta. Another needle is inserted through the guide needle for cell sampling.

After the examination, you may experience some vaginal bleeding. While this shouldn't be a cause for alarm, you should report any bleeding to your physician.

Keep in mind that even though CVS offers much earlier diagnostic testing than amniocentesis, there is a slightly higher risk of miscarriage. The exact figures vary according to which study you look at, but the average increase is about 1 percent—double that of amniocentesis. The risk is lower when you seek out a practitioner who has extensive experience with CVS.

What's more, the test results can sometimes be inconclusive. If this is the case, a follow-up amniocentesis may be recommended to clear up any confusing results.

Finally a handful of recent studies (most of them from hospitals and medical centers overseas) have associated CVS with an increased risk of limb malformations, including shortened fingers and toes, missing digits, and missing nails. In response to these findings, the National Institute of Child Health and Human Development and the American College of Obstetricians and Gynecologists (ACOG) in April 1992 convened a panel of international experts to review the safety of this prenatal test. The panel concluded that, to date, clusters of CVS–associated limb malformations have occured at certain centers, but many centers report no apparent increased frequency of such problems among babies born to thousands of women receiving the test. Until we know more, ACOG recommends that you discuss fully the risks and benefits of this and all prenatal tests with your physician.

It's normal to worry about whether your baby will be born healthy. For most women, the diagnostic tests described here will bring good news and take much of the worry out of midlife pregnancy. Still, the whole process of fetal diagnostics can be nerve-racking. It's a good idea to discuss the procedures, your feelings, *and* your options with both your physician and your partner even before undergoing the various tests. You may also want to consider consulting with a genetic counselor. Trained counselors can review your family history and put into perspective your risk of passing on a genetic defect to your baby. Most major hospitals have genetic counselors. For a referral to a counselor in your area, contact the National Society of Genetic Counselors, c/o Executive Director, 233 Canterbury Drive, Wallingford, PA 19086.

Even if terminating a pregnancy is not an option for you, you should consider undergoing some of the various prenatal tests. Knowing in advance that your child may be born with a birth defect can help prepare you emotionally. It also allows you and your physician to plan for any special medical needs the baby may have after delivery.

A Final Word

While midlife pregnancy does carry certain risks, the odds are still largely in your favor that you'll give birth to a healthy baby. This is particularly true if you take good care of yourself (eat right, exercise, avoid most drugs and environmental toxins, and see your doctor regularly) throughout your pregnancy. (See Suggested Reading below.)

You may want to consider taking part in the latest advance *in obstetrics: preconception care*. Essentially this means practicing good prenatal habits while you're actively trying to conceive. Many women don't know they're pregnant until up to eight weeks after conception. Yet this is a crucial time in your baby's life, when most of its major organ systems are forming. Eating nutritiously, exercising, and avoiding potentially harmful substances during this time can boost your odds of having a healthy baby. In fact, studies now show that neural tube defects can be prevented by taking a prenatal vitamin and mineral supplement containing folic acid *before* you conceive. Preconception tests, such as glucose-tolerance and blood-pressure screening, can also help you nip any problems in the bud and boost your odds of having a healthy pregnancy *and* delivering a healthy baby.

····································
Suggested Reading
····································

PREGNANCY AND PRENATAL CARE

American College of Obstetricians and Gynecologists. *Planning for Pregnancy, Birth and Beyond*. New York: Dutton, 1992.

Eisenberg, Arlene, Heidi E. Murkoff, and Sandee E. Hathaway, B. S. N. *What to Eat When You're Expecting*. New York: Workman Publishing, 1986.

Eisenberg, Arlene, Heidi E. Murkoff, and Sandee E. Hathaway, B. S. N. *What to Expect When You're Expecting*. New York: Workman Publishing, 1991.

PREGNANCY LOSS

Friedman, Rochelle, and Bonnie Gradstein. *Surviving Pregnancy Loss*. New York: Little, Brown, 1992.

Pizer, Hank, and Christine O. Palinski. *Coping with a Miscarriage*. New York: NAL–Dutton, 1986.

Scher, Jonathan, and Carol Dix. *Preventing Miscarriage: The Good News*. New York. HarperCollins, 1991.

Senchyshyn, Stefan, and Carol Coleman. *How to Prevent Miscarriage and Other Crises of Pregnancy: A Leading High-Risk Doctor's Prescription for Carrying Your Baby to Term*. New York: Macmillan, 1990.

INFERTILITY

Carson, Stephen L. *Conquering Infertility: A Guide for Couples*. New York: Prentice Hall, 1991.

....
Resources and Support
....

American College of Obstetricians and Gynecologists, Resource Center, 409 12th St., SW, Washington, D.C. 20024. The college provides free brochures on pregnancy after age thirty-five, amniocentesis, and a wide range of other pregnancy-related subjects. Send a stamped self-addressed business envelope along with your request for information.

American Fertility Society 1209 Montgomery Highway, Birmingham, AL 35216-2809. Phone: (205) 978-5000. This professional society for health-care workers provides information on all aspects of fertility and problems of infertility. The staff can also refer you to local fertility centers and specialists.

C/SEC, Inc. (Cesareans/Support, Education and Concern), 22 Forest Road, Framingham, MA 01701. Phone: (508) 877-8266. This organization provides information about recovery from cesarean birth and also about cesarean prevention and vaginal birth after a C-section. Send a self-addressed, stamped business envelope for a list of publications and support groups in your area.

National Down Syndrome Society (NDSS), 666 Broadway, New York, NY 10012. Phone: (800) 222-4602. The NDSS provides information on Down's syndrome and referrals to local support groups.

National Society of Genetic Counselors, c/o Executive Director, 233 Canterbury Drive, Wallingford, PA 19086. This professional organization of more than one thousand genetic counselors provides referrals to genetic counselors in your area. The NSGC does not maintain or disseminate information about specific genetic disorders. Please allow up to six weeks for a response.

Resolve, 1310 Broadway, Somerville, MA 02144-11731. Phone: (617) 623-0744. Resolve is a national non-profit organization with more than fifty-five local chapters providing information, counseling, and emotional support to couples with fertility problems. Publications include *Infertility: A Guide for the Childless Couple* ($10.95) and *Understanding Artificial Insemination: A Guide for Patients* ($4.00). The organization also offers more than fifty fact sheets on such topics as infertility, adoption, miscarriage, surrogate parenting, and pregnancy.

....

Chapter 11

PMS and Other
Menstrual Problems:
How to Manage
Them
in Midlife

One of the most common and bothersome reproductive problems to many premenopausal women is a cluster of symptoms known as premenstrual syndrome, or PMS. Actually, premenstrual syndrome may be as perplexing to the medical community as it is to women who suffer from it. There are several reasons why PMS has often confounded even the experts. To begin with, the symptoms are broad—up to 150 different symptoms, ranging from bloating and breast tenderness to irritability and depression, have been associated with PMS. The exact cause (or causes) remains elusive, and, because of this, there is no definitive way to diagnose or treat the condition.

In spite of our general lack of knowledge about PMS, many women *can* be helped and a majority of their symptoms relieved, often with such simple measures as making minor changes in diet and exercising regularly. However, you'll have to work closely with your physician and possibly try many different treatment regimens until you find one that brings relief.

During your premenopausal years, you may begin to notice changes in your menstrual cycle or in your periods themselves. Many of these changes are simply your body's signals that menopause is approaching. Others, however, could be red flags possibly signaling a medical problem that should be treated. We'll discuss the symptoms, diagnosis, and treatment of some of the more common menstrual problems in this chapter, as well.

Premenstrual Syndrome

Once tossed off as a nervous condition or dismissed simply as a "woman's" problem, PMS is now recognized as a very real disorder. The syndrome affects only women in their reproductive years. This includes women who have had their uterus removed before experiencing a natural menopause but who still have their ovaries intact.

Literally hundreds of symptoms have been associated with PMS. Some of the classic physical symptoms include breast tenderness, water retention (swelling of the abdomen, fingers, ankles), fatigue, food cravings, nausea, headaches, backaches, and clumsiness. Women may also suffer from such emotional symptoms as mood swings, impaired concentration, irritability, hostility, anxiety, and depression.

However, it is not so much the type or severity of the symptoms as their *timing* that characterizes them as PMS. Generally speaking, symptoms associated with PMS usually worsen the week or two before menstruation and let up or disappear altogether within one or two days after the start of your period. Some women even experience a surge of energy the week of menstruation. On the other hand, a minority of women may experience some or all of these symptoms the week *after* their menstrual periods. Indeed, the key may not be so much *when* during your menstrual cycle that symptoms appear but the fact that they appear *cyclically* during your menstrual cycle, which is why PMS might more aptly be named cyclic-disorder syndrome.

What Causes PMS?

Experts are still debating whether PMS is an emotional disorder or a physiological one. The truth probably lies somewhere in between. Several different theories have been developed, implicating everything from hormonal imbalances to psychological disorders.

•   **Hormonal imbalances:** Since symptoms correspond with the menstrual cycle, it's logical to assume that reproductive hormones are somehow responsible. However, it's still not clear what role hormones play in PMS. When David Rubinow, M.D, and other researchers at the National Institutes of Health compared hormonal levels of women with PMS with those of another group of women who don't suffer from the syndrome, they found no detectable excesses or deficiencies in estrogen, progesterone, follicle-stimulating hormone, luteinizing hormone, testosterone, or other androgens that would set PMS sufferers apart.

The researchers also measured levels of the hormone prolactin, involved in the development of the breasts and in breast-milk production and believed to be responsible for the breast tenderness that many women experience just before their periods. The group found that while prolactin levels do fluctuate throughout a woman's menstrual cycle, there were no significant differences in levels of prolactin between PMS sufferers and nonsufferers. Nevertheless, one drug that suppresses prolactin secretion (*bromocriptine,* brand name Parlodel) is effective in relieving breast tenderness, possibly as a result of *other* effects of the drug that haven't yet been identified.

Still other researchers have found that one of the most widely used treatments for premenstrual syndrome, progesterone suppositories, is no more effective overall than a placebo (sugar pills) in alleviating premenstrual symptoms.

In spite of these findings, a hormonal basis for PMS still can't be discounted altogether. For example, some women, particularly those who experience such symptoms as premenstrual spotting and menstrual cramps, *do* benefit from natural progesterone in the form of a *pill* (micronized oral progesterone). It's entirely possible, too, that women with PMS may simply be more sensitive to relatively minor fluctuations in normal levels of hormones than other women. However, the current technology for measuring blood hormone levels is not yet sophisticated enough to test this theory.

Other hormones that have not yet been thoroughly investigated may also be at least partly responsible for PMS symptoms. One new focus of research is on *inhibin,* a hormone secreted by the ovaries only during the second half of the menstrual cycle. Inhibin signals the pituitary gland to stop producing follicle-stimulating hormone.

Estrogen is suspected of playing a role in increased edema during pregnancy and may possibly contribute to premenstrual fluid retention, as well. Although the exact mechanisms are poorly understood, estrogen may directly affect the transport of sodium through the kidneys, which play a key role in the body's sodium-fluid balance. Estrogen also increases blood flow throughout the body, leading to dilation of blood vessels in estrogen-responsive tissues. In women with PMS, sodium and water are known to accumulate in the breasts, hands, and feet, and it's possible that they can also accumulate in the brain, causing irritability and headaches.

• **Neurotransmitters:** The brain hormone serotonin and natural pain-relieving chemicals known as *endorphins* increase as levels of progesterone and estrogen rise. Some researchers speculate that PMS may be a result of the abrupt withdrawal of these neurohormones before menstruation. In this way, reproductive hormones may play a "supporting" role in triggering the symptoms of PMS.

• **Hypoglycemia:** The symptoms of hypoglycemia, or low blood sugar, are similar to many symptoms associated with PMS: shakiness, sweating, dizziness, headache, irritability, anxiety, and fatigue. Researchers are now looking into whether some symptoms of PMS may actually be caused by abnormalities in carbohydrate metabolism. Some scientists have found, for instance, that insulin receptors (specialized parts of cells that attract and bind insulin to the cell, where it helps the cell absorb blood sugars) are doubled in concentration during the first half of the menstrual cycle among women with PMS. This could result in impaired glucose tolerance during the second half of the menstrual cycle, when premenstrual symptoms typically appear. Salt and sugar binges may exacerbate the hypoglycemic effect. Dieting to offset the fluid retention and bloating associated with PMS may make the problem even worse.

• **Nutritional deficiencies:** Several studies have suggested that nutritional deficiencies may influence PMS symptoms. A possible deficiency in vitamin B_6 has received the most attention. This vitamin helps the body manufacture the brain chemicals dopamine and serotonin. A deficiency of these neurotransmitters has been implicated as a cause of naturally occurring depression. Lower dopamine levels also result in an excess of the hormone aldosterone in the body, which may lead to salt and fluid retention. So a deficiency in dopamine or serotonin might explain the PMS symptoms of anxiety, irritability, depression, and fluid retention.

It's still not clear exactly how vitamin B_6 deficiency may come about. Women with PMS may not absorb the vitamin as efficiently or may have a problem converting the vitamin into a form the body can use. Or they simply may not eat a balanced diet: Vitamin B_6 is often lost in the processing of whole grains, cereals, and rice. Moreover, excessive sugar intake, alcohol consumption, and stress all increase the body's need for vitamin B_6.

Another nutrient receiving increased scrutiny for a possible role in PMS is magnesium. Studies have found lower blood levels of magnesium in women with PMS, particularly those who crave sweets. And a recent study has shown that magnesium supplements may help ease some PMS symptoms. No one is certain how magnesium works. A magnesium deficiency may cause lower levels of the neurotransmitter dopamine, which may in turn impair dopamine's ability to induce relaxation and increase mental alertness.

• **Psychological disorders:** Still other theories focus on a possible link between premenstrual syndrome and other psychological problems. In one study, about 30 percent of women with primary recurrent depression experienced their first depressive episode during a period of reproductive hormonal change, such as after pregnancy. And symptoms associated with such psychological disorders as anxiety and depression are known to worsen during the latter half of the menstrual cycle among affected women.

• **Prostaglandins:** These substances, produced in such tissues as the brain, breasts, gastrointestinal tract, kidney, and reproductive tract, are thought to interact with other hormones and possibly influence symptoms associated with PMS. Levels of the breast milk–producing hormone prolactin, for instance, are influenced by prostaglandins that cause dilation of the blood vessels and breast tenderness. Prostaglandins produced in the central nervous system act like neurotransmitters to modify thirst, appetite, temperature, mood, and certain hormones. In the kidney, blood flow and fluid balance are tied to prostaglandin actions. And prostaglandins produced in the uterine lining are believed to be responsible for premenstrual cramping, diarrhea, and nausea.

Although research on the possible causes of PMS remains elusive, one thing is certain: Women with PMS are not overemotional or imagining their problems. They are suffering from a very real disorder related to biological changes.

Making a Diagnosis

With the exception of one blood test—a test for levels of follicle-stimulating hormone, which can differentiate between PMS and early menopausal symptoms—there are no specific laboratory tests to diagnosis PMS. Usually, a diagnosis is made only after other possible psychological and physiological causes have been ruled out. If you suspect you have PMS, we recommend the following work-up to help make a diagnosis.

• **Menstrual Symptoms Questionnaire:** Since the main criteria for a diagnosis of PMS is the timing of your symptoms, you may be asked first to chart your symptoms for several months. According to the National Institutes of Health, a diagnosis of PMS can be made only after you have charted your symptoms for at least three months. However, most women have already experienced their symptoms for a long time and usually don't want to wait any longer to get relief from them.

If you suspect you suffer from PMS, start by filling out the Menstrual Symptoms Questionnaire on the opposite page. The first part of the form will help you determine what your main symptoms are and whether they occur cyclically. (If you score higher in the "Week Before Period" column than the "Week After Period" column, then you're a good candidate for PMS and should be further evaluated.)

The second part of the form will help you target your most troublesome symptoms, which, as you'll see in the next section, will be useful in determining the best mode of treatment for you.

• **Menstrual Symptoms Diary:** Once you have identified your worst symptoms, you should begin charting them monthly—even before you begin treatment for PMS. Some women find the process of filling out the charts to be therapeutic in itself. Charting your symptoms helps you become more aware of them, and this often improves your ability to cope with them. Using the Menstrual Symptoms Diary on page 223, rate each of your worst symptoms on a scale of one to four every day of the month. Don't forget to weigh yourself every day, as well, which will help gauge your body's propensity to retain fluid.

Once you've begun treatment, charting your symptoms will be useful in determining how effective the treatment regimen is. If symptoms don't improve after three or four months (you may experience a placebo effect when you first begin treatment, which usually wears off after a month or two), you and your physician may want to try a different approach.

• **Medical evaluation:** You should undergo a complete physical examination if you are suspected of having PMS. The physical can help rule out other medical disorders that can cause symptoms similar to those of PMS. A pelvic exam will be performed to check for ovarian cysts, fibroid tumors of the uterus, pelvic inflammatory disease, and endometriosis. (These conditions don't *cause* PMS but may occur coincidentally.)

You should have blood tests, including a fasting blood-glucose test to rule out hypoglycemia. Remember, some of the physiological symptoms associated with PMS, such as increased appetite, carbohydrate craving, and fatigue are also symptoms of hypoglycemia. (You should note that while the fasting blood-glucose test doesn't always detect hypoglycemia, it's the best method we've got for the moment.) Your physician may want to test your thyroid function, too, since hypothyroidism may contribute to an estrogen-progesterone imbalance and depression. Your physician may also test your blood levels of follicle-stimulating hormone (FSH) to determine whether your symptoms are early signs of menopause, which respond to an entirely different approach to treatment.

• **Nutritional evaluation:** Deficiencies or excesses in your diet may make premenstrual symptoms worse. For instance, too much sodium may result in excessive fluid retention just before your period. Women suffering from PMS have also been reported to consume more refined sugar, refined carbohydrates, dairy products, caffeine, and protein, and less vitamin B, iron, zinc, and magnesium than healthy women. A registered dietitian or qualified nutritionist can evaluate your diet and eating habits and guide you to better food choices to help alleviate any dietary-related symptoms.

Menstrual Symptoms Questionnaire

Grade your symptoms for last menstrual cycle only.

Grading of symptoms:
0 = None
1 = Mild, does not interfere with activities
2 = Moderate, interferes with activities, not disabling
3 = Severe, disabling, not able to function

	Week after period	*Week before period*
1. Weight Gain		
2. Ankle Swelling		
3. Swelling of Fingers		
4. Abdominal Bloating		
5. Breast Heaviness		
6. Breast Tenderness		
7. Increased Desire for Sweets		
8. Increased Desire for Salty Foods		
9. Appetite Increased/Compulsive Eating		
10. Appetite Decreased		
11. Thirst Increased		
12. Alcohol Cravings		
13. Constipation		
14. Diarrhea		
15. Sweats, Flushes, Heart Pounding		
16. Faintness/Lightheadedness		
17. Headaches (tension)		
18. Headaches (migraine)		
19. Stiffness of Joints		
20. Tense/Agitated		
21. Outbursts Over Small Irritants		
22. Mood Swings		
23. Depressed/Cry Easily		
24. Sleeping Difficulties/Insomnia		
25. Forgetful or Distractable		
26. Difficulty in Making Decisions		
27. Unable to Concentrate		
28. Clumsy or Accident-prone		
29. Impulsive/Impatient		
30. Feel Lonely/Neglected		

	Week after period	Week before period
31. Feel unappreciated	_____	_____
32. Neutral Mood	_____	_____
33. Energetic/Euphoric	_____	_____
34. "At War with the World"	_____	_____
35. Need for Greater Self-control	_____	_____
36. Dissatisfied with Look or Feel	_____	_____
37. Feeling More Affectionate	_____	_____
38. Feeling Less Affectionate	_____	_____
39. Tendency to Nag	_____	_____
40. Increased Physical Activity	_____	_____
41. Lack of Pep and Energy	_____	_____
42. Increased Ambition	_____	_____
43. Avoid Social Activity	_____	_____
44. Stay at Home and Avoid People	_____	_____
45. Tendency to Use Sick Time	_____	_____
46. Thoughts of Suicide	_____	_____
47. Decreased Work/School Performance	_____	_____

Other symptoms

Acne	_____	_____
Fever Blisters	_____	_____
Bladder Infection	_____	_____
Other	_____	_____

In any given month, which of the above symptoms do you find to be the *most troublesome*? Rank in order of highest priority.

A. _____

B. _____

C. _____

D. _____

E. _____

F. _____

G. _____

Menstrual Symptoms Diary

Using the symptoms scale here, rate each of your five worst symptoms according to how you feel *each day*. Use the Menstrual Grading Scale to record the amount and severity of menstrual bleeding and related symptoms. Don't forget to record your weight, as well (weigh yourself on the same scale and at the same time every day).

SYMPTOM SCALE
1 = Slight
2 = Moderate
3 = Severe
4 = Extreme

MENSTRUAL GRADING SCALE
0 = None
1 = Slight (spotting)
2 = Moderate
3 = Heavy
4 = Heavy and cramps
C = Cramps
D = Low Back Pain

Sunday	*Monday*	*Tuesday*	*Wednesday*	*Thursday*	*Friday*	*Saturday*
Wt _____ Menses _____	Wt _____ Menses _____	Wt _____ Menses _____	Wt _____ Menses _____	Wt _____ Menses _____	Wt _____ Menses _____	Wt _____ Menses _____
Wt _____ Menses _____	Wt _____ Menses _____	Wt _____ Menses _____	Wt _____ Menses _____	Wt _____ Menses _____	Wt _____ Menses _____	Wt _____ Menses _____
Wt _____ Menses _____	Wt _____ Menses _____	Wt _____ Menses _____	Wt _____ Menses _____	Wt _____ Menses _____	Wt _____ Menses _____	Wt _____ Menses _____
Wt _____ Menses _____	Wt _____ Menses _____	Wt _____ Menses _____	Wt _____ Menses _____	Wt _____ Menses _____	Wt _____ Menses _____	Wt _____ Menses _____
Wt _____ Menses _____	Wt _____ Menses _____	Wt _____ Menses _____	Wt _____ Menses _____	Wt _____ Menses _____	Wt _____ Menses _____	Wt _____ Menses _____

- **Fitness evaluation:** Several studies have shown that exercise can significantly reduce some symptoms of PMS. If you're over forty and want to begin a meaningful exercise program to alleviate PMS symptoms, you should consider undergoing a fitness evaluation (see Chapter 5).

- **Psychological evaluation:** A psychological evaluation can help differentiate between PMS and underlying environmental (work/home) or psychological problems, some of which may be made worse by the menstrual cycle. Your physician may refer to you a mental-health professional (either a psychiatrist or psychologist) for the evaluation.

- **Creating a temporary menopause:** If you suffer from severe symptoms, your physician may recommend that you try taking GnRH agonists (Lupron, Synarel) for several menstrual cycles. These drugs block the secretion of *gonadotropin-releasing hormone* by the hypothalamus, which ultimately halts pro-

---

Should You Have a Hysterectomy to Treat PMS?

Having a hysterectomy (surgical removal of the uterus) alone won't cure PMS, since your ovaries continue to function, and women with PMS who have had a hysterectomy usually continue to experience symptoms. The only real cure for PMS is surgically to remove the *ovaries along with the uterus,* an operation known as *hysterectomy with bilateral oophorectomy.* This operation alleviates symptoms altogether by inducing a "surgical" menopause. However, this type of surgery should be considered a last resort for women with severe PMS that seriously interferes with their lives, *and only after all other therapeutic measures have failed to relieve their symptoms.*

Removal of the ovaries to treat PMS should always be weighed against the risks associated with this surgery, including an increased risk of heart disease and osteoporosis later in life. (For more on the benefits and risks of hysterectomy with bilateral oophorectomy, see Chapter 13.)

To determine whether surgery may be an option for you, your physician will first recommend that you take GnRH agonists (Lupron, Synarel) for three to six months. Remember, these drugs induce an artificial menopause in premenopausal women who take them (see text above). If your PMS symptoms improve dramatically or disappear altogether while taking the drugs, you may want to consider surgery. (If your symptoms *don't* subside while taking the drug, surgery won't help them, either.) However, you should also discuss with your physician the ways in which you will manage the long-term health risks associated with this type of surgery. Taking postmenopausal estrogens is one of the best ways to protect yourself (see Chapter 20), but, for a variety of reasons, many women never fill their first prescription. Moreover, some women (particularly those with a family history of breast cancer) may be advised *not* to take postmenopausal estrogens, and a very small subgroup of women are so sensitive to synthetic estrogen that the remedy is worse than the condition it was meant to treat.

224

duction of estrogen and progesterone by the ovaries, inducing an artificial menopause. If symptoms don't abate while you're taking the drug, they're probably *not* caused by PMS. If symptoms do clear up while taking this medication and you have debilitating PMS, you may want to consider having a hysterectomy with removal of both ovaries. (See Should You Have A Hysterectomy to Treat PMS? on the opposite page.) The drug itself should not be used for longer than six months unless it is taken along with estrogen (either in the form of birth control pills or postmenopausal hormone therapy) because it has been associated with bone-loss.

Developing a PMS Treatment Plan

There's no cure for PMS, so the goal of your treatment plan will be to find ways to control your symptoms. No one treatment works for all women. You and your physician should work closely to discover your worst symptoms and develop a treatment regimen tailored to your needs. (See A Symptoms Guide to Treating PMS below.) However, by first changing some of the factors under

---

A Symptoms Guide to Treating PMS

Predominant Symptoms	Recommended Evaluation and Treatment
Psychological (mood swings, depression, irritability, insomnia)	• Psychological assessment (How are things at home?) • Stress management (see Chapter 6) and improving home and work environments Aerobic exercise twice a day during premenstrual phase for 30 minutes per session • Micronized oral progesterone (has a sedative effect) once or twice a day beginning on day 14 of menstrual cycle for 12 to 14 days • Psychotropic drugs that increase brain levels of serotonin (Buspar, Sinequan): as recommended by your physician
Somatic (fluid retention, breast tenderness, bloating, diarrhea, cramps)	• Gynecologic evaluation • Tailor treatment to predominant symptom: - Fluid retention: low-salt diet, diuretics (Aldactone) twice daily for 12 to 14 days beginning on day 14 of your menstrual cycle - Breast tenderness: evening primrose oil (Efamol) twice daily for 12 to 14 days beginning on day 14 of your menstrual cycle

---

Predominant Symptoms	Recommended Evaluation and Treatment
	- Diarrhea and cramps: prostaglandin inhibitors (Ponstel) 4 times per day for 12 to 14 days beginning on day 14 of your menstrual cycle
Dietary (low blood sugar, food cravings)	• Nutritional evaluation, including glucose-tolerance test
	• Eat small, frequent meals; cut back on refined sugars, salt, and caffeine
Gynecologic (premenstrual spotting, menstrual cramps, midovulatory pain)	• Gynecologic evaluation
	• Tailor treatment to predominant symptom:
	- Spotting: micronized oral progesterone twice daily for 12 to 14 days beginning on day 14 of your menstrual cycle
	- Cramps: prostaglandin inhibitors (Ponstel) four times daily for 12 to 14 days beginning on day 14 of your menstrual cycle
	- Midovulatory pain: low-dose oral contraceptives

Note: Many older premenopausal women may be menopausal. Your doctor may recommend that you undergo a blood test for levels of follicle-stimulating hormone (FSH). If FSH levels are over 40 mIU/ml, your symptoms may improve by taking postmenopausal hormone therapy using micronized estrogen and progesterone.

If your symptoms are severe and don't respond to any of the treatments here, your doctor may recommend that you try taking GnRH agonists (Lupron, Synarel). If your symptoms improve while taking these drugs, you may want to discuss with your physician the pros and cons of having your ovaries surgically removed to treat your PMS (see page 224).

your own control, such as your diet, exercise habits, and how you handle stress, you should experience a real improvement overall. Other benefits to this non-drug approach are that there are no side effects and you feel more in control of your own body.

Nutritional Therapy
A good sound nutrition strategy can help bring certain physical symptoms under control, particularly food cravings, fluid retention, and breast tenderness. Research on food and mood now suggests that what you eat may also help control such emotional symptoms as depression, anxiety, and mood swings. Try a Prudent Diet for PMS on the opposite page.

Most women find that a diet designed to help control hypoglycemia is beneficial for PMS symptoms, as well. A sensible eating plan usually incorporates the following guidelines:

• **Eat small, frequent meals.** By eating three scaled-down meals per day and nibbling on nutritious snacks in between, your blood-sugar levels will be less likely to seesaw and trigger symptoms. Ideally, no more than three hours should pass without eating. Since studies have shown that women with PMS have an increased appetite during the second half of the menstrual cycle, eating regularly throughout the day may also help take the edge off a heartier-than-normal appetite.

• **Eat foods high in complex carbohydrates and protein, such as vegetables, whole grains, fish, and poultry.** These foods take longer than others to be converted into glucose, which helps keep blood-sugar levels on a more even keel. These foods are also high in vitamins, minerals, and fiber.

While in the past, women with PMS have been advised to cut back on carbohydrates, research now suggests that eating carbohydrate-rich meals just before your period may help alleviate such symptoms as depression, anger, tension, fatigue, confusion, and sleepiness.

Carbohydrates raise levels of serotonin in the brain. Low levels of serotonin have been associated with depression, and some researchers speculate that the carbohydrate cravings common among women with PMS during the week before their period may be the body's way of trying to alleviate depression. So if you have a craving for carbohydrates and are not overtly hypoglycemic, indulge. But be sure the carbohydrates you consume are *complex* carbohydrates (starchy foods such as whole-wheat pasta, brown rice, potatoes, and fresh fruits and vegetables) and *not* sticky buns and candy bars. Try keeping a variety of high-carbohydrate snacks on hand, such as apples, dried fruit, yogurt with fresh fruit, and peanut butter on crackers.

• **Cut back on sodium during the week or two preceding your period.** A high-sodium diet can cause you to retain water. (Tips on cutting back on sodium can be found on page 74.)

• **Avoid refined sugar, flour, pasta, and prepackaged or canned foods.** Refined sugar can send your blood sugar soaring, then cause it to come crashing down an hour or two later. Most of the vitamins and minerals in refined flour and pasta have been removed, leaving them with little nutritive value. And prepackaged and canned foods are usually high in sugar and salt.

• **Avoid caffeine.** Caffeine has been implicated in causing breast tenderness and can aggravate symptoms of tension and anxiety.

• **Avoid alcohol during the premenstrual phase of your cycle.** Women in general have a lower tolerance to alcohol than men, and this tolerance may be further reduced in the last half of your menstrual cycle. Drinking alcohol can also cause rebound hypoglycemia, which may further intensify the symptoms of PMS.

What About Vitamin Supplements?

Deficiencies in vitamin B$_6$ and magnesium have been associated with PMS, and there's even evidence to suggest that taking vitamin B$_6$ and magnesium supplements may help alleviate certain PMS symptoms. However, study results—particularly those dealing with the effectiveness of vitamin B$_6$—have been inconclusive.

Remember, vitamin B$_6$ is instrumental in the body's manufacture of serotonin and dopamine, and a B$_6$ supplement is thought to raise levels of serotonin in the brain, possibly improving depression, anxiety, and irritability. Another benefit of vitamin B$_6$ is that it is a natural diuretic, working in part by suppressing the hormone aldosterone, which may contribute to water retention.

If you do take Vitamin B$_6$, be sure to take it as part of a B-complex vitamin. Taking B$_6$ alone can deplete other B vitamins. You also should not take more than 50 to 100 milligrams of vitamin B$_6$ daily. Women who have taken 500 milligrams or more of B$_6$ for two months or longer have developed burning, shooting or tingling pains or numbness in their hands and feet, clumsiness, or an unstable gait—a condition known as *sensory neuropathy*. (At least one study has found that these symptoms occur in sensitive women taking as little as 50 milligrams per day.) The condition usually clears up when you stop taking vitamin B$_6$.

Magnesium, on the other hand, is fairly safe to take. In the study we mentioned earlier, women took 360 milligrams three times daily.

Exercise

There's some evidence to suggest that regular aerobic exercise can help relieve such PMS symptoms as anxiety and depression, possibly by stimulating the endorphin system in the brain and helping to offset the sudden drop in endorphin levels as menstruation begins. Aerobic exercise also relieves muscle tension and improves sleep. Exercise has been shown to help relieve premenstrual bloating and breast tenderness, too.

To reduce premenstrual tension and ease other PMS symptoms, we recommend that you participate in an aerobic activity (such as walking, jogging, or bicycling) twice a day (once in the morning and once in the evening) for thirty minutes per session during the premenstrual phase of your cycle. The endorphin-stimulating effects of exercise wear off after a while. By exercising twice a day, you get a double dose.

Stress Management

A general-treatment regimen should include stress management techniques as well as diet and exercise. Stress can exacerbate the symptoms of PMS. There's some evidence that women may experience an exaggerated response to stress during the last half of the menstrual cycle, including increased heart rate, blood pressure, and higher levels of the "stress" hormones epinephrine and norepinephrine.

One stress-reducing technique that has been shown to improve emotional symptoms is the relaxation response (described on page 132). In a five-month study of 107 women conducted at Harvard Medical School, those who elicited the relaxation response for fifteen to twenty minutes every day experienced a significant improvement in such symptoms as hostility, irritability, anger, and anxiety. (Improvements were measured by daily charting of the women's symptoms.) Fifty-eight percent of the women with the most severe symptoms experienced a decrease in their symptoms when they practiced the relaxation response, compared with 17 percent of women who only charted their symptoms.

The researchers speculate that the relaxation response may help reduce premenstrual tension by decreasing your responsiveness to norepinephrine, a neurotransmitter believed to influence such moods and behaviors as aggression and anxiety.

You should also do what you can to de-stress your home and/or work environment. Inform your colleagues at work that you suffer from PMS and educate your family members about your condition. Family, friends, and co-workers are often just as bewildered by your premenstrual personality changes as you are. With a clear understanding of the problem, the people closest to you will be better able to offer support during your premenstrual period.

Try not to overcommit yourself during this time. Even a little stress can aggravate symptoms; taking on more than you can handle will only add to the stress—and exacerbate your symptoms.

Drug Therapies

Women with severe symptoms may also be helped by certain medications. However, you should try medications only if the self-help measures discussed earlier don't significantly improve your symptoms. You should note that drug therapies should be tailored to your individual symptoms. Not *all* women will benefit from diuretics, but women who experience fluid retention will. Keep in mind, too, that *all* drugs have side effects. Some medications that have been found to be helpful include the following:

• **Progesterone:** Progesterone has a sedative effect and may be appropriate for women with severe emotional symptoms, such as mood swings, depression, irritability, and insomnia. Many women experience feelings of euphoria after taking it. Those who benefit most from progesterone are women who have emotional symptoms *along with* such gynecological symptoms as premenstrual spotting and menstrual cramps. These symptoms are indicative of lower levels of progesterone in the body.

For PMS symptoms, we recommend that you take *micronized oral progesterone,* a natural form of the hormone, since some types of synthetic progestogens have been associated with *increased* moodiness among women who take them and since progesterone suppositories may not be as effective. Plus, while synthetic progestogens have been associated with such side effects as decreased levels of protective HDL cholesterol and decreased glucose tolerance (see page 440), micronized oral progesterone doesn't appear to have these effects.

Your doctor may prescribe from 100 to 300 milligrams per day for the week or two before your menstrual period, depending on the severity of your symptoms. The dosage may be taken from one to three times per day. Taking your progesterone twice a day—100 milligrams in the morning and 200 milligrams before bedtime—may be optimal. The morning dosage calms you for the better part of the day and the evening dosage helps you sleep better at night. Your doctor may have to adjust the dosage of medication to suit your particular needs.

• **Diuretics:** A mild diuretic may be helpful for women who experience excessive fluid retention and bloating. However, not *any* diuretic (including many over-the-counter brands) will do. Many diuretics actually produce a rebound effect; that is, after you stop taking them, you gain even more water weight than before you started using them. For this reason, your physician will likely prescribe a diuretic that works by inhibiting the hormone aldosterone, such as *spironolactone* (Aldactone), *triamterene* (Dyazide, Dyrenium, Maxide), or *amiloride* (Midamor). These types of diuretics don't have the rebound effect associated with other diuretics and may be safely taken cyclically by women whose chief symptoms are premenstrual weight gain and those symptoms attributed to water retention. The typical dosage is 25 milligrams four times a day from three days prior to your expected symptoms until menstruation.

If you suffer from mild edema and are tempted to take a nonprescription diuretic, you should be aware that restricting the salt in your diet during the two weeks before your period can be equally effective as a diuretic.

• **Prostaglandin inhibitors:** Women with diarrhea and abdominal cramps may benefit from taking aspirin, ibuprofen (Advil, Motrin IB), or mefenamic acid (Ponstel). Your physician may prescribe 250 milligrams of Ponstel (or the equivalent) three times a day for the week before your period, increasing the dosage to four times a day during your period, if necessary.

• **Oral contraceptives:** A low-dose oral contraceptive may be prescribed for women who experience midovulatory pain, those who are sensitive to minor hormonal fluctuations, and those with heavy and/or painful periods—particularly if these women also need a reliable method of birth control. (For more on oral contraceptives, see Chapter 9.)

• **Evening primrose oil (Efamol, Vita-Glow):** Women who experience breast tenderness and abdominal bloating may find this nutritional supplement helpful. The supplement contains an oil from the seeds of evening primrose, as well as vitamin E. (Vitamin E supplements have also been reported to relieve breast tenderness.) The usual dosage is 500 milligrams four times a day for the two weeks before your period. Evening primrose oil can be found in some health food stores. However, because the health claims on the labels of these products (including relief from a wide range of PMS symptoms) have not been substantiated by their manufacturers, the U.S. Food and Drug Administration has banned the sale of the supplements in this country.

• **Psychotropic drugs (BuSpar, Sinequan):** Women with severe emotional symptoms may benefit from antianxiety drugs. These drugs increase brain levels of serotonin, which has a calming effect. The decision to use these drugs and the dosage should be individualized and determined by your physician.

• **Postmenopausal hormone therapy:** Many older premenopausal women may actually be menopausal. Women with FSH levels over 40 mIU/ml may benefit from postmenopausal hormone therapy using a low dose of micronized estradiol and progesterone. Some women at our clinic, particularly those with premenstrual hot flashes, have improved by using the Estraderm skin patch (0.05 mg). (For more on postmenopausal hormone therapy, see chapters 20 and 21.)

Other Menstrual Problems

If you've had fairly predictable menstrual periods throughout your reproductive years, you may be surprised when you note a sudden change in the regularity of your menstrual cycles, as well as in the quantity and duration of menstrual flow. These changes are usually signs that you are entering the menopausal transition years and that your ovaries' production of the hormones estrogen and progesterone are declining. (Changes may be more apparent by keeping a record of your menstrual cycles as well as recording the amount of blood flow you experience during menstruation. Use the Menstrual Symptoms Diary on page 223.) These disturbances in the regularity of your menstrual cycle and blood flow may last anywhere from two to eight years. A typical pattern: Levels of estradiol begin to fall first, resulting in a gradual shortening of the second half of the menstrual cycle. You may experience more frequent periods as a result. This may be followed by a gradual drop in progesterone, which increases the length of the cycle, resulting in heavier periods.

Although menstrual irregularities and increasingly long periods of *amenorrhea* (cessation of menstruation) are normal during the pre-and perimenopausal years, you should still promptly report to your physician *any* changes in your menstrual cycle or in the amount of blood flow you experience. Menstrual irregularities can have many different underlying causes, some of which may require medical attention.

Spotting, Light Bleeding, and Skipped Periods

Experiencing an unusually light blood flow or even a day or two of spotting around the time you would normally expect your period is often a sign of *anovulation*—a menstrual cycle in which your ovaries did not release an egg. Skipping a period altogether is another indication that you are not ovulating. As we mentioned earlier, these irregularities are a perfectly normal part of the menopausal transition and may occur with increasing frequency as you approach menopause. Nevertheless, you should report them to your doctor when they first begin to occur, since such medical conditions as pregnancy (remember, you can still get pregnant until you are past menopause) could also be responsible. When amenorrhea lasting more than six months is *not* related to pregnancy, breast-feeding, or menopause, your body releases only the hormone estrogen, which, over time, may overstimulate your uterine lining and possibly increase your risk of developing endometrial cancer. Long-term amenorrhea during your childbearing years may also increase your risk of developing breast cancer *after* menopause. In addition, studies have shown that women of reproductive age who aren't ovulating often have low estrogen levels and *may experience the same pattern of bone loss as postmenopausal women,* putting them at increased risk of osteoporosis later in life. Bone loss is more rapid in the first few years, so early diagnosis and treatment is a must.

If you miss a period altogether, your physician will first want to rule out one of the main causes of amenorrhea among premenopausal women: pregnancy. If you are not pregnant and have not had a period for two to three months, your doctor will probably administer a blood test for levels of follicle-stimulating hormone to determine whether you are approaching (or past) menopause. He or she will also perform a pelvic examination to check for ovarian cysts or other ovarian masses that could temporarily interfere with menstruation.

Once your physician has ruled out the obvious, he or she may look for other causes of amenorrhea, including thyroid problems, stress, extreme weight changes (either a gain or a loss), and strenuous exercise.

- **Stress:** A stressful situation at work or at home may cause temporary or prolonged bouts of amenorrhea. No one is sure exactly how stress affects the menstrual cycle. However, studies on monkeys suggest that a pituitary hormone known as *corticotropin*, which increases during times of stress, may inhibit the release of hormones secreted by the hypothalamus that stimulate ovulation.

- **Extreme weight loss:** Severe weight loss can also shut off the menstrual cycle's main controls in the hypothalamus. Women who go on a crash diet may experience temporary amenorrhea. Those with the eating disorder anorexia nervosa may experience prolonged amenorrhea, even after regaining weight.

- **Extreme weight gain:** Obesity may lead to amenorrhea in several ways: (1) body fat can convert androgens into estrogen, resulting in elevated estrogen levels; (2) obesity depresses a binding protein known as sex hormone–binding globulin, which leads to higher blood levels of the more biologically active "free" estrogen and testosterone; (3) obesity is usually associated with increased insulin levels, which appear to stimulate the ovaries to produce more androgens. Higher levels of estrogens and androgens can suppress ovulation. Losing weight usually reverses the condition.

- **Strenuous exercise:** Women who exercise strenuously may experience more menstrual irregularities and amenorrhea, partly because these women have low levels of body fat. Generally speaking, a drop in body fat below 22 percent may result in amenorrhea.

But the sheer stress of strenuous workouts may also contribute to the problem. Amenorrheic ballerinas have been known to begin menstruating again during periods of rest, even if they experience no change in body weight or percentage of body fat.

The majority of women with exercise-induced amenorrhea begin ovulating again when they ease up on exercise or stop working out altogether. However, many women are not willing to give up their routine. And since regular moderate exercise is associated with numerous health benefits (see Chapter 5), few women should be discouraged from stopping altogether.

Hormone therapy is recommended for strenuous exercisers with low estrogen levels to protect against a loss of bone mass. However, you should be aware that you may begin ovulating again when taking hormone therapy, and the postmenopausal hormones prescribed *will not* protect against pregnancy. For this reason, low-dose oral contraceptives should be prescribed both to replace the missing estrogen and protect against pregnancy. Excellent preparations include Loestrin, Ovcon-35, and Nordette.

If you experience exercise-induced amenorrhea and don't want to take hormone therapy or birth-control pills, you should at least take a calcium supplement.

- **Postpill amenorrhea:** Although it was once believed that birth-control pills continued to suppress the ovaries even after usage of them ceased, this doesn't appear to be the case. Most women start menstruating within three months after they stop taking birth-control pills. If you haven't started menstruating by this time, your physician may recommend that you take progestogens for one week out of every month to keep your uterine lining from being overstimulated and to help you start menstruating again. If you are still amenorrheic after six months, your physician will probably look for an underlying cause.

- **Thyroid problems:** Your doctor may measure levels of *thyroid-stimulating hormone* in your blood to determine whether you are suffering from an underactive thyroid (*hypothyroidism*).

Heavier-than-Normal Bleeding, Prolonged Bleeding, and/or More Frequent Periods

These changes, too, are a normal part of the menopausal transition. Some 75 percent of women in their late thirties and forties who experience these symptoms have what is known as *dysfunctional uterine bleeding* (DUB), which is typically caused by a hormonal imbalance associated with anovulation. In these women, estrogen stimulates the uterine lining unopposed by progesterone. As a result, the endometrium thickens and may shed irregularly, especially if estrogen levels drop.

Again, however, these menstrual irregularities may be signs of other medical problems, such as benign fibroid tumors of the uterus, miscarriage (threatened or incomplete), ectopic pregnancy (a potentially life-threatening condition in which the embryo implants in the Fallopian tubes), or, less frequently, early endometrial cancer. Diabetes, thyroid problems, and kidney disease may also interfere with the normal menstrual cycle. For this reason, *all* types of abnormal bleeding should be evaluated by your physician.

Your doctor will perform a physical examination and Pap smear, as well as various laboratory tests, including a complete blood count, blood coagulation tests (when relevant), thyroid-function tests, and a fasting blood-glucose test. In addition, your physician will probably want to obtain a small sample of the uterine lining through endometrial sampling (see page 401) to rule out *endometrial hyperplasia* (overstimulated uterine lining) or endometrial cancer. Dysfunctional uterine bleeding is diagnosed only when no secondary causes for the bleeding (except monthly anovulation) are found.

Treatment of DUB depends on your age and the extent of the bleeding. Your doctor may recommend that you take a progestogen for ten days every month for three months.

Some women may benefit by taking combination (estrogen-progestogen) birth-control pills for episodes of heavy bleeding. Rather than taking one pill every day, you start by taking one pill two to four times a day for five to seven days. Usually, this type of hormone therapy will stop bleeding within twelve to twenty-four hours. You should be aware, however, that within two to four days after you stop this short course of birth-control pills, you may experience a heavy, crampy period. *This is not a recurrence of the problem or a failure of hormone therapy.* Rather, it is a result of a buildup of endometrial tissue over time that is reacting to withdrawal of estrogen and progestogen in the normal way: by shedding. (Taking Anaprox, Ponstel, or another prostaglandin inhibitor will help reduce cramps and bleeding.) On the fifth day of your period, you will again begin taking birth-control pills in the usual way—once a day for three weeks, followed by a medication-free week in which you can expect to have a regular period. You should experience a decrease in the amount of bleeding and pain with each successive cycle. After three such cycles, the uterine lining should have been restored to normal and you may be advised to stop taking birth-control pills for a few cycles to see whether you begin menstruating more regularly.

If heavy bleeding does not abate even after hormone therapy, your physician may recommend that you undergo a *hysteroscopy*, in which an endoscope (a thin, lighted tube) is inserted through the vagina and into the uterus to inspect the uterine lining, or a *dilatation and curettage*, an operation in which the cervix is dilated and the endometrial lining removed with a curette, a small instrument with a rounded, sharp cutting edge.

Two relatively new surgical options for women with severe bleeding include *laser ablation*, which involves destroying the uterine lining with a laser beam and leaving the thick uterine wall intact, and *roller-ball electrocoagulation*, a similar operation in which a specially designed heated probe is used to destroy the uterine lining (see page 267). Hysterectomy is also an option for recurrent episodes or if bleeding is associated with other symptomatic problems, such as uterine prolapse (see Chapter 13).

Headaches

Headaches are a common complaint around the time of menstruation. Some women however, suffer from "menstrual migraines"—severe headaches often accompanied by nausea, vomiting, and sensitivity to light or sound that typically occur during the week before or the week of menstruation. Some women may experience menstrual migraines around the time of ovulation, as well. The headaches are believed to be triggered by fluctuating estrogen levels—particularly a drop in estrogen after a period of several days' exposure to high estrogen levels. Prostaglandins may also play a role in the development of these headaches. Studies have shown that injections of prostaglandin E-1 can produce migrainelike headaches in people who don't normally suffer from migraines. (Low levels of this prostaglandin can constrict blood vessels, while high levels can dilate blood vessels.) We know that estrogen stimulates the manufacture of prostaglandins in the body, possibly triggering a headache.

Treatment of menstrual migraines is similar to that of common migraines. If you develop a migraine, your physician may prescribe drugs that constrict the blood vessels in the brain (dilation of blood vessels is what usually causes the pain of a migraine), such as *ergotamine* (Bellergal, Cafergot, Ergomar, Ergostat, Wigraine) or *isometheptene* (Isocom, Midrin). These drugs are the treatment of choice, but they must be taken at the first sign of a headache (the prodromal phase) to be most effective. One drawback to these medications is that they may cause nausea and vomiting. For this reason, your doctor may also prescribe an anti-nausea medication. The anti-nausea medication *prochlorperazine* (Compazine suppositories) helps control nausea and, if taken early enough, will abort the headache, too.

To prevent menstrual migraines, you should first try to eliminate as many of the other triggers of migraine headaches as you can (including prolonged stress, waking up later than you normally do in the morning, and skipping meals), particularly in the week before and during your period. Certain foods and beverages that can precipitate a headache should also be avoided, including alcohol, chocolate, foods with nitrates (such as hot dogs), and foods containing monosodium glutamate. If you regularly consume caffeine—found in coffee, tea, cola, chocolate, and some aspirin compounds—and want to cut back, you should do so gradually, since sudden withdrawal from caffeine can trigger a migraine. (You'll find tips for gradually weaning yourself from caffeine on page 92.)

Some women find they can control their headaches by taking postmenopausal estrogens. Depending on the type of headaches you have, the estrogen patch, taken either continuously or only during the second half of your menstrual cycle, may help reduce the number of headaches you have. If a higher dosage of estrogen is needed, Estrace, taken orally or vaginally, may be prescribed.

Some of the most useful medications for the prevention of menstrual migraines are prostaglandin-inhibiting nonsteroidal anti-inflammatory drugs, such as *naproxen* (Naprosyn). If your menstrual cycles are regular and the time of your migraine is easily predicted, you may be able to take these drugs for about a week before the time you expect your period and through the week of menstruation. Low doses of aspirin have also been found to help prevent migraines.

Other drugs that may be prescribed to help prevent menstrual migraine include Bellergal, a tranquilizer that contains ergotamine and the narcotic phenobarbital; beta-blockers and calcium channel blockers, normally used to treat hypertension and heart disease; or the antidepressant amitriptyline (Elavil, Endep, Etrafon, Limbitrol, Traivil).

Painful Periods

More than 50 percent of menstruating women suffer from *dysmenorrhea,* the medical term for painful periods. Dysmenorrhea occurs only during menstrual cycles in which you ovulate. The pain is believed to be caused by the release of prostaglandins from the endometrium just prior to and during your period. The prostaglandins produce painful uterine contractions, which may be accompanied by nausea, diarrhea, headaches, and emotional changes. However, such medical conditions as endometriosis and pelvic inflammatory disease may also cause painful periods, which is why you should be evaluated by a physician.

If you suffer from painful periods that *aren't* caused by any underlying conditions, your physician will prescribe prostaglandin inhibitors, such as *naproxen* (Naprosyn), *ibuprofen* (Motrin), or *mefenamic acid* (Ponstel).

If pain is still severe, your doctor may recommend that you take oral contraceptives to inhibit ovulation and limit the release of prostaglandins.

A Final Word

You will inevitably experience more menstrual irregularities as you approach menopause, and some women may notice a worsening of premenstrual symptoms. Most of these problems can be managed by promptly reporting them to your doctor and working closely with your physician to develop an effective treatment plan tailored to your needs.

Chapter 12

....

Menopause: The
Hard Facts
and the Good News

If you're lucky, you won't even know you've experienced menopause until a year *after* your last menstrual period—the medical definition of menopause. Most women, however, will experience one or more of the classic symptoms, such as hot flashes and vaginal dryness, sometimes *before* they've stopped menstruating. A minority will have symptoms severe enough to seek medical treatment.

Perhaps more important are the "silent" changes in your body that often accompany menopause. As we've mentioned earlier, estrogen appears to have a protective effect on both your heart and your bones. When estrogen levels fall after menopause, you lose that built-in biological protection. As a result, your risk of heart disease and the bone-thinning disorder osteoporosis rises.

Even if you have *none* of the overt symptoms of menopause, or if symptoms are relatively mild, you should be monitored closely by your physician during the menopausal years to ensure that the silent changes don't take a toll on your health. The good news is that virtually *all* of the changes associated with the change of life can be managed and their impact on your health and the quality of your life minimized.

Making a Diagnosis

As you've already seen, the chief role of estrogen and progesterone is to help regulate your menstrual cycle and prepare your uterus for pregnancy. But like all hormones, these chemical messengers circulate throughout your body, interacting with other hormones and with your body's metabolism. Estrogen *receptors* (specialized parts of cells that allow various hormones to lock into the cell and influence its activity) have been found in many tissues throughout the body, including your mucous membranes, your bladder, your breasts, your bones, and your skin. For this reason, when estrogen levels fall around the time of menopause, you may experience a number of physical (and sometimes psychological) changes. Some are nuisance symptoms that let you know you're close to (or just past) menopause. Others, as we mentioned earlier, are "silent" changes—and are more serious.

The type of symptoms and changes you have depends on whether you are in the early part of your menopause (pre- and perimenopausal) or past menopause. Generally, hot flashes and mood swings are experienced by pre- and perimenopausal women, while symptoms of the vagina and bladder occur in postmenopausal women. The silent changes occurring to your heart and bones may not become problematic until many years after menopause, but changes can (and should) be monitored throughout this time in your life.

A thorough physical examination is recommended around the time of your menopause (see Chapter 3), particularly if you are suffering from bothersome symptoms associated with menopause, such as hot flashes. Your physician may want to confirm that you are menopausal by administering a blood test for FSH levels. Increasing FSH levels are an important clinical sign that you are approaching (or have already experienced) menopause. If you are still menstruating, the test is administered during the second half of your menstrual cycle— about a week before your anticipated period. Levels above 40 mIu/ml (except at the time of ovulation) indicate that you are menopausal.

Your physician can also help you determine whether your menopausal symptoms are serious enough to warrant treatment. While there are several "objective" ways to measure many menopausal symptoms (for instance, hot flashes can be measured by gauging the temperature of your finger or skin), these methods are used mostly for research purposes. In our clinic, we've found that the best judge of whether you should be treated for hot flashes and related menopausal symptoms is *you*. Fill out the Menopausal Symptoms Questionnaire on the opposite page to help determine which menopause-related symptoms you may be experiencing and which may require treatment.

Abnormal Bleeding

You may recall that fluctuating hormone levels as you approach menopause cause irregular menstrual cycles and bleeding patterns. Again, the FSH blood test is one way to differentiate between abnormal bleeding related to menopause and other problems. Your physician will probably want you to undergo other tests as well as a complete physical examination if you have abnormal bleeding patterns in the years just preceding menopause (see Chapter 11). *Any bleeding you experience after a natural menopause (provided you're not taking postmenopausal hormone therapy) is abnormal and should immediately be brought to your doctor's attention.* Among the conditions that could cause postmenopausal bleeding is endometrial cancer. Your physician can perform a series of diagnostic tests, including ultrasound and endometrial sampling, to help determine the cause of the bleeding (you'll find a description of these tests in Chapter 18).

Menopausal Symptoms Questionnaire

Grading system: Please assess symptoms listed below according to the following symbols:

A = No symptoms
B = Mild; symptoms experienced but not severe enough to warrant treatment
C = Moderate; symptoms make you feel uncomfortable to the extent that you would like treatment
D = Severe; symptoms interfere with your daily living style; you feel you need treatment

SYMPTOMS

Hot flushes _____   Vaginal discharge _____
   How many/day? * _____   Dryness _____
   How many/week? * _____   Intercourse:
Perspiration _____   Painful _____
Palpitations _____   Difficult _____
Insomnia: Frequency/week _____
   Difficulty getting to sleep _____   Increased [†] _____
   Early A.M. awakening _____   Decreased [†] _____
Mood change _____   Interest in sex:
Irritability _____   Same [†] _____
Depression _____   Increased [†] _____
Vaginal itching _____   Decreased [†] _____
   Burning _____

OTHER SYMPTOMS

_____

_____

_____

_____

FACTORS THAT AGGRAVATE OR IMPROVE SYMPTOMS
1. Are the above symptoms made worse by stress?   Yes ___ No ___

   If yes, type of stress: _____

    * Please write in the appropriate number.
    [†] Check the appropriate category.

2. Are the above symptoms made worse by any other
   events?   Yes ____ No ____

   If yes, briefly note: _____

3. Are you on or have you recently been on hormones
   or other treatment?   Yes ____ No ____

4. Did your symptoms improve/worsen during treatment?

   Symptoms: Increased _____ Decreased _____ Same _____

5. Symptoms that were improved/worsened. Use same grading as before.

   Symptom   *Grade before treatment*   *While on treatment*

   _____   _____   _____

   _____   _____   _____

6. Remarks regarding symptoms not mentioned above:

   _____

   _____

   _____

   _____

   _____

   _____

   _____

Hot Flashes

Hot flashes are sometimes called the "badge of menopause" because they're so common among menopausal women. About 85 percent of perimenopausal women experience hot flashes (also known as hot flushes, night sweats, or vasomotor symptoms). Indeed, what was once chalked up as "all in your head" has finally become recognized as a real biological phenomenon that has a great impact on many women.

For some women, hot flashes may be nothing more than an occasional fleeting sensation of warmth. Others may experience hourly waves of heat, drenching sweats, and a racing heart. Sleep may be disrupted several times a night by night sweats. The lack of sleep causes fatigue, irritability, and impaired memory.

The sensations may last anywhere from thirty seconds to up to thirty minutes. Some women experience as few as several hot flashes a year, while others with very severe hot flashes may suffer up to fifty per day. Daily hot flashes appear to be the norm. According to Ann M. Voda, R.N., Ph.D., professor and director of the Tremaine Trust Women's Health Research Program at the University of Utah in Salt Lake City, hot flashes most frequently occur between the hours of 6:00 and 8:00 A.M. and again between 6:00 and 10:00 P.M. However, every woman's pattern of hot flashes differs, so don't be alarmed if you have hot flashes only at night or only during the day.

For many women, hot flashes begin *before* menopause and are a telltale sign that it is approaching. However, hot flashes are most prevalent in the year or two following menopause and, for the majority of women (64 percent), last from one to five years. Another 25 percent of women experience hot flashes for six to ten years. A minority of women (10 percent) have hot flashes for ten years or more.

Hot flashes are more severe in surgically menopausal women, at least for the first year after having their ovaries removed. This is probably because the drop in estrogen among these women is so abrupt. Surgically menopausal women are also more likely to suffer unrelenting hot flashes for years after menopause.

Hot flashes may feel worse in summer months and/or in hot, humid climates. And while many women report feeling hot flashes in the upper part of their body, the sensations can occur elsewhere, as well. Dr. Voda asked patients to document where on the body they experienced hot flashes. Some had heat sensations only in the hands, thighs, or other parts of the body.

It's hard to predict who will suffer hot flashes. It appears to be an equal-opportunity phenomenon: Researchers have found no relation between hot flashes and employment status, social class, age, marital status, domestic work load, or number of children. They've also found no connection between hot flashes and the age a woman experiences her first menstrual period, age at menopause, number of pregnancies, height, or medical problems. Indeed, the only factor that correlates with frequency of hot flashes in menopausal women is body weight: Women with hot flashes tend to weigh less and have less body fat than asymptomatic women.

Anatomy of a Hot Flash

To understand how a hot flash occurs, it helps to know a little bit about your body's temperature-regulating system. This remarkable system, which involves your skin and underlying fat tissues, your blood vessels, and central nervous system, allows your body to maintain a constant "core" temperature (that is, the temperature of the deep tissues of your body)—even when you are exposed to vast changes in the outside temperature. Except when you have a fever, your core temperature doesn't fluctuate more than one degree day in and day out.

The master controls, or thermostat, for your body's temperature-regulating system reside in the hypothalamus, the part of your brain that governs such basic needs as hunger and thirst, sex drive, and certain emotions. The hypothalamus contains large numbers of heat- and cold-sensitive neurons that increase their activity when they sense a rise or fall in temperature. Still other neurons in the hypothalamus become excited in response to signals transmitted to the brain from cold and heat receptors in the skin and certain deep tissues in the body.

When the hypothalamus detects that your body temperature is too hot, it sends out signals to dilate the blood vessels, increasing blood flow to the skin. This allows excess body heat to be transferred to the skin and out of the body. The hypothalamus also activates sweat glands (located just under the skin), which help cool your body.

If the hypothalamus senses that your body temperature is too cold, it signals the blood vessels to constrict, which helps keep body heat from escaping. The hypothalamus also signals your body to generate more heat by shivering and by increasing your rate of metabolism.

When you have a hot flash the hypothalamus somehow gets its signals mixed. Thinking your body temperature is too warm, it suddenly sets in motion the mechanisms to cool you off.

Studies have shown that immediately prior to the onset of a hot flash (five to sixty seconds), many women experience a premonition, or *aura*, of an impending hot flash. It's during this time that your heart rate and blood flow to the skin (particularly the hands and fingers) accelerate.

At the start of a hot flash, your skin becomes cold and clammy. Blood flow to your extremities increases four- to thirty-fold, and your heart rate continues to accelerate (from eight to sixteen beats per minute over normal). Your finger temperature rises and you begin to sweat. As a result of these cooling mechanisms, your core body temperature drops, reaching a low about five to nine minutes after the onset of the hot flash. When your body temperature drops significantly, your blood vessels constrict, your metabolism increases, and you begin to shiver. This helps return your body temperature to normal.

What Causes a Hot Flash?

No one knows what causes this sudden, temporary downward resetting of the body's thermostat, although we have some clues.

• **The role of estrogen:** It's natural to assume that estrogen plays a major role in hot flashes, since hot flashes occur when estrogen levels drop around menopause. The abrupt onset of hot flashes after surgical removal of the ovaries and the relief of hot flashes with estrogen therapy appear to clinch the argument.

But the exact role of estrogen is still a mystery: Throughout your post-menopausal years, estrogen levels remain low; yet some women never experience hot flashes, while others have only sporadic hot flashes. Preteenage girls have low estrogen levels and they don't experience hot flashes. And hot flash—like episodes have been reported during pregnancy, when estrogen levels are high.

Apparently, hot flashes are more a consequence of estrogen withdrawal rather than low estrogen levels. Obese women are less troubled by hot flashes, probably because their increased body fat converts androgens into estrogen. And women who are born without ovaries and who have never had normal estrogen levels typically don't suffer hot flashes until *after* they've been given estrogen therapy that is later stopped.

Exactly how estrogen withdrawal triggers hot flashes isn't known yet, either. Animal studies have shown that estrogen increases the activity of warm-sensitive neurons in the hypothalamus and decreases the activity of cold-sensitive neurons. Estrogen also increases blood flow throughout your body.

Estrogen works in several ways to enhance the activity of epinephrine and norepinephrine, two neurotransmitters that also interact with the hypothalamus and help control body temperature. Estrogen withdrawal may reduce the activity of these neurotransmitters, thus leading to hot flashes.

• **The role of progesterone:** Progesterone also appears to play a role in hot flashes. The rise in progesterone during the second half of the menstrual cycle raises the set point of the hypothalamus—and raises your body temperature—making you feel warmer. When you take progestogen (a synthetic form of progesterone), hot flashes may *feel* less severe because your body's thermostat has been adjusted to a higher setting.

• **Other reproductive hormones:** High levels of follicle-stimulating hormone and luteinizing hormone were initially thought to play some role in triggering hot flashes. But hot flashes often decline or stop after menopause, in spite of continued high levels of gonadotropins. And hot flashes may persist even when LH and FSH levels are reduced by drugs such as danazol, used in the treatment of endometriosis.

On the other hand, when women who never had hot flashes take drugs that block gonadotropin-releasing hormone (GnRH) receptors in the pituitary gland, they experience hot flashes for the first time. Although GnRH is not the immediate trigger of hot flashes, some people believe that it may be involved somehow in causing them.

• **Catecholamines:** The neurotransmitters epinephrine and norepinephrine help control the dilation and contraction of blood vessels, particularly those in the fingers. Studies have demonstrated increases in epinephrine and decreases in norepinephrine during hot flashes. A decrease in circulating norepinephrine could help explain the rise in blood flow to the fingers.

Norepinephrine may also help trigger hot flashes. In the brain, norepinephrine influences both the body's temperature-regulating system and the endocrine system. Animal studies have shown that when a part of the hypothalamus in monkeys is stimulated with norepinephrine, they experience dilation of the blood vessels in their fingers and toes and a drop in their core body temperature similar to changes occurring in women during hot flashes. And as we mentioned earlier, estrogen may influence the activity of norepinephrine in the brain.

• **Beta-endorphins and other opiates:** The symptoms of menopausal hot flashes—visible flushing of the neck and face, perspiration, goose bumps and shivering, and sleep disturbances such as insomnia and intermittent awakening—are also signs of narcotics withdrawal. This has led researchers to believe that beta-endorphins and other *opiates*, naturally occurring narcotics in the body that are responsible for pain relief and feelings of euphoria, may play a role in hot flashes, too.

Estrogen and progesterone have been found to alter the activity of these naturally occurring opiates. It's possible that lower levels of estrogen and progesterone cause a withdrawal of opioids from parts of the hypothalamus, triggering some of the same withdrawal symptoms that drug addicts experience.

Handling Hot Flashes: What You Can Do

If you experience mild to moderate hot flashes, there are several ways to increase your comfort level without resorting to drugs.

• **Keep a record or diary of your hot flashes.** Hot flashes are not necessarily random occurrences that always take you by surprise. According to Dr. Voda, many women find that certain substances or circumstances act as triggers—a hot cup of coffee, for instance. Other common triggers are other hot beverages, such as tea, highly seasoned, spicy foods, and alcohol. By keeping a record for two weeks every year, you may discover some of your own triggers and may be better able to manage your hot flashes by avoiding these triggers. You'll find a Hot Flash Diary on page 483, as well as diagrams (Figure A.1) to track your hot flashes on page 484.

• **Wear layers of thin clothing that can be removed during a hot flash.** Clothes of 100 percent cotton are best because they absorb moisture, dry quickly, and allow heat to escape. Avoid wearing polyester, which traps heat and may even aggravate your hot flashes.

• **Keep your home and work environments cool.** As we mentioned earlier, a warm climate can make your hot flashes *feel* worse. Some women find that a hot environment acts as a trigger. To avoid this, set your office or home thermostat at 65 degrees Fahrenheit—lower if possible. Keep a hand fan in your purse and sit next to the air conditioner (or away from heat ducts) at meetings or social gatherings. To reduce nighttime awakenings, keep your room temperature at 65 degrees Fahrenheit or lower. Open the windows in winter. Turn on the air conditioner in summer.

• **Avoid emotionally charged or stressful situations.** Stress may trigger hot flashes in some women. (For help coping with stress, see Chapter 6.)

• **When a hot flash occurs, run cold water over your wrists or splash water on your face to cool off.** If possible, take a cold shower.

• **Exercise regularly.** Regular physical activity may help alleviate hot flashes. Swedish researchers have found that among 634 women who had experienced a natural menopause and were not taking hormones, physically active women reported fewer and less severe hot flashes than inactive women. The researchers suspect that exercise helps counter hot flashes by raising the level and activity of beta-endorphins in the body.

• **Try biofeedback.** You may be able to train your body to (at least partially) override a hot flash through the use of biofeedback. Of eight women we trained in the use of biofeedback, all reported fewer and less severe hot flashes after the training. Essentially, the women were told to "think warm" throughout the day to keep the thermostat in their bodies at a higher set point. At the onset of a hot flash, the women were instructed to "think cold" to help return their body temperature to normal. Ask your physician or other health professional about biofeedback training.

Handling Hot Flashes: What Your Doctor Can Do

If your hot flashes are so severe that they interfere with daily living and the quality of your life, you may want to consider one of several drug treatments available. Keep in mind, however, that *all* drugs have side effects.

• **Estrogen:** Estrogen reduces the frequency of hot flashes by more than 95 percent in most women. Several different forms of estrogen therapy are available for relief of hot flashes, and these are discussed in more detail in Chapter 20. Keep in mind that it may be two weeks before you start feeling relief from hot flashes, and up to four weeks before you experience the maximum effect of the drug.

Remember, too, that estrogen is not a permanent cure for hot flashes; they may return when treatment is discontinued. Your physician may wean you from the drug by tapering the dose of estrogen over a number of weeks or months to avoid the return of intense hot flashes.

• **Progestogen:** Researchers accidentally discovered that progestogen can be used to treat hot flashes when women with endometrial cancer who were taking progestogen also experienced relief of their hot flashes. The higher the dose of progestogen, the greater the relief. Like estrogen, you need to take progestogen for a couple of weeks before hot flashes abate, and up to four weeks before you experience maximum relief.

Progestogen may be useful for women who can't take estrogen. One type of progestogen, megesterol acetate (Megace), is often prescribed to help control hot flashes in women who have had breast cancer. But the drug may cause weight gain, irregular bleeding, abdominal bloating, breast tenderness, and mood changes. Progestogen also may adversely affect blood-lipid levels. (The types of progestogens and dosages will be discussed in Chapter 21.)

• **Androgens:** These drugs are effective in controlling hot flashes when used with estrogen. When used alone, higher doses may be needed, leading to more severe side effects, including growth of facial hair and a deepening voice.

• **Clonidine (Catapres, Combipres):** This drug, usually prescribed to lower blood pressure, also relieves hot flashes, but not as effectively as estrogen. We're not sure exactly how the drug works. We know that it blocks the neurotransmitters epinephrine and norepinephrine and it appears to stabilize the temperature-regulating center of the hypothalamus. Clonidine may also block the dilation of blood vessels in the arms and legs, which occurs during a hot flash.

In the largest studies, clonidine reduced the frequency of hot flashes from 12 to 40 percent among women who took it, depending on the dosage. However, higher doses were related to bothersome side effects, including dry mouth and dizziness.

Clonidine works best when delivered via a skin patch worn on your shoulder. The skin patch is changed once a week.

• **Methyldopa (Aldomet):** This is yet another blood pressure medication that works the same way as clonidine. Studies have shown that Aldomet reduces the frequency of hot flashes by 20 percent compared with a placebo. However, side effects such as dry mouth, fatigue, and headache limit its use.

• **Bellergal:** This tranquilizer has been found to reduce the frequency of hot flashes by 50 percent, but no one's sure which of its ingredients, including *phenobarbital*, is responsible for its effectiveness. The drug is particularly effective if your most prominent symptom is perspiration. However, it may cause constipation and dry mouth in some users.

As for the phenobarbital, the levels in Bellergal are not very high, so addiction is not a big problem. The drug is a good choice for women with breast cancer, who are usually advised not to take estrogen.

Bellergal comes in time-released tablets that can be taken once before bedtime or, if hot flashes are severe, once in the morning and again at night.

• **Other drugs:** There's some evidence that the analgesic *naproxen* (Anaprox), a nonsteroidal antiinflammatory agent, reduces hot flashes. Beta-blockers, drugs used to treat high blood pressure and other heart problems, appear to be effective in treating hot flashes, as well, although these drugs are less effective in treating other menopausal symptoms, such as anxiety and insomnia.

Sleep Disruptions

A primary complaint of women with hot flashes is that their sleep is disrupted. For a while, experts believed these sleep disruptions were chiefly caused by night sweats. But studies have shown that sleep disturbances are not always a result of hot flashes, and not all hot flashes disrupt sleep. Indeed, while most hot flashes are associated with waking episodes, 40 percent of waking episodes are not associated with hot flashes.

Taking over-the-counter or prescription sleeping pills won't necessarily guarantee you a good night's sleep since these medications do nothing to treat the underlying problem. For occasional insomnia, specialists in sleep disorders recommend that you first try to improve your sleep habits (see page 131). If menopause-related insomnia is severe enough to interfere with daily living, the best treatment is estrogen therapy. Women who take estrogen fall asleep faster, sleep longer, have fewer episodes of wakefulness, and have more periods of dream sleep (also known as rapid-eye-movement, or REM, sleep) than women who take a placebo. (If you're using estrogen therapy to help relieve sleep, you should take your estrogen just before bedtime. This way, blood-estrogen levels will peak during the night and help you sleep better.)

Of course, sleep disturbances and early-morning awakenings are also signs of major depression. (Other symptoms of depression can be found on page 134.) If you suffer from sleep disturbances, we recommend you undergo a complete physical *and* psychological profile to rule out other possible causes.

Emotional Changes
(The "Menopausal Syndrome")

Although many women fear that menopause will make them "go crazy" or "fall apart," new research is challenging this long-held belief. You may recall from Chapter 1 that recent studies have found no increased incidence of depression among menopausal women. And rather than having regrets about losing their ability to bear children, most women today express *relief* that they don't have to worry about contraception anymore.

Nevertheless, a minority of women may experience emotional ups and downs related to the hormonal changes of menopause. Mood changes such as irritability, depression, insomnia, impaired memory, and crying jags frequently precede and follow menopause. In many instances, these changes are hormone-related.

How can hormones influence your mood? To begin with, irritability, impaired memory, and anxiety are typical signs of chronic sleep disturbances— particularly dream sleep (see Sleep Disruptions on the opposite page). Hot flashes and night sweats often disrupt sleep.

Estrogen and androgens (the "male" hormone testosterone) also appear to have a "mental tonic" effect among women taking them. Apparently, estrogen in doses conventionally used to treat menopausal symptoms enhances the mood of women who aren't suffering from clinical depression. Moreover, women who take estrogen and testosterone together feel more composed, elated, and energetic than women who take estrogen alone.

This feeling of well-being may stem from a direct effect of these hormones on the brain. Estrogen receptors have been found in parts of the brain that govern emotions. Estrogen may also affect a number of different neurotransmitters that have been tied to feelings of depression and elation. For instance, estrogen is believed to reduce levels of the brain chemical monoamine oxidase (MAO). The lower levels of MAO, in turn, *increase* catecholamines in the brain, including norepinephrine, serotonin, and tryptophan. (Certain depressions have been associated with decreased levels of catecholamines, especially norepinephrine.) Estrogen appears to *increase* levels of other catecholamines, notably the more biologically active "free" tryptophan, a precursor of serotonin.

Whatever the mechanism that causes mood swings and other psychological symptoms, women whose symptoms are *hormone-related* often find relief with estrogen therapy. Aside from the "mental tonic" effect that estrogen has, it also helps you sleep better at night and in this way may improve your sense of well-being.

Of course, hormones won't help women who are suffering from true clinical depression or other serious psychological problems. Also, trouble on the homefront or at work could trigger bouts of insomnia, irritability, depression, and mood swings, which won't be influenced by hormone therapy.

How can you tell the difference between hormone-related symptoms and those that are not related to hormones? It's often not easy. You should start by undergoing a thorough physical and psychological evaluation. We make a point of asking, "How are things at home?" during our patients' physical examination to ensure that other possible causes of these symptoms aren't overlooked.

If the cause of the symptoms is still not clear after a complete medical and psychological work-up, you may want to try taking hormones. (We'll discuss the types of hormone therapy available for these symptoms in Chapter 21.) If you feel better after starting hormone therapy, you simply continue the treatment. If your symptoms are the same or become worse after taking hormones, you and your physician should look for another cause—and treatment regimen.

Anxiety

While it's comforting to learn that menopause is not associated with any increase in mental illness, it doesn't necessarily mean that at times you won't *feel* as though you're falling apart. Our patients frequently complain of anxiety. Your physician should first rule out any physical problems that can cause a feeling of anxiety, such as mitral valve prolapse (see page 335), thyroid problems, or even hot flashes, which are often accompanied by heart palpitations and a feeling of anxiety or dread.

If a physical problem is not the cause, remember that you have plenty to be anxious about. Your body is undergoing tremendous changes at this time in your life. And while studies show that a majority of women feel *relieved* about their menopause, it's not unusual to have mixed feelings about the end of your childbearing years. Some women may fear that they will lose a reminder of their femininity with the loss of menstruation. If you're one of a growing number of women who opted not to have children, you may suddenly find you have nagging doubts about your decision now that it's final.

Menopause is also a reminder that you're growing older. Feelings about aging may influence the way you feel about yourself, and may feed your anxiety. Your partner's feelings about your menopause can influence your feelings about yourself, as well.

A key to easing anxiety is to understand the physical changes you're going through by reading as much as you can on the subject (which is why we wrote this book). You'll need to make an extra effort to keep the lines of communication open with the important people in your life, too, including your partner and your physician. Support groups can be enormously useful in helping you to recognize that you're not the *only* one who feels the way you do. Individual or group counseling is beneficial, too. (For more on support groups and counselors, see Chapter 6.)

Headaches

Many women who suffer from "menstrual migraines"—migraine headaches that coincide with hormonal changes, such as menstruation, ovulation, and use of birth-control pills (see page 235), may find that their headaches improve or remit during menopause. Such headaches are believed to be triggered by fluctuating estrogen levels—particularly a drop in estrogen after a period of several days' exposure to high levels of estrogen. The constant lower levels of estrogen after menopause may help explain why headaches improve.

For reasons we don't fully understand, migraine headaches continue and even accelerate for some women during menopause. These women may be helped by continuous estrogen therapy. Estrogen raises levels of pain-relieving opioids in the brain and stabilizes certain mood-altering catecholamines (dopamine and serotonin), which may be why estrogen often eliminates migraines.

If oral estrogens don't improve your migraines, often the estrogen patch or estrogen pellets will, since these forms of estrogen therapy are associated with more steady blood-estrogen levels. On the other hand, cyclic therapy, in which you take estrogen for three weeks, then stop taking the medication for a week, results in a period of estrogen withdrawal that has been associated with an increase in migraine headaches. You and your physician may have to experiment with various forms of estrogen therapy before finding one that works for you.

Adding an androgen to postmenopausal estrogen therapy appears to help, too. In one study by R. Don Gambrell, Jr., M.D., a gynecologist at the Medical College of Georgia in Augusta, 20 percent of patients who had headache reported improvement after treatment with estrogen pellets alone. However, 60 percent reported improvement with the combination of estrogen plus testosterone.

Progestogens, which are usually given along with estrogens to protect against overstimulation of the uterine lining, may aggravate migraines. Some women whose headaches are relieved with continuous estrogen therapy alone find that the migraines and mood swings return when they take a progestogen cyclically along with the estrogen. If progestogens are a problem, your physician may first recommend that you change the type of progestogen you're taking. If that doesn't work, he or she may reduce the dosage of progestogen to the lowest possible amount needed to protect the uterine lining. If headaches persist, switching to micronized oral progesterone may solve the problem.

Estrogen doesn't *always* relieve menopausal migraines. If after trying different types of estrogen therapy, your headaches have *worsened*, you may have to try a different treatment approach. Ask your physician about other possible therapies.

For the most part, women who suffer menopausal migraines have a long history of migraines. If you suddenly begin experiencing severe, debilitating migrainelike headaches after menopause, you should undergo a complete physical examination to rule out other possible causes. Often, migraine headaches that develop after menopause are *not* hormone-related.

Vaginal Dryness (Atrophic Vaginitis)

As estrogen levels fall during menopause, estrogen-sensitive tissues in the vagina respond. Capillaries in the vaginal walls shrink, reducing blood flow and nutrients to these tissues. The outer folds of the vagina shrink as a result, causing the skin to sag and become dry. The vaginal lining (*epithelium*) becomes pale and thin, making the vagina susceptible to irritation and infection. These changes decrease the thickness of epithelium, increase the pH (acid-base balance) of the vagina, and change the bacterial flora in your vagina. As a result, many postmenopausal women experience vaginal dryness, or a discharge (which is often confused with infection), itching, burning, and—perhaps most important—pain during intercourse (*dyspareunia*).

These may seem like minor irritations, but they can have major consequences: When symptoms interfere with sexual performance they can lead to anxiety and a decrease in desire, and self-esteem. Your symptoms may even affect the sexual performance of your partner, who may worry about hurting you. Indeed, these symptoms are often the ones about which postmenopausal women are most concerned.

Making a Diagnosis

Once again, you will probably be the best judge as to whether you have atrophic vaginitis. Don't delay reporting *any* vaginal irritation or painful intercourse to your physician. Pain during intercourse is often one of the first signs of atrophic vaginitis. Too often, women wait until the problem escalates and begins to interfere with sexual relations.

Your physician will first exclude other possible causes of vaginitis, such as infection. Sometimes, during the physical examination, your doctor may actually be able to see thinning of the vaginal walls. A pH test using secretions from the side walls of the vagina may also provide clues. (A pH of less than 4.5 is considered normal; any values above 4.5 mean the vaginal pH has become too alkaline—a sign of atrophic vaginitis.) Finally, your doctor may perform a test to determine the vagina's *maturation index*, in which a sample of cells is gently scraped from the vaginal walls and viewed under a microscope to determine the percentage of *parabasal cells*. If 20 percent or more of the cells are this type, a diagnosis of atrophic vaginitis will be made.

The maturation index and pH test can also be used over time to monitor treatment. As treatment progresses and the condition of the vagina improves, your pH should return to normal and the parabasal cells should be replaced with intermediate and superficial cells.

Coping with Vaginal Dryness

There are several things you can do to lessen the impact of vaginal dryness on your sex life.

• **Keep sexually active.** Surprisingly, one way to keep vaginal walls healthy is to stay sexually active. Studies by the noted sex experts William Masters and Virginia Johnson have found that women who engage in sexual activity at least once a week have significantly lower pH values and maintain better vaginal health than those who don't. This is because sexual arousal does produce some natural lubrication, chiefly by increasing blood flow to the vagina, which aids in the secretion of lubricating fluid through the vaginal lining. (The vagina has no glands.) Any sexual activity—even self-stimulation—helps improve blood flow and keep tissues supple.

• **Take your time.** When you do make love, do so in a relaxed, unhurried atmosphere. Recognize that it may take longer for your vagina to become lubricated. Sometimes, taking a warm bath before lovemaking helps to relax your muscles and stimulate vaginal secretions.

• **Use a lubricant.** Some women use a water-based lubricant, such as K-Y jelly, during intercourse. However, these lubricants don't provide long-lasting relief of vaginal symptoms, nor do they appear to lower vaginal pH.

A promising new lubricant called Replens contains the compound *polycarbophil*, which appears to work even better than water-based lubricants. Indeed, the new lubricant may be almost as effective as estrogen in lowering vaginal pH and restoring a more normal vaginal milieu. In the study we conducted along with Gloria Bachmann, M.D., at the University of Medicine and Dentistry of New Jersey in New Brunswick, we compared the effects of Replens and a water-based lubricant on women complaining of vaginal itching, burning, irritation, pressure, and dyspareunia. While both the water-based lubricant and the polycarbophil-based moisturizer improved vaginal moisture, only the polycarbophil moisturizer lowered pH, increased the quantity of vaginal secretions, and decreased the fragility of the vaginal lining. And while more than 80 percent of the women in the study reported improved symptoms with nonhormonal therapy, 61 percent preferred the new vaginal moisturizer. One application of Replens lasts from 48 to 72 hours, so you don't have to use this type of lubricant just before intercourse or every time you have intercourse.

• **Change the sexual script.** There's no rule dictating that making love means having intercourse. If intercourse is just too painful, try other means of stimulation, such as oral sex or even self-stimulation.

• **Discuss the use of postmenopausal estrogen creams with your doctor.** The most effective way to relieve vaginal dryness is with estrogen. Estrogen (particularly vaginal creams) can actually *reverse* some of the menopause-related changes in the vaginal tissues. Estrogen increases blood flow to the vagina and thickens the vaginal epithelium. Estrogen also improves the acid-base (pH) balance of the vagina, which may reduce your risk of developing vaginal infections.

A note of caution: You should *not* use vaginal estrogen creams as a lubricant before having intercourse. At least one report in the medical literature traced one man's breast enlargement to his wife's liberal use of estrogen creams. We subsequently conducted a study to see how well estrogen creams were absorbed through a man's penis and into his bloodstream. Study participants applied estrogen cream to their penises, and blood samples were taken hourly for six hours and then again twenty-four hours later in order to monitor estrogen levels in the men's bloodstreams. After two hours, blood-estrogen levels more than doubled. Levels of the "male" hormone androgen fell by more than 50 percent, as well. After twenty-four hours, however, the men's blood-hormone levels had returned to normal.

We still don't know what impact, if any, a woman's use of estrogen creams will have on her partner's health. But given the penis's ability to absorb estrogen, it's probably better *not* to use estrogen creams as a lubricant.

Is This a Normal Discharge or a Vaginal Infection?
It's easy to confuse the normal vaginal discharge of menopause with a vaginal infection. However, there are a few ways you (and your physician) can tell the

Some Common Causes of Vaginal Irritation			
Condition	Symptom	Discharge	Treatment
Atrophic vaginitis	Dryness, burning	Watery gray	Estrogen cream
Bacterial vaginosis	Fishy odor	Creamy gray/yellow	Metronidazole (Flagyl, Metrogel); ampicillin
Yeast vaginitis	Itching, burning	Thick, cheesy white	Nystatin (Mycostatin); Miconazole (Monistat); Clotrimazole (Gynelotrimin)
Trichomonas	Itching	Frothy yellow/green	Metronidazole (Flagyl)

difference. Generally speaking, any discharge that has a strange color (white, cheesy, bloody, or one that stains your clothing), has an odor, or causes itching or irritation is a sign of infection. A normal vaginal discharge is translucent or gray and odorless. (See Some Common Causes of Vaginal Irritation above.)

If you're not sure whether your vaginal discharge is normal or if you suspect you have an infection, see your doctor, who can culture a sample of vaginal secretions or examine it under a microscope for signs of infection.

More Frequent Urination

The bladder and urethra develop from the same tissues as the vagina in the growing embryo, so it's not surprising that the hormonal changes of menopause have an effect on them.

As with the vagina, the cells lining the urinary tract respond to hormonal changes by becoming thinner and more easily inflamed. As a result, you may experience an increase in the frequency and urgency of urination, as well as abdominal pressure during urination. When no bacterial cause for these symptoms can be found, you are most likely suffering from what's known as the *urethral syndrome*. These changes in your urinary tract also increase the risk of bacterial urinary tract and bladder infections. Stress urinary incontinence (loss of bladder control, especially when you sneeze, cough, or laugh) may worsen after menopause, too.

If you experience symptoms suggestive of a bladder infection (urgency and frequency of urination), your physician will probably ask you to collect a urine sample so it can be checked for bacteria. If no infection is found, your doctor can confirm the diagnosis of urethral syndrome with a urethroscopy, in which an *endoscope* (a thin, lighted tube) is used to view the inside of the urethra.

Because the underlying cause of urethral syndrome is low estrogen levels, it makes sense that hormone therapy would help the condition. Indeed, some studies show that up to half of all postmenopausal women who suffer from urethral syndrome improve after taking estrogen. Estrogen helps thicken the urethral lining and improves blood flow to the area. Estrogen also improves the tone of the urethra, all of which result in better bladder control. (For more on hormone therapy and other treatments for urethral syndrome, see Chapter 19.)

Heart Disease

Postmenopausal women are more than twice as likely to develop heart disease as premenopausal women. This fact leads us to suspect that women are somehow protected against heart disease before menopause and that they lose this protection in the postmenopausal years.

We're still not sure why your risk of heart disease rises after menopause. We do know, however, that estrogen affects blood-cholesterol levels, a major risk factor for cardiovascular disease. Total cholesterol levels of postmenopausal women are about 25 mg/dl higher than those of premenopausal women. And total cholesterol levels fall between 10 and 18 percent among postmenopausal women who take estrogen.

The drop in estrogen also affects the levels of artery-clogging low-density lipoproteins (LDLs), the "bad" cholesterol that raises your risk of heart disease, and high-density lipoproteins (HDLs), the "good" cholesterol believed to protect against heart disease. Postmenopausal women are also more prone to develop atherosclerosis, or narrowing of the arteries—perhaps as a result of higher LDL and lower HDL cholesterol levels.

But not everyone is convinced that the drop in estrogen after menopause is the main culprit. One study involving 121,700 women found no increased cardiovascular risk associated with menopause. Other studies, including the famed Framingham Heart Study, have shown that premenopausal women who've had a hysterectomy are at much greater risk of developing heart disease than women who haven't had the surgery—*even when they haven't had their estrogen-producing ovaries removed.* Plus, changes in blood lipids account for only about 30 percent of the protection conferred by estrogen.

Because cholesterol levels do tend to rise after menopause, we recommend that *all* women undergo a *lipid profile* at the time of menopause. If your blood lipids are normal (see page 311), you should have the test repeated every other year after menopause. If you have high blood cholesterol or if you are being treated with progestogen (which may adversely affect blood-cholesterol levels—see page 312), you should undergo a lipid profile every year. The test involves having blood drawn from your arm after an overnight fast. The blood is sent to a laboratory, where total cholesterol, triglycerides, low-density lipoproteins, and high-density lipoproteins are measured and the ratio of total cholesterol to HDLs is calculated. The test gives a general idea of your risk of heart disease. Having the lipid profile done regularly helps to monitor any menopause-related changes in your cholesterol. You can keep your risk of heart disease down and counter the menopause-related rise in blood cholesterol by following the program for prevention of heart disease outlined in Chapter 16.

Osteoporosis

We all lose bone mass as we age. However, the drop in estrogen after menopause results in a rapid loss of bone mass. Weakened bones increase the risk of fractures of the hip, wrist, and the arm. The weight-bearing bones of the spine may collapse, as well. This condition is known as osteoporosis, and the resulting fractures are a major cause of disability and death in a woman's later years.

Fortunately, there's much you can do to slow (and possibly reverse) the rapid loss of bone mass associated with menopause. (Chapter 17 describes our complete program for the prevention of osteoporosis.) Probably the most important thing you can do is to have your bone density tested either before or just after menopause. These measurements indicate how much bone you have to begin with, how rapidly you are losing bone after menopause, and whether you should consider taking postmenopausal hormones to protect your bones from further loss. (The tests are also described in Chapter 17.) Regular bone-density testing can also help monitor your treatment and ensure that it is working.

A Final Word

Being menopausal doesn't mean you have to be miserable. For a majority of women, menopausal symptoms are quite manageable without any medical intervention. If your symptoms *are* severe enough to interfere with daily living, there are a number of ways your physician can help make you more comfortable—and postmenopausal hormone therapy is just one of many options available to you.

Regardless of the severity of your symptoms, you should regularly see your physician so that you can be monitored for the "silent" changes that accompany menopause. Regular checkups help reduce your risk of developing the more serious menopause-related risks to your health: heart disease and osteoporosis.

Suggested Reading

Midlife Wellness: A Journal for the Middle Years, c/o The Women's Medical and Diagnostic Center, 222 Southwest 36th Terrace, Gainsville, FL 32607.

North American Menopause Society, c/o University Hospitals Department of OB/GYN, 2074 Abington Road, Cleveland, OH 44106. This organization provides information on menopause and maintains a list of menopause clinics around the country.

....

Chapter 13

*Hysterectomy and
Surgical Menopause:
Understanding
the Risks
and Alternatives*

About 600,000 women undergo a hysterectomy (removal of the uterus) each year, making it the most frequently performed major surgical procedure in the United States aside from cesarean sections. The most common age at which hysterectomy is performed is forty to forty-five.

Because of the sheer number of women involved, hysterectomy has also become one of the most controversial procedures. While a hysterectomy can save your life if you have cancer of the reproductive organs, it is more often performed to treat such benign conditions as fibroid tumors of the uterus, heavy periods (dysfunctional uterine bleeding), uterine prolapse, and endometriosis—conditions for which viable alternatives often exist.

There are several reasons for the dramatic increase in hysterectomies in the last few decades. Advancements in surgical procedures, anesthetics, and antibiotics have made hysterectomy a safe and effective procedure. Equally important was the thinking in the 1960s and 1970s that once a woman had completed her family, her uterus was nothing but a useless, troublesome organ that should be removed.

For some time now, however, experts have questioned the wisdom of that school of thought, particularly when the risks of hysterectomy, including possible serious long-term risks to your health, are taken into account. Since hysterectomy is so prevalent and so many hysterectomies today are "elective," it is essential that you become informed. This includes knowing *all* of the benefits and risks of the surgery, as well as other options.

What Is a Hysterectomy?

There are actually many different kinds of hysterectomy:

- **Hysterectomy, or simple hysterectomy:** The removal of the uterus and, sometimes, the attached Fallopian tubes. Your hormone-producing ovaries are left intact; if you undergo a hysterectomy before menopause, you will still experience a natural menopause, with one exception: You won't have the cessation of menstruation to tip you off.

- **Total hysterectomy:** Contrary to popular belief, this term does not mean that the ovaries are removed along with the uterus. Rather, it refers to the removal of the uterus and cervix. As with simple hysterectomy, you will still have your ovaries intact.

- **Subtotal, or partial, hysterectomy:** these terms are used to describe the removal of the uterus above the cervix. The cervix and ovaries are left in place.

- **Oophorectomy:** The medical term for the removal of one ovary. If you are premenopausal when you lose one ovary, the other ovary will take over, ovulating every month and producing the estrogen and progesterone necessary to regulate your menstrual cycle. You will be able to bear children and you will experience a natural menopause at the same genetically preprogrammed time as long as you have one functioning ovary.

- **Salpingo-oophorectomy:** This means the loss of a Fallopian tube and an ovary on one side. Again, if only one ovary is removed before you experience a natural menopause, the other will compensate for the loss.

- **Bilateral oophorectomy:** This term refers to the removal of both ovaries. When performed before you experience a natural menopause, the procedure results in instantaneous, or "surgical," menopause, regardless of whether your uterus is left intact.

- **Bilateral salpingo-oophorectomy:** The removal of both ovaries and Fallopian tubes. Again, this operation results in surgical menopause among premenopausal women.

- **Hysterectomy with bilateral salpingo-oophorectomy:** This is the medical term for removal of the uterus, both Fallopian tubes, and both ovaries—what most women refer to as a total or complete hysterectomy. The operation results in surgical menopause.

- **Radical hysterectomy:** This operation, usually performed to treat invasive cancer of the cervix or endometrium, involves removing the cuff of the vagina, the supporting tissues around the uterus, and the lymph glands that drain the pelvis.

Also, there are three ways to perform a hysterectomy.

- **Vaginal hysterectomy:** This operation involves removing the uterus through the vagina. It is usually reserved for uncomplicated conditions involving only the uterus (or cervix), such as endometrial hyperplasia (precancerous lesions of the uterine lining), dysfunctional uterine bleeding (DUB), and uterine prolapse. Because the uterus is removed through the vagina, there's no incision, no scar, less pain, and a slightly shorter hospitalization (four to five days) and recovery time.

On the other hand, vaginal hysterectomy carries a greater risk of post-operative infection.

•   **Abdominal hysterectomy:** This procedure, performed through an incision across your abdomen, is used when a medical condition such as cancer, endometriosis, large fibroids, adhesions (scar tissue) from previous abdominal or pelvic surgery, or chronic infections may involve the Fallopian tubes or ovaries as well as the uterus.

As with vaginal hysterectomy, this procedure carries certain risks, too, depending on the reason for the operation and the extent of the surgery. Generally speaking, patients undergoing abdominal hysterectomies are more likely to receive blood transfusions during their hospital stay.

•   **Laparoscopically assisted vaginal hysterectomy:** In this new procedure, the uterus is detached through one or two tiny abdominal incisions with the help of a laparoscope (a device much like a small lighted telescope), then removed through the vagina. The laparoscope provides the surgeon with a close-up view of the abdomen and uterus, giving the doctor much more control over the surgery than if the entire operation were performed vaginally. Postoperative pain and recovery time are similar to that of a vaginal hysterectomy.

Laparoscopically assisted vaginal hysterectomy may not be appropriate for all women. And because the procedure is relatively new, it may not be available everywhere. The procedure will probably become more widely available over the next several years as more physicians are trained in the technique.

Who Needs a Hysterectomy?

If you develop cancer of the ovaries, uterine lining, or invasive cervical cancer (cancer that has spread beyond the cervix), a hysterectomy can potentially save your life. Chronic pelvic infections and large fibroid tumors that press on and endanger nearby organs may also require a hysterectomy. When you are not faced with a life-threatening condition, the amount of pain and suffering your condition causes (endometriosis can be extremely painful; fibroid tumors can cause heavy bleeding) will also factor into the decision. Some of the most common indications for hysterectomy include the following:

•   **Fibroid tumors of the uterus:** The most common cause of hysterectomy is benign fibroid tumors, also known as *myomas*. These tumors of the muscle cells usually develop on or inside the uterus (and occasionally on the cervix). Fibroid tumors can be found in three general locations in the uterine wall: *Submucosal* fibroids grow just under the endometrial lining and protrude into the uterine cavity; *intramural* fibroids are located in the middle of the muscular wall of the uterus; *subserosal* fibroids grow directly beneath the peritoneum, or outer lining of the uterus. Sometimes, subserosal fibroids become *pedunculated,* meaning that they grow outside of the uterus and are attached to the uterine wall by a stalklike growth. Although some women may have only one fibroid, most women have multiple tumors.

Fibroid tumors usually grow slowly (it may take twenty years for the tumor to grow to the size of an orange) and are rarely cancerous. The majority of them cause no symptoms and require no treatment. However, some fibroid tumors can grow quite large and cause problems, including pelvic pain, heavy bleeding, and infertility. If fibroids enlarge the uterus beyond the size of a sixteen-week pregnancy, your physician cannot palpate your ovaries.

• **Endometriosis:** The most dramatic increase in the hysterectomy rate in recent years has been for the treatment of *endometriosis,* a condition in which parts of the uterine lining grow outside of the uterus. Between 1965 and 1984, the hysterectomy rate for this condition rose by a whopping 121 percent, compared with an increase of 1.2 percent for cancer-related hysterectomies and a *decline* of 7.2 percent for uterine fibroid–related hysterectomies, and 14 percent for uterine prolapse–related hysterectomies. We're not sure whether the rise in the hysterectomy rate for endometriosis is a result of an increase in the prevalence of the condition or a result of better diagnosis through the more widespread use of laparoscopy.

While endometriosis is *not* a life-threatening condition, it can significantly erode the *quality* of life for some women. Endometrial growths respond to the hormonal changes of the menstrual cycle in the same way that the uterine lining does: by swelling and bleeding. Endometriosis can cause pelvic pain, painful periods, pain during intercourse, and difficulty in defecating. When endometrial implants grow on the Fallopian tubes and ovaries, they can cause infertility.

• **Prolapse (or pelvic relaxation):** Although the overall number of hysterectomies performed to correct prolapsed, or "sagging," pelvic organs has declined, the number of women over age sixty-five who have a hysterectomy for this reason has *increased,* mostly because the number of women in this age group has risen.

Prolapse of the uterus, vagina, bladder (*cystocele*), intestine (*enterocele*) or rectum (*rectocele*) (see Figure 13.1) occurs when the ligaments and tissues supporting these organs weaken and stretch, causing the organs to change their position within the pelvis and, in severe cases, even to protrude out of the vagina.

Prolapse may cause a variety of symptoms. A telltale sign is pressure in the vagina and a feeling that "everything is falling out," which usually worsens during the day and feels better if you lie down. Other symptoms may include urinary incontinence (loss of bladder control), which may actually improve as the prolapse worsens; repeated bladder infections; constipation; difficulty having a bowel movement; and difficulty achieving penetration during intercourse. Some women experience back pain. Low back pain may be caused by tension on the ligaments caused by a prolapsed organ; high back pain may be a result of pressure on the kidneys or *ureters* (the tubes leading from the kidneys to the bladder). Some women with vaginal prolapse may also experience vaginal dryness and in rare instances may develop ulcers on the exposed area of the vagina. *Menorrhagia,* or heavy menstrual bleeding, may be another sign of prolapsed organs.

Women at highest risk of developing prolapsed organs are:

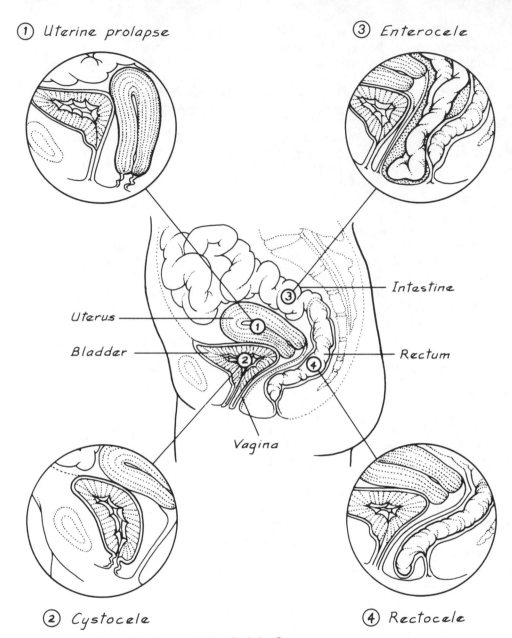

① Uterine prolapse   ③ Enterocele

Intestine

Uterus

Bladder

Rectum

Vagina

② Cystocele   ④ Rectocele

Figure 13.1   Prolapse of the Pelvic Organs

1. Those who have experienced physical trauma to the pelvic floor during childbirth. Prolonged labor, particularly the second stage of labor, when you are pushing the baby out, increases the risk of later developing prolapse of the pelvic organs. Having a forceps delivery may also increase your risk, for it is a sign of a difficult labor. A rapid

second stage of labor may also be an early sign of prolapse potential; the lack of resistance by the pelvic-floor muscles suggests that these muscles, which help support the pelvic organs, may be weak.

2. Postmenopausal women who aren't taking hormone therapy. Estrogen affects the connective tissues that help support the pelvic organs, and the drop in estrogen levels after menopause may further weaken these tissues.

3. Women with a genetic predisposition to develop prolapsed organs. The pelvic anatomy of some women, inherited from their mothers, may make them more likely to develop prolapsed organs.

Increased abdominal pressure, caused by obesity, coughing due to chronic bronchitis or asthma, and constipation may also make you more prone to prolapse.

• **Cancer:** Hysterectomy is often a necessary and potentially life-saving procedure in patients with ovarian cancer, endometrial cancer, and *invasive* cervical cancer, in which the cancer cells have spread beyond the cervix (for more on these conditions, see Chapter 18).

Although sterilization was an indication for hysterectomy as recently as twenty years ago, it is no longer considered a valid reason for having a hysterectomy, since simpler, safer, and cheaper methods of sterilization are now available (see page 181–186).

Keep in mind that these are the most common indications for having a hysterectomy. But unless you have a life-threatening condition, such as cancer, the decision is most emphatically up to you. Alternative therapies *are* now available for many of these conditions. Your job will be to become as informed as you can about *all* of your options. This means weighing the benefits and risks of hysterectomy against those of the newer alternative therapies. First, let's look at some of the risks associated with hysterectomy.

Risks Associated with Hysterectomy

As safe as hysterectomy is today, like *any* surgical procedure, it is not without risks. The most frequent (and usually reversible) complications arise from anesthesia, bleeding during surgery, postoperative infection, and, rarely, from perforation of the bladder or bowel. Vaginal hysterectomy carries a slightly greater risk of postoperative infection than abdominal hysterectomy. For this reason, physicians now routinely prescribe antibiotics to prevent such infections in women undergoing a vaginal hysterectomy.

Of even greater concern, however, are the long-term effects on your health and well-being. These include:

• **Hormonal changes:** If one or both ovaries are left intact after a hysterectomy, you should not experience a premature menopause, since the ovaries and not the uterus are responsible for the production of estrogen. However, some studies suggest that in a minority of women the blood supply to the ovaries may be affected by surgical removal of the uterus, which may cause these women to experience hot flashes and other symptoms of estrogen deficiency.

Premenopausal women who have *both* ovaries removed experience a sudden severing of the hormones estrogen and progesterone and experience what is known as *surgical menopause*. Because the drop in those hormones is immediate rather than gradual, surgically menopausal women often experience more and more severe symptoms of menopause, such as hot flashes and vaginal dryness. These women are also at a greater risk of heart disease and osteoporosis if they don't take postmenopausal estrogens. Usually, menopausal symptoms and long-term health risks in these women can be managed with postmenopausal estrogens (see Chapter 20).

• **Depression:** A few researchers have suggested that women who undergo a hysterectomy may be more prone to depression, anxiety, and sexual problems after surgery—what has become known as *posthysterectomy syndrome*. These problems are more prevalent in women who experience a decline in estrogen after surgery, women who had sexual problems *before* surgery, and those who believe that hysterectomy somehow detracts from their femininity. Women who have a definite estrogen deficiency and who do not suffer from clinical depression may find postmenopausal estrogens helpful (see page 246). Counseling may be beneficial for women with sexual problems and those who feel they have suffered a loss of their femininity.

• **Heart disease:** Surgically menopausal women are at a much greater risk of developing heart disease. As mentioned in Chapter 12, the drop in estrogen after menopause is associated with an increase in total cholesterol and the detrimental LDL cholesterol and a decrease in protective HDL cholesterol, all of which can raise your risk of heart disease.

However, blood cholesterol isn't the *only* risk factor for heart disease (see Chapter 16). And some studies, including the Framingham Heart Study, suggest that even women whose ovaries remain intact after hysterectomy may be at increased risk of heart disease. Other researchers have found that having a hysterectomy without having your ovaries removed is only marginally associated with an increased cardiac risk.

Until we know more about the effects of hysterectomy on your chances of developing heart disease, it wouldn't hurt to take steps to *protect* yourself from any increased risk if you've had a hysterectomy. (You'll find a complete program outlined in Chapter 16.) If you've experienced surgical menopause, postmenopausal estrogens can reduce your risk by up to 50 percent. Other lifestyle measures, such as eating a low-fat diet and exercising regularly, can also significantly reduce your risk of heart disease.

• **Osteoporosis:** At least one study has shown that women who've had a hysterectomy but who have retained their ovaries have lower bone mass than women who've never had a hysterectomy. And surgically menopausal women who *don't* take postmenopausal estrogens are definitely at a much greater risk of developing osteoporosis, since they lose the protective effects of estrogen on bone mass years earlier than women who undergo a natural menopause.

One of the most effective ways to offset this risk is for surgically menopausal women to take estrogen. Exercise and adequate calcium are important, too. Indeed, we found that surgically menopausal women who took estrogen *and* regularly performed muscle-strengthening exercises experienced an 8 percent increase in bone mass. A comparison group of women who took hormone therapy and didn't exercise neither gained nor lost bone mass during the twelve-month study.

How "Useless" Is Your Uterus?

Some physicians recommend hysterectomy to their patients even when there is no strong pathological reason for having the operation. They argue that you can live without your uterus and that by having a hysterectomy you won't have to worry about monthly menstruation, unwanted pregnancy, or the possible development of benign or malignant (cancerous) diseases of the uterus. Some women are lured by the promise of "better sex"—a shaky promise at best, since some women report having *more* sexual problems *after* hysterectomy. This line of reasoning, sometimes called the "useless uterus syndrome," became popular in the 1960s but has since come under fire for a number of reasons.

To begin with, the surgery is expensive and, as you've already seen, potentially risky. Moreover, hysterectomy is one type of contraception that is *totally* irreversible (tubal ligation is much safer and cheaper, and can *sometimes* be reversed). For the most part, there are no prescreening tests that can identify those women who would benefit most from an elective hysterectomy and eliminate those who would be better off without one. (One exception would be *GnRH agonists*—drugs that suppress the body's production of estrogen and progesterone—which may be used to help determine whether women with endometriosis or severe PMS would benefit from having their ovaries removed; if symptoms are relieved by the drug, these women may benefit from a hysterectomy with bilateral oophorectomy.)

As for having your uterus removed to *prevent* cervical or uterine cancer, the practice simply can't be justified. Both of these cancers can be easily screened for, detected, and treated early, with a nearly 100 percent cure rate.

We now know, too, that the uterus is involved in prostaglandin production and possibly vitamin D synthesis, which is important in bone formation. These findings suggest that the uterus *is* a viable hormone-producing organ whose usefulness *doesn't* end with the end of your childbearing years.

For these reasons, recommending a hysterectomy for the sake of having one is no longer considered a justifiable medical practice.

Should You Have Your Ovaries Removed to Prevent Cancer?

From 1965 to 1984, about 36 percent of women who underwent a hysterectomy also had both ovaries removed. (Women ages forty-five to sixty-four were most likely to have both their uterus and ovaries removed.) In some cases, the ovaries were removed because they were diseased or damaged by pelvic inflammation or endometriosis, but a significant number of women had perfectly normal, healthy ovaries removed.

263

Some physicians routinely recommend that ovaries be removed at the time of hysterectomy, particularly if the patient is around the age of menopause. They reason that since the woman can no longer have children and the ovaries will soon lose their function at menopause anyway, the surgery will prevent the possibility of ovarian cancer developing at a later date. Although cancer of the ovaries is not common, when it does occur it is often fatal because early diagnosis is difficult.

While this argument may at first appear sound, it must be placed into perspective. The chances of developing ovarian cancer after a hysterectomy vary from one in one hundred to one in ten thousand depending on which study you look at. By comparison, breast cancer affects one in nine women, and colon cancer affects one in twenty-five. How many physicians recommend removal of these tissues as a means of preventing future cancer?

Removal of the ovaries to prevent ovarian cancer should also be weighed against the long-term health risks associated with this surgery: As we mentioned earlier, surgically menopausal women are at a significantly greater risk of developing heart disease. And 25 to 50 percent of women who have had both ovaries removed prior to a natural menopause will develop osteoporosis at a relatively early age if they do not receive postmenopausal hormone therapy. Does the "benefit" of preventing unlikely ovarian cancer outweigh the very real risks of heart disease and osteoporosis?

This is the question you must ask your physician *before* surgery. Discuss the pros and cons of leaving your ovaries alone if they are healthy. Ask your doctor about the use of ultrasound screening for ovarian cancer. If your ovaries must be removed, discuss how you will go about offsetting the long-term health risks associated with a surgical menopause. (Keep in mind that one of the best ways to minimize these risks is to take estrogen. However, many surgically menopausal women who are advised to take estrogen don't comply with their doctor's advice for one reason or another. One way to improve your own compliance is to have your physician monitor your blood-cholesterol levels and bone density while you're taking estrogen; see Chapter 21.)

Some Alternatives to Hysterectomy

Alternative therapies now make it possible for many women with benign conditions such as fibroid tumors, endometriosis, and dysfunctional uterine bleeding to avoid hysterectomy. Even some precancerous conditions can be cured without resorting to hysterectomy. Here's a brief look at some of your options.

• **Fibroid tumors:** Myomectomy, surgical removal of the fibroids through an abdominal incision, may be an option for women with small symptomatic tumors. However, the operation itself usually takes longer than a hysterectomy and often results in heavy bleeding.

Depending on the type of fibroid and its size and location, some tumors can be removed using *hysteroscopy* or *laparoscopy*. These procedures involve the use of an endoscope, which allows the physician to peer into the uterus or abdominal cavity, along with specially designed surgical instruments that fit into the endoscope.

The hysteroscope is inserted into the uterus through the vagina, where lasers or electrocautery (a heated probe) are used to excise fibroid tumors embedded within the inner walls of the uterus (submucosal fibroids). This type of surgery is particularly attractive because there are no incisions or scars, bleeding is minimal, and the patient can often go home on the day of the operation.

Small, painful fibroids growing on stalks outside of the uterus (subserosal) can sometimes be removed with laparoscopic surgery. A laser is used to sever the fibroid at the stem while controlling bleeding. The tumor is then cut into small pieces and removed through the laparoscope.

A word of caution: Although the laser and electrocautery do cut down on the amount of bleeding associated with myomectomy, patients undergoing these procedures are still at potential risk and should be prepared for major abdominal surgery if bleeding becomes a problem. Moreover, these procedures generally are not recommended for women with fibroid tumors larger than a twelve-week pregnancy.

However, a new class of fibroid-shrinking drugs is offering hope for women who want to preserve their fertility (or uterus) but whose fibroids are too large to remove surgically without damaging the uterus. The new drugs, called GnRH agonists (Lupron, Synarel), indirectly stop the body's production of estrogen, which stimulates the growth of fibroids. In clinical trials at universities around the country, the drugs have been shown to reduce the size of troublesome fibroids from 20 to 60 percent. The drugs probably won't take the place of surgery, but they can often shrink fibroids to a point where they can be more easily removed by surgery.

So far, no long-term side effects associated with GnRH agonists have been reported, although women who took the drugs did experience symptoms typical of menopause, such as hot flashes and vaginal dryness. Other possible side effects include decreased sex drive, depression (particularly among women with a past history of depression), fatigue, headaches, insomnia, irregular bleeding, and weight gain. Some studies suggest the drugs also may accelerate bone loss while being used. For this reason, it's wise to have your bone mass tested before and during treatment. And because GnRH agonists may cause you to lose bone mass, taking these drugs for more than six months is not advised. Women generally resume menstruating within eight to twelve weeks after stopping the drug.

Some women who have small symptomatic fibroids and who are close to menopause may simply want to wait it out, since fibroids often shrink after menopause. These women should be monitored by their physicians every six months and should periodically undergo vaginal ultrasound screening to ensure the fibroids aren't growing any larger.

• **Endometriosis:** Some women with endometriosis may be able to skip surgery altogether, thanks to new drug therapies being developed. *Danazol* (Danocrine) a form of the "male" hormone testosterone, GnRH agonists (Lupron, Synarel), oral contraceptives, and progestogen are often effective in relieving pain and, in some cases, restoring fertility.

If surgery is necessary, lasers and the laparoscope have proven to be powerful tools. Unlike the scalpel or electrocautery, the high-precision laser can destroy endometrial growths on the ovaries, Fallopian tubes, and uterus without damaging the organs themselves. The laser also reduces the chances of postsurgical scars, or *adhesions*, developing on these organs, which can cause or compound infertility. Studies have shown that pregnancy rates in women after this procedure range from 40 to 70 percent, depending on the severity of the disease. Pregnancy rates were highest among women who took Danazol after the surgery to shrink any endometrial growths that might have been missed by the surgery.

Another plus: Laser laparoscopy can be used to treat endometriosis at the time of diagnosis (laparoscopy is the only way to make a definitive diagnosis of endometriosis), thus sparing the woman another hospital stay and further surgery.

• **Prolapse:** Surgery is the only truly effective treatment for prolapsed organs. Although exercises to strengthen the pelvic floor muscles (Kegel exercises) are sometimes prescribed for women suffering from prolapse, these exercises strengthen only these muscles; they do nothing to strengthen (or shorten) the ligaments supporting the uterus, bladder, and other pelvic organs nor can the exercises repair muscles damaged by a hernia (in which the organs have slipped between separated muscles).

The type of surgery you undergo depends on the type and degree of prolapse you have.

Degree I: organs have "fallen" midway down the vagina

Degree II: organs have prolapsed to the vulva

Degree III: organs protrude beyond the vulva

Uterine prolapse: Some physicians now repair a prolapsed uterus by shortening and restructuring the supporting ligaments of the uterus (and any other prolapsed organs) rather than removing the uterus altogether. However, if the prolapse is severe, this type of reconstructive surgery may not be able to restore the uterus to its normal position. In addition, prolapse can recur after reconstructive surgery.

Prolapse of the bladder: To repair a prolapsed bladder, the connective tissues that surround the bladder are brought together across the midline (where the incision is made).

Prolapse of the intestines: Enteroceles are treated by surgically removing the pouch of the peritoneum into which the small intestine bulges.

Prolapse of the rectum: For mild cases with minimal symptoms, your physician may recommend exercises to strengthen the muscles around the rectum and anus. You will also be advised to avoid straining when having a bowel movement. If a high-fiber diet, plenty of fluids, and exercise don't help relieve constipation, your physician may recommend that you take a stool softener.

If surgical treatment is necessary, the procedure involves bringing the pelvic-floor muscles together in the midline (where the incision is made) between the vagina and the rectum.

Prolapse of the vagina: Pessaries (instruments placed in the vagina to support the uterus or rectum) are only temporary measures your physician may recommend until surgery can be scheduled. Surgical treatment includes shortening the ligaments supporting the vagina to restore the vaginal vault to its normal position and, in some cases, vaginal hysterectomy. The most drastic treatment—surgically closing the vagina—is rarely used.

Estrogen therapy is recommended for postmenopausal women before surgery to repair a prolapsed organ. Vaginal estrogen creams increase the collagen content of the connective tissues supporting the pelvic organs, increase blood flow, normalize the bacterial flora of the vagina, and may also influence the *fascia* (covering of the muscle), all of which enhance healing and result in a better surgical outcome.

•   **Dysfunctional uterine bleeding:** Dysfunctional uterine bleeding usually occurs just before menopause as a result of a hormone imbalance. Usually, the bleeding responds to hormone therapy (progestogen). If it doesn't, the next step has often been a hysterectomy. Now, however, some women may benefit from two alternative procedures. One, called *laser ablation,* involves destroying the uterine lining with a laser beam, leaving the thick uterine wall intact. The other, called *roller-ball electrocoagulation,* is essentially the same, except a specially designed heated probe is used to destroy the uterine lining.

Before you undergo either procedure, you must have a thorough workup to determine the cause of the bleeding. This may include diagnostic hysteroscopy (which may be performed in your doctor's office) to rule out fibroids or precancerous lesions of the endometrium. The procedures themselves are done in the hospital under general or spinal anesthesia and take about thirty to forty minutes. Since the operations are performed through a hysteroscope, there's no incision and no scar. Pain is usually limited to two to three hours of postoperative cramping, and the recovery time is short: Most women are in and out of the hospital on the same day, and many can return to work the next day. The major drawback is that the surgery renders you sterile. Keep in mind, too, that no long-term studies have been conducted on these procedures, so long-term risks associated with the operations, if any, aren't known yet.

•   **Precancerous cervical changes:** Precancerous lesions of the cervix (*cervical intraepithelial neoplasia, or CIN*) and *cervical carcinoma in situ* (cancer cells that are localized and haven't spread) can be treated with cryotherapy (freezing the cells), laser surgery, or with a recently developed technique known as LEEP (loop electrosurgical excision procedure). Success rates for cryosurgery and laser surgery are around 90 percent. The LEEP procedure, which involves scooping the cancerous cells out of the cervix with a thin wire loop that's been charged with a high-frequency radio wave, may enjoy an even greater success rate because it removes all of the cancerous cells in one fell swoop. (For more information on these procedures and the prevention, diagnosis, and treatment of cervical cancer, see Chapter 18.)

A Final Word

If you've been told you need a hysterectomy for anything other than cancer, be sure to discuss *all* the options with your physician before agreeing to the surgery. If you're still not sure whether you need a hysterectomy, get a second opinion. In fact, most insurance companies now *require* a second opinion.

....
Suggested Reading
....

Cutler, Winnifred B. *Hysterectomy: Before and After.* New York: Harper & Row, 1988.

Harris, Dena E., M.D., and Helene MacLean. *Recovering From a Hysterectomy.* New York: HarperCollins, 1992.

....
Resources and Support
....

The Endometriosis Association, 8585 North 76th Place, Milwaukee, WI 53223. Phone: (800) 962-ENDO. This self-help organization acts as a clearinghouse for information and referrals. The association publishes a newsletter for members and has produced a videotape, *You're Not Alone: Understanding Endometriosis,* available for $15.95.

Chapter 14

....

Sexuality in the Middle Years: A Discussion for Women and Men

We tend to think of lovemaking as the most natural act in the world. But even the closest couples can encounter difficulties. Problems—for both men and women—tend to escalate in the menopausal years. Only 7 percent of women younger than age twenty report a sexual problem. The number increases to 18 percent in women ages twenty to thirty-four, 22 percent in women ages thirty-five to fifty, and 28 percent in women older than age fifty.

There are several reasons for the decline in sexual activity and increase in sexual problems as you grow older, but there's no reason why you *can't* have a fulfilling sex life after age fifty. Knowing what to expect, keeping the lines of communication open with your partner, and being open to new alternatives can help keep you sexually active throughout your middle and later years.

Both you and your partner are undergoing physical changes that may affect lovemaking. With a little knowledge, a lot of reassurance, and medical treatment, if necessary, these changes don't have to bring an end to your sex life.

What a Woman Can Expect

Orgasms

Although you won't lose your ability to have an orgasm as you grow older, the number of involuntary contractions of the uterus during orgasm does decrease by 50 percent. As you grow older, the clitoris retracts and shrinks faster after orgasm, too. But these changes should in no way detract from sexual satisfaction.

Remember, too, that it's perfectly normal *not* to have an orgasm *during* intercourse. In fact, a majority of women don't. The reason is that the vagina simply doesn't have an abundance of nerve endings. The clitoris, on the other hand, does contain numerous sensitive nerve endings that respond to sexual stimulation. Most women need direct stimulation of the clitoris to achieve orgasm. Telling your partner this or even stimulating the clitoris yourself can often solve a major sexual problem.

Some women find that applying a small amount of testosterone cream to the clitoris helps it respond to stimulation and enhances the quality of an orgasm. This, in turn, may also stimulate your sex drive by making orgasms more intense and enjoyable.

Vaginal Atrophy

After menopause, sharply declining levels of estrogen result in physical changes that affect the vagina. Many women experience thinning and drying of the vaginal walls, which may cause the vagina to become less elastic. Vaginal blood flow decreases and the pH balance of the vagina becomes more alkaline. As a result, you may experience delayed or reduced vaginal secretions during sexual stimulation. Whereas it may have taken a minute for your vagina to become lubricated at age twenty-five, now it may take you fifteen minutes or longer. Lack of lubrication can make lovemaking painful, a condition physicians call dyspareunia. Some women may even bleed after intercourse as a result of trauma to the fragile vaginal walls. You may first notice the itching and burning of vaginal atrophy only after sexual encounters. Later, you may notice a dry feeling in the vagina throughout the day.

Low estrogen levels also may affect your urinary tract (see page 252), which can result in urinary frequency or urgency, and sometimes in loss of bladder control (urinary incontinence). Some women may be embarrassed about losing control of their bladder during intercourse.

Vaginal dryness can be easily remedied and its impact on your sex life minimized (see Coping with Vaginal Dryness on page 250). Too often, however, couples don't seek help until this seemingly minor problem has become a major headache. Be sure to report painful intercourse or other symptoms of atrophic vaginitis to your doctor without delay.

Sexual Desire

When it comes to sexual desire, the role of hormonal changes that menopause brings is less clear-cut. Some women feel greater sexual desire because their children are out of the house or because they no longer have to worry about unwanted pregnancy. Others may experience a decrease in desire as a result of painful sex. Symptoms of menopause—hot flashes, fatigue, and irritability—may temporarily suppress desire, as well.

Interestingly, high levels of the "male" sex hormone testosterone have been linked to greater feelings of desire and more frequent sexual fantasies among postmenopausal women who take testosterone (see page 444). In our study on menopause and aging supported by the National Institute on Aging, we found that while testosterone levels *do* decline somewhat after a natural menopause, levels of the more biologically active "free" testosterone remain essentially unchanged by menopause. *So there appears to be no biological reason why sexual desire should decline after menopause.*

If you *do* feel a decrease in sexual desire after menopause, particularly because of bothersome menopausal symptoms, be sure to reassure your partner that your lack of sexual desire isn't a lack of desire for *him*. Remember, too, that often when troublesome menopausal symptoms are treated with postmenopausal hormone therapy, sexual interest and satisfaction are restored.

What a Man Can Expect

Men may take longer to achieve an erection as they grow older and the erection may be less turgid in older men than younger ones. An eighteen-year-old can attain a full erection in three seconds. At age forty-five, the average time is still only eighteen to twenty seconds. But by age seventy-five, it may take five minutes or more, and this will still be a perfectly normal amount of time. Also, while a younger man may be able to achieve an erection again shortly after orgasm, it may take an older man much longer.

The amount of sperm decreases with age, as well. Sometimes, no semen is ejaculated at all. Other times, semen may be ejaculated back into the bladder, where it is later passed in the urine, a condition known as *retrograde ejaculation*. No harm occurs in any of these situations and they need not interfere with the enjoyment of sex for either partner.

Recognizing that these changes are normal helps ease performance anxiety that can sometimes put a damper on sex. Be patient and expect to spend a little more time directly stimulating the penis. Remember that after orgasm, your partner may not be ready again for a while. Keep in mind that not every sexual experience must end with orgasm. Focusing solely on achieving climax may make you and your partner anxious and could result in bouts of impotence. Instead, agree with your partner on occasion *not* to have orgasm during sex. Rather, concentrate on hugging, kissing, and gentle caressing.

Medical Problems That Sometimes Lead to Sexual Problems

Any major physical illness may depress sexual interest. Usually, the decline in sexual desire is temporary and interest is aroused again once you start feeling better. However, some illnesses are more likely than others to trigger chronic sexual problems.

Heart Disease

Heart disease doesn't directly affect either partner's sexual responsiveness or their ability to achieve climax. However, men and women with heart problems often fear that strenuous sexual activity may trigger another heart attack (a "coital coronary") or bout of angina—even after receiving reassurances to the contrary from their doctors. While orgasm does increase your heart rate and blood pressure, it rarely leads to a heart attack. If this fear continues to get in the way of your enjoyment of sex, you may want to seek regular counseling from your physician or a family or sex therapist.

Diabetes

One of the most common biological causes of impotence is diabetes. Indeed, impotence is often one of the first symptoms of undiagnosed diabetes in men. Impotence occurs when uncontrolled or poorly controlled diabetes damages the blood vessels and nerves involved in achieving and sustaining an erection.

After a complete physical and psychological evaluation to determine the cause of impotence, the first step in treating diabetes-related impotence is to make sure the patient's diabetes is well controlled. Any medications and excessive alcohol intake that may contribute to or cause impotence should be discontinued or changed. Often, counseling with a sex therapist or marital counselor is advised to help the man overcome the performance anxiety that often accompanies impotence. Men who have irreversible diabetes-related impotence are good candidates for any of a number of penile implants now on the market. Success rates for the implants are approximately 90 percent.

Arthritis

The joint pain and reduced range of motion of both osteoarthritis and rheumatoid arthritis can interfere with the mechanics of having sexual intercourse. There may be a need to experiment with new positions (either having the woman on top or having both partners lie on their sides facing one another—see figures 14.1 and 14.2). Sometimes a firmer support, such as a board under the mattress or prop-up cushions under the pelvis, can help if arthritis pain or decreased range of motion limits you or your partner.

Osteoporosis

If you have osteoporosis, there's no reason why you *shouldn't* have intercourse. You should, however, have your physician check to see that you don't have a problem with vaginal lubrication. This will help ensure that the use of excessive force is avoided when your partner enters you.

Figure 14.1

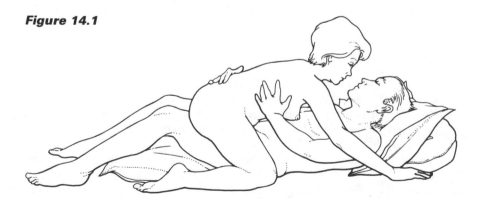

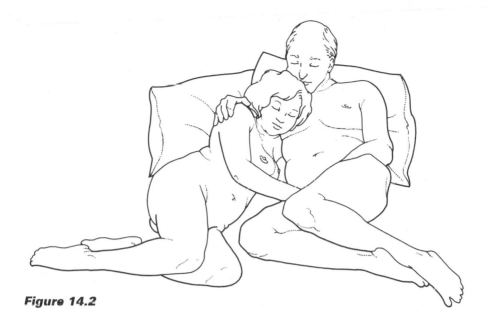

Figure 14.2

Since it's best to avoid putting any excessive pressure or weight on your bones, the missionary position is not recommended. The safest way to have intercourse is with your partner positioned behind you (see Figure 14.3). Lying on your sides facing one another or positioning yourself on top of your partner works well, too.

Medications

Several types of medications may interfere with sexual desire and, in particular, with a man's ability to attain and sustain an erection. Tricyclic antidepressants may restore a man's sexual desire but impair his ability to have an erection. *Thioridazine* (Mellaril), an antipsychotic often prescribed for older patients

Figure 14.3

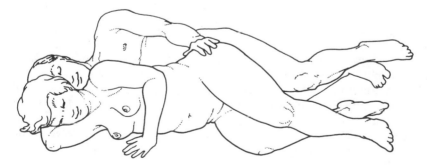

can cause retrograde ejaculation. Certain antihypertensive drugs, such as beta-blockers and *guanethidine* (Esimil, Ismelin), may also cause impotence.

Sexual problems are usually resolved after the medication is stopped. In the case of antihypertensive drugs, you may want to ask your doctor about switching to another medication that doesn't have this side effect.

Surgery and Sexuality

Understandably, after major surgery you probably won't feel much like having sex, and most times you *shouldn't*. Once you have fully recovered, you will probably feel well enough to resume an active sex life. However, some operations may indirectly have an impact on your sex life.

Hysterectomy

Some women say their sex lives *improve* after having a hysterectomy. Others report that removal of the uterus has an adverse effect on their ability to have sex.

The physical changes resulting from a hysterectomy may directly affect sexual function by contributing to vaginal dryness, shortening and narrowing of the vagina, vaginal scarring, and decreased sensation in the genital area. Some women report a reduction in libido and in their ability to achieve an orgasm after a simple hysterectomy (in which the ovaries are left intact). It's still not clear whether removal of the cervix affects sexual function, but the cervix has been reported to act as a trigger for orgasm.

When a premenopausal woman's ovaries as well as her uterus are removed, sexual problems—particularly vaginal dryness—may be severe, since production of estrogen and testosterone are abruptly halted by the loss of the ovaries. Even in postmenopausal women, hysterectomy with removal of the ovaries may adversely affect sexuality, since the ovaries would have continued to produce testosterone (which has been associated with increased sex drive) after menopause.

Some studies have suggested that sexual difficulties after hysterectomy may be a result of a preexisting depression or the psychological fear that hysterectomy will lead to diminished sexual satisfaction and loss of attractiveness, which for some women becomes a self-fulfilling prophecy.

Postmenopausal hormone therapy and other means of easing the physical symptoms associated with surgical menopause may help put your sex life back on track. Counseling with a sex or family therapist may also prove helpful.

Mastectomy

Women with breast cancer who have a mastectomy (removal of one or both breasts) may not be as sexually active as they were before the operation. While the loss of a breast in itself doesn't cause sexual problems in a direct physical sense, it may dampen a woman's desire for sex if she feels self-conscious about her physical attractiveness.

Often, if breast cancer is caught early, physicians may use a less disfiguring procedure called *lumpectomy*, involving removal of the tumor rather than the entire breast (see page 386), followed by radiation therapy. Another option is to undergo breast reconstruction, which often helps a woman adjust more comfortably to mastectomy.

Prostate Surgery

Some men experience impotence after prostate surgery. If an abdominal incision is used for surgery, nerve damage is a likely cause. The most common procedure, however, transurethral resection of the prostate (TURP), which doesn't involve an abdominal incision, is also associated with impotence. Usually, the problem is psychological in nature and can often be resolved with counseling.

Some Common Sexual Problems

Impotence

One of the most common problems for men in the middle and later years is impotence. The good news is that research in recent years has shown that in the majority of cases physical problems are the culprits, accounting for up to 65 percent of impotence. Middle-aged and older men are more prone to impotence simply because they are more susceptible to physical illnesses that can cause it, including hypertension (or, more often, the drugs used to treat it) and diabetes.

When impotence can be traced to physical causes, such as medication or disease, all that may be needed to cure it is a change in medication or treatment of the disease. If those measures don't work, penile implants and other devices that increase blood flow to the penis may be used. For those cases in which physical problems *aren't* the cause, sex therapy may be necessary.

Inhibited Sexual Desire

For years, scientists believed that low sexual desire—one of the most common complaints among couples seeking sex therapy today—was caused chiefly by emotional conflicts, anger, and frustration between two partners. New research shows that a loss of sexual desire may have important chemical roots, too. Much of the research today focuses on the "male" hormone testosterone and other androgens, which some experts now refer to as "libido" hormones. Several studies have shown that menopausal women who take androgens report more feelings of desire and arousal and have more frequent sexual fantasies (see also page 444).

Still other research suggests that the brain chemical dopamine, a neurotransmitter that's also instrumental in the production of testosterone in men and women, may influence desire, as well. Animal studies suggest that dopamine plays a major role in sex drive. What's more, when patients with Parkinson's disease are given synthetic dopamines to treat their condition, they report an increase in sexual arousal. These studies suggest that certain drugs may one day serve as modern-day love potions to boost sexual desire in patients who suffer from a biochemical imbalance.

However, it's difficult to separate purely physical causes of low sexual desire from psychological ones. To complicate matters, any major physical illness, disability, or surgical procedure may temporarily dampen desire. Mental illnesses, such as depression; chronic use of alcohol, marijuana, and cocaine; and major life stresses, such as loss of a job, divorce, or death of a spouse, can all result in a temporary loss of sexual desire. As promising as the new research is, most cases of decreased sexual desire still respond best to counseling.

Lack of a Partner

One of the most overlooked sexual problems faced especially by older women is lack of a partner. When sexually active and inactive women of the same age are asked how often they would make love under ideal circumstances, there is no difference in the frequency reported by the two groups. Apparently, the decision to stop being sexually active stems from lack of a partner or lack of a capable and willing partner. This needn't stop you entirely from engaging in sexual activity. And you shouldn't rule out self-stimulation as a means of sexual gratification when you don't have a partner.

Getting Help

If you think you have a sexual problem, begin with a visit to your physician. Communicate the problem as clearly as you can to the doctor and make sure he or she is comfortable talking about it. The doctor should give you an answer based on the same kind of scientific facts that he or she would use to answer a question about an infection. If your doctor tells you to buy a new nightgown, ask for a referral.

When complaints are long-standing, you may want to consider seeing a sex therapist. Sex therapists can help couples whose problem isn't resolved simply by treating physical causes; they may also be able to help couples overcome a problem that has psychological roots. Ask your physician for a referral or send a stamped, self-addressed envelope to the American Association of Sex Educators, Counselors and Therapists, Suite 1717, 435 North Michigan Avenue, Chicago, IL 60611. This association can provide information and a list of sex therapists practicing in your state.

Whatever you do, don't put off seeking help for *any* sexual problem. Often, the solution is as simple as having your physician write a prescription.

Sexually Transmitted Diseases

Another type of sexual problem that crops up even in the middle years is sexually transmitted diseases. For the most part, sexually transmitted diseases are a problem primarily for sexually active single men and women under age thirty, particularly those with more than one sexual partner. But sexually transmitted diseases know no age limits. If you are sexually active with more than one partner today, you are at risk *regardless of your age*. That's why it's important to protect yourself from sexually transmitted diseases even in your middle years. Prevention is particularly important in light of the fact that the human immunodeficiency virus, which is believed to cause acquired immune deficiency syndrome (AIDS), can be transmitted through sexual intercourse. In addition, untreated or poorly treated bacterial infections can lead to *pelvic inflammatory disease* (PID), a potentially serious infection of the reproductive organs. Moreover, one sexually transmitted disease, which is caused by the *human papilloma virus*, has been linked to an increased risk of developing cervical cancer.

Gonorrhea

This bacterial infection is one of the most common sexually transmitted diseases: More than 1 million new cases are reported each year. Symptoms in men include a yellowish discharge and pain when urinating. Symptoms in women may include a foul-smelling vaginal discharge or abnormal menstrual bleeding. However, about half of the women infected with gonorrhea have no symptoms or so few that they don't seek treatment. The danger is that many of these women will develop pelvic inflammatory disease. Indeed, about half of the estimated 500,000 annual cases of PID in the United States are caused by gonorrhea. Many of these women will develop tubal scarring and infertility.

Gonorrhea can be diagnosed by having your physician take a gonorrhea culture, which involves using a swab to collect vaginal secretions from the vaginal walls and cervix. Penicillin is the treatment of choice. Since some strains of gonorrhea have become resistant to penicillin, a repeat culture may be performed after you've been treated. If penicillin fails to cure the infection, another antibiotic will be prescribed.

Syphilis

This bacterial infection, perhaps the oldest known sexually transmitted disease, is not the health scourge it was before the advent of antibiotics. However, the number of infected men and women today is on the rise, a trend that appears to be somehow associated with the AIDS epidemic.

The main symptom of *primary syphilis* is the development of a chancre, or lesion, in the genital area, which may appear between ten and ninety days after exposure to an infected partner. (Some patients may develop more than one chancre.) Since the chancre is often painless, a woman may not even notice a lesion that has developed inside the vagina.

If left untreated, the chancre heals within three to six weeks, but the infection itself remains in the body, and, about four to ten weeks later, symptoms of *secondary syphilis* appear. These include flulike symptoms, such as aching muscles and joints, malaise, and low-grade fever. Some people may develop enlarged lymph nodes. The most prominent symptom is a rash that appears on the body, including the palms of the hands and the soles of the feet.

If the infection is not treated, symptoms go away between three to twelve weeks, followed by a latent stage of the disease in which no symptoms are apparent. In the later stages of syphilis, the infection may damage the skin, joints, bones, heart, or central nervous system.

Because the bacteria that causes syphilis is difficult to grow in a laboratory dish, a blood test that detects syphilis antibodies is used to diagnose the infection. A three-week regimen of oral penicillin or two separate injections of penicillin are usually used to treat syphilis. (Tetracycline or Doxycycline may be used for those who are allergic to penicillin.) Repeat testing at three, six, and twelve months following treatment is also recommended, since some patients suffer a relapse after treatment of early syphilis.

Chlamydia

This sexually transmitted disease is caused by the bacteria *chlamydia trachomatis,* which invades the mucous membranes of the human body, particularly the cells lining the sexual organs. Once it enters a cell and begins to multiply, the bacteria can be difficult to detect. In women, chlamydia takes up residence in the cervix. Left untreated, it can travel up into the uterus, ovaries, and Fallopian tubes and, like gonorrhea, develop into pelvic inflammatory disease.

When symptoms do occur, they typically appear seven to twenty-seven days after infection. With men these include a mild discharge and pain during urination; in women, symptoms include a heavier-than-normal vaginal discharge that's often yellow in color, pain or burning during urination, a dull, vague pain in the lower abdomen, or pain during intercourse. Women taking oral contraceptives may experience breakthrough bleeding. Others may have some vaginal bleeding during intercourse. But many women experience no symptoms whatsoever.

Your physician can detect chlamydia with a number of simple diagnostic tests that have been recently developed. Treatment involves a seven- to fourteen-day course of antibiotics. Tetracycline is the antibiotic of choice. (Penicillin is not effective against chlamydia.)

Herpes

These painful lesions of the genital area are caused by a virus known as herpes simplex virus Type II. (Herpes simplex virus Type I typically causes fever blisters or cold sores around the mouth.) Usually, the first outbreak is the worst, causing fever, headache, malaise, and achiness that's accompanied by genital pain, itching, pain with urination, vaginal and urethral discharge, and tenderness in the groin, as well as lesions that blister and then crust over. It usually takes two to three weeks for the lesions to heal, during which time the disease can be transmitted.

Unlike bacterial STDs, there's no permanent cure for herpes, and infected people can break out again and again. Subsequent outbreaks are generally more mild but just as infectious as the first. And while it was once believed that herpes could be transmitted only by an infected person with open lesions, there's evidence that some people may shed the virus even when they have no symptoms.

Treatment of active cases involves using acyclovir (Zovirax), either in the form of a topical cream or pill.

Genital Warts

These sexually transmitted warts may appear on the cervix, penis, or in the vaginal or rectal area and are caused by the *human papillomavirus.* Their appearance can vary from a barely visible lesion to a soft, velvety, flat bump or a cauliflowerlike growth, ranging in color from pale to dark pink. These highly infectious warts are particularly important to treat because some strains of HPV (HPV strains 11 and 16) are associated with an increased risk of cervical cancer in women.

Although warts generally develop an average of two to three months after exposure to a person with HPV infection, many infected people may be completely asymptomatic. Nevertheless, you can still develop complications, such as cervical cancer. This is just one more reason why you should have regular Pap smears.

A physician can often diagnose genital warts by simple observation. An abnormal Pap smear may be the first clue that women have genital warts on the cervix. Many men report an unusual discharge or the need to urinate often.

Treatment involves freezing the warts with liquid nitrogen or cryosurgery, burning them off with caustic chemicals or electrocautery, and, in severe or persistent cases, using laser treatment, loop electrosurgical excision procedures (LEEP), in which the infected part of the cervix is removed with a thin wire loop that's charged with high-frequency radio waves (see page 397), or interferon. Treatments may have to be repeated several times, sometimes over several months. Sometimes warts reappear even after treatment, so repeat reexaminations are often recommended even after the warts appear to go away. And because of the increased risk of cervical cancer associated with certain strains of HPV, once you have had genital warts you should be sure to have an annual Pap smear.

AIDS

Human immunodeficiency virus, which is believed to cause AIDS, is without a doubt the most frightening of all sexually transmitted diseases because it is always fatal and there is no cure. The chance that you have contracted AIDS is slight if you aren't in a high-risk group (hemophiliacs, intravenous-drug users, those who've had sex with bisexual or homosexual males or with intravenous-drug users, and people who have had a blood transfusion between 1979 and 1985). Nevertheless, if you are not in a mutually monogamous relationship with an uninfected partner, you should *always* practice safe sex (see Protecting Yourself from Sexually Transmitted Diseases below). The virus is capable of being transmitted by heterosexuals, and it is possible that your partner may not know he is infected.

If you *do* fall into a high-risk group, you should consider having your blood tested for the HIV virus.

Protecting Yourself from Sexually Transmitted Diseases

There are several ways you can protect yourself from virtually all of these sexually transmitted diseases. One of the best ways is simply to limit the number of sexual partners you have. You should also avoid having intercourse if you or your partner(s) have or suspect you have a sexually transmitted disease.

Several studies suggest that barrier methods of birth control may help protect against sexually transmitted diseases. We know, for instance, that nonoxynol-9, the most widely used spermicide, kills all of the major sexually transmitted bacteria and viruses, including gonorrhea, syphilis, chlamydia, herpes, trichomonas, and possibly the AIDS virus.

Latex condoms appear to offer the most protection, particularly when used together with a spermicide containing nonoxynol-9. Latex condoms can protect the woman from contact with infected semen, which can spread gonorrhea, trichomoniasis, AIDS, hepatitis B, and chlamydia. Latex condoms can also protect both partners against lesions that may harbor syphilis. However, condoms don't provide complete protection: Areas of the skin not covered may be infectious or vulnerable to infection. And not all condoms protect equally well. High-quality latex condoms are the best. Natural-membrane condoms contain pores that may allow passage of very small particles, such as the human immunodeficiency virus (HIV) and hepatitis B virus.

There's also some evidence that the diaphragm and spermicide-saturated contraceptive sponge protect against sexually transmitted diseases, particularly gonorrhea and chlamydia, which invade the cells of the cervix.

Another way you can protect yourself is to perform monthly genital self-examinations (see page 52). While GSE won't *prevent* you from getting a sexually transmitted disease, it will help alert you to possible symptoms, allowing you and your partner to seek treatment early.

Finally, if either you or your partner discovers that you have a sexually transmitted disease, *both* partners should be treated. To help reduce the risk of reinfection, you should avoid having sexual intercourse during treatment and until a follow-up examination confirms that you are cured.

A Final Word

Whether you have an active sex life in your middle and later years depends on a number of different factors, including how sexually active and satisfied you are in your premenopausal years. A key is for both partners to know what changes to expect and to know each other's problems and desires. Only through mutual knowledge and understanding will you be able to adjust to many of the aging changes that can affect your sex life.

You may also have to reexamine some of your own attitudes about sex (some people have an aversion to touching their genitals and to self-stimulation) and some of your sexual practices. Often, this means putting a premium on physical affection, tenderness, and intimacy.

Keep in mind, too, that if you are sexually active with more than one partner (or if you are involved with someone who has multiple sexual partners), you should also be sure to take measures to protect yourself from contracting a sexually transmitted disease.

Overall, if you're willing to communicate openly with your partner and change the sexual script when necessary, there's no reason why you can't be sexually active *and* satisfied throughout your middle years and well into your later years.

Suggested Reading

Brecher, Edward M. *Love, Sex and Aging.* Mount Vernon, NY: Consumers Union, 1984.

Masters, William H., Virginia E. Johnson, and Robert Kolondy. *Masters and Johnson on Sex and Human Loving.* New York: Little, Brown and Company, 1986.

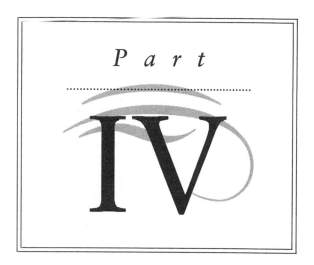

Part

IV

*Coping with
Common Medical
Problems
in Midlife and
Beyond*

C h a p t e r   1 5

....

Obesity and a
"Throw Away the
Scales"
Approach to Weight
Control

If you've got a weight problem, you're not alone. The middle years have been dubbed the "fat years" because so many women tend to gain weight during this time in their lives. According to the National Center for Health Statistics, one in four American women ages thirty-five to sixty-four is overweight (more than 20 percent over her ideal weight for her height). And unlike men, whose weight gain peaks between ages thirty-four and sixty-four, many women continue to gain weight even beyond the middle years.

If you're overweight, now's the time to take action. Several studies now suggest that *when* and *where* you put on pounds may be more important to your overall health than how many pounds you gain.

As you may have already discovered, however, the dieting patterns you relied on when you were younger don't seem to work anymore. Either the weight fails to come off altogether or, when the diet's over, the bathroom scale begins its slow, steady ascent back up to your previous weight, or beyond.

Over the years, we've developed a much more sensible approach to weight control for the middle years—one that emphasizes losing body fat and improving your body composition rather than just losing weight. During this weight-loss regimen, you needn't ever step on a bathroom scale to measure your progress. In fact, we recommend that you stay away from the scales altogether. It's possible to become too dependent on a scale, which may not always reflect the true measure of your progress. First, let's take a look at what fat is, how it affects your health and well-being, and how you came to be overweight in the first place.

What Is Fat?

What you refer to as fat is medically known as *adipose tissue*. About half of the fat in your body is located just under the skin and consists of billions of fat cells, engineered to store large amounts of energy and water. Some experts estimate that the average adult has about 30 billion adipocytes (fat cells), which hold about 135,000 calories—enough energy to live for forty to fifty days without food. Fat also provides heat insulation for the body.

Obesity (excess body fat) occurs when the calories you take in regularly exceed the calories you burn during your daily activities. The excess energy is stored as fat.

While this explanation may sound simple, anyone who's tried to lose weight knows that obesity is much more complicated than calories in equals calories out. In fact, obesity is probably caused by a combination of genetic, metabolic, environmental, psychological, and sociological factors that we're just beginning to sort out.

Actually, it's more accurate to talk about "obesities" rather than obesity, since there appear to be several types. People with enlarged fat cells are said to have *hypertrophic obesity*. (The fat cell itself is capable of storing up to 80 to 95 percent of its volume as pure *triglyceride*, which is simply a form of fat your body can use.) People with an excess number of fat cells have *hyperplastic obesity*.

The size of your fat cells changes more readily than the number, and most overweight people have enlarged fat cells, which is good, because overfilled cells can be shrunk to the point of invisibility as the fat stored in them is used up. When your fat cells are full, however, your body will make new ones. No one's sure how new fat cells are made, although high glucose and blood-insulin levels (which occur when existing fat cells are full) seem to prompt their production. We also don't know how fat you must be before your body makes new fat cells. One theory holds that biochemical differences cause some people to make new fat cells more readily than others.

Once your body makes new fat cells, you're stuck with them for life. While you can reduce the size of existing cells, you can't reduce their number (unless, of course, you have them surgically removed with a procedure called liposuction). This procedure is generally not recommended for obesity that can be treated with diet and exercise.

Obesity can also be categorized by its distribution pattern on your body, which has important implications for your health. Some people—particularly women—are more likely to accumulate fat in the buttocks, hips, and thighs, what's known as gynecoid, gluteal, or pear-shaped obesity (see Figure 15-1). Men are more prone to accumulate fat around the middle or abdomen. This pattern of obesity, known as android obesity, or having an apple-shaped body, is associated with a higher risk of hypertension, diabetes, high cholesterol, and early death. Apple-shaped women are just as likely as men to share the increased health hazards that accompany android obesity.

Good Fat, Bad Fat

Although we tend to think of fat as inherently bad, we all need a certain amount of body fat to survive. Fat allows us to store large amounts of water and energy. Women need a certain amount of body fat to menstruate, conceive, and carry a pregnancy to term. Girls need at least 20 percent of weight as body fat before they begin menstruating, which helps explain why some budding

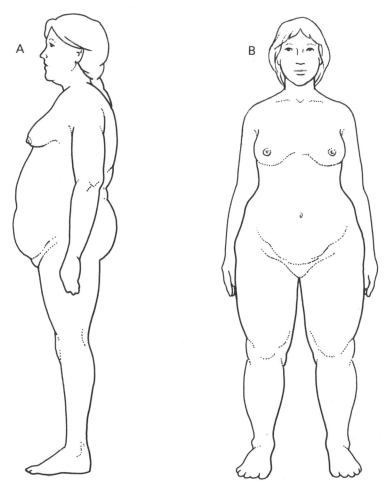

Figure 15.1   "Apple" and "Pear" Fat Distribution
(A) Apple (B) Pear

ballerinas and teenage track stars often start menstruating an average of one or two years after their nonathletic peers.

Too little body fat may also cause women to lose bone mass. And in studies investigating the relationship of body fat to longevity, severely underweight people don't fare much better than the obese.

On the other hand, too much body fat is clearly a health hazard. Most studies show that leaner people live longer. One reason for the higher mortality rate among obese people may be the increase in disease risks associated with obesity, including:

•   **Heart disease:** Your risk of heart disease increases with your weight. During one eight-year study, Harvard University researchers found that even mildly to moderately overweight women had an 80 percent increased risk of heart disease compared with the leanest women in the study.

Obesity is associated with high levels of LDL cholesterol and triglycerides and lower levels of HDL cholesterol, which helps explain the increased risk of coronary heart disease.

• **Hypertension:** People 20 percent or more overweight are three times as likely as normal-weight people to develop hypertension.

• **Diabetes:** At least 80 percent of people with Type II (noninsulin-dependent, or adult-onset) diabetes are more than 15 percent over their ideal body weight at the time of diagnosis. And the risks of diabetes—heart disease and stroke, kidney disease, blindness, and amputations due to infection—increase with the amount of body fat and its distribution.

• **Cancer:** Some population studies have shown a link between obesity and an increased risk for cancers of the breast, colon, kidney, and endometrium. Experts speculate that chemical carcinogens may be stored in body fat and somehow released into the bloodstream and transported to other tissues in the body. Hormones may play a role, too: Androgens secreted by the adrenal gland can be converted to estrogen in fat tissue, and the higher levels of estrogen in obese women may stimulate the development of breast and uterine cancers.

• **Low self-esteem:** Obesity can take a toll on your emotional well-being, too.

It's Not How Much You Weigh, but When and Where You Put on Weight

New research now shows that it's not so important how much you weigh but when and where you put on the weight that determines how risky it is to your health. And gaining weight in adulthood appears to be particularly risky. For instance, the Harvard researchers found that women who gained weight after age eighteen had about double the coronary risk of women who were heavy as teenagers but whose weight remained steady through adulthood.

As you may recall, people with apple-shaped bodies are more likely to have high blood-cholesterol levels, high insulin levels, and high blood pressure. One reason may be that abdominal fat is simply less reactive to insulin and other metabolic processes than gluteal fat and more insulin is therefore readily released into the bloodstream, where it can raise cholesterol levels.

Why Do Women Get Fat?

As we mentioned earlier, several factors working together probably contributed to your weight problem. Here's a brief look at some of the influences on your weight.

• **Your gender.** It's a biological fact: Women simply have more body fat than men (an average of 25 percent, compared to 15 percent for men.) This makes it easier for a woman to gain weight, and somewhat harder for her to lose weight, than a man.

• **Your genes.** Although no genes or genetic markers for obesity have yet been found, some people apparently inherit a genetic predisposition to obesity from their parents.

• **Your metabolism.** Over the last ten years, researchers have pinpointed several mechanisms that help regulate metabolism and that could help explain why some people may be fatter than others. These include the following:

Brown fat. This specialized type of fat cell is responsible for keeping your vital organs warm. Brown fat appears to become more or less metabolically active in response to other factors, such as cold temperatures and exercise, and because the major source of fuel for brown fat is white fat (the fat storage cells in your body), it is thought to play a role in regulating your weight.

Muscle. Muscle tissue burns calories faster and more efficiently than does fat tissue, and, generally speaking, the more muscle you have, the more active is your metabolism. This is why it is crucial that you retain as much muscle mass as you can when dieting, and lose only fat.

Enzymes. Several recent studies have shown that the activity of an enzyme in fat cells known as *lipoprotein lipase* (LPL), which takes triglycerides from the bloodstream and packs them into fat storage cells, increases after dieting. These findings suggest that your body may be programmed to refill depleted fat cells after dieting.

• **Your hormones.** Although true glandular obesity is rare, several hormones do have an impact on your weight. For instance, some researchers now believe that insulin, a hormone produced by the pancreas, may be part of an internal regulating system designed to help keep rampant obesity in check. Studies have shown that insulin directly stimulates the sympathetic nervous system, which in turn makes brown fat metabolically more active. Insulin is also known to increase heat production in your body. The researchers suspect that in these ways, insulin may help your body burn off some excess calories as heat, thus protecting against further obesity. The price you pay for this protection, however, is high insulin levels.

Thyroid hormones, which help regulate metabolism, are influenced by what you eat. Fasting decreases T4, the metabolically active thyroid hormone, which may help explain why your metabolism slows when you're fasting. When you overeat, the thyroid excretes more T4, and metabolism increases. In spite of the connection between the thyroid gland and metabolism, problems with the thyroid gland are *rarely* a cause of obesity. Moreover, while in the past thyroid medications have been given to some dieters to speed up their metabolism and help them lose weight, the treatment has potential side effects, including heart problems and increased calcium excretion, which could lead to osteoporosis.

The reproductive hormones estrogen and progesterone may also influence your weight. Estrogen causes you to deposit increased quantities of fat, particularly in the breasts, hips, buttocks, and thighs. Progesterone may somehow stimulate your appetite; studies have shown that women tend to eat more during the second half of the menstrual cycle, when progesterone levels rise.

• **Your age.** For reasons that are not entirely clear, your metabolism slows as you grow older. One reason may have to do with certain physical changes associated with aging—in particular, the loss of muscle mass. (The average woman can expect to lose about one percent of muscle mass per year after age 30, which is usually replaced with fat.) Since muscle is more metabolically active than fat, metabolism may slow as muscle mass declines.

•   **Your appetite.** The controls for hunger and satiety, or the body's *appestat*, may be somehow short-circuited in overweight people. Hunger and satiety are regulated by the hypothalamus (the part of the brain that controls such basic needs as hunger, thirst, and sex drive); certain neurotransmitters in the brain (particularly norepinephrine, which stimulates appetite, and serotonin, which suppresses it); the stomach, which signals the brain that you've had enough to eat via several chemical messengers; the liver; and fat itself, which may somehow indirectly communicate a feeling of fullness to the brain. Of course, if your mouth has ever started watering at the sight or smell of food, you know that external cues can trigger your appestat, as well.

If you are beginning to feel that your weight problems are beyond your control, don't despair. Neither your gender, your genes, nor any of these other contributing factors mean that you are necessarily fated to be fat. In fact, sensible eating habits (ones that don't deprive you *too* much) combined with a regular exercise program can help counteract most of the forces that may have contributed to your weight problem. Remember: Even if your parents were overweight and you have inherited their "fat genes," your environment—specifically, your diet and exercise patterns—combined with your genetic makeup, will ultimately determine how much you weigh. And while you can't choose your parents, you can certainly choose what you eat and how much you exercise. Exercise can also help counter the loss of muscle mass associated with aging (and chronic dieting), and even the postdieting effects of lipoprotein lipase. Some people find exercise to be an effective appetite suppressant, as well. Before we tell you more about the ways in which you can lose weight, take a few moments to size up the problem and set some sensible goals for yourself.

How Fat Are You and How Much Should You Weigh?

How do you know whether you have a weight problem? Until now, you probably weighed yourself on a bathroom scale (or your doctor's) and compared your total weight for your height against the "ideal" weights in standard height and weight tables (see page 472). While it's a start, traditional scales and weight tables don't distinguish between overweight and overfat. And as you've already seen, excessive body fat, not weight per se, is associated with increased health risks of heart disease, high blood pressure, diabetes, and some cancers.

Remember, too, that it's possible to be normal weight and still be overfat. It's also possible to lose weight on a diet without losing fat. And if you combine dieting with exercise, you may gain muscle and lose fat without seeing a change in your total weight on the scale.

The most accurate way to assess your weight—and monitor the effectiveness of your weight-loss efforts—is to determine your percentage of body fat.

Start by determining your body-mass index (page 29). A health professional may also use skin-fold calipers or one of the other methods described in Chapter 3 to determine your body composition. Now compare your percentage of body fat with the norms for women your age (see Table A.1 on page 472) to determine your ideal percentage of body fat.

You'll notice from this table that as you grow older, your percentage of body fat rises somewhat. This means that even with your best efforts, you probably *won't* get your total weight down to the level it was, say, in your twenties or thirties. If you accept this fact right from the start, you're likely to set more realistic weight-loss goals. You'll be much more likely to succeed at your effort, too.

Remember, too, that your bone size and the amount of muscle you have (which are genetically determined) also factor into your overall weight and your percentage of body fat. If you have large bones and quite a bit of muscle, you may not be able to reach the ideal weight suggested in weight tables. Genetics may make it difficult for some women to reach their ideal percentage of body fat, too. Keep in mind that if you don't reach your goal, *even a 10 percent drop in your weight will improve your overall health*. So don't be discouraged; *almost any weight loss is better than none.*

Before beginning your weight-loss regimen, check with your physician or another qualified health professional (such as a registered dietitian) to ensure that your goals are realistic.

There's much we don't know about the causes of obesity. We know for certain that your body follows the basic laws of thermodynamics—energy in equals energy out—in other words, excess body fat almost always results from chronically consuming more calories in a day than you use during your normal activities. These excess calories are stored as fat. To lose weight, you'll need to create a calorie deficit, in which you take in fewer calories than you expend. This forces your body to draw on existing fat stores to meet its energy needs. To do this, you can either take in fewer calories by eating less food, burn more calories by increasing your physical activity, or both.

Cutting Calories

By far, the most popular way to lose weight is to cut calories. It's also one of the fastest ways to lose weight. But as you'll soon see, dieting alone is not the best way to maintain your weight once you've lost it. Indeed, dieting in itself can ultimately be a setup for failure. When you starve yourself, your body undergoes a series of adaptive changes that tend to conserve energy, glucose, and protein to prolong survival. Frequent crash diets lead to improvements in your body's adaptive responses, so with each dieting episode, the rate of weight loss is slower and, once you return to your normal eating habits, the rate of weight gain is more rapid. Crash dieting also may lead to changes in your body's appestat (appetite-regulating mechanisms), resulting in a tendency to overeat after the diet's over.

Nevertheless, dieting can be a powerful weight-loss tool—particularly when combined with exercise. The dieting approach you take depends on how overweight you are (see How Fat Are You and How Much Should You Weigh? on the opposite page).

If You Are Mildly Overweight

In some sense, it's harder to lose a little weight than a lot. The weight often comes off more slowly when you have less to lose. If you've become a chronic dieter, you may find you gain weight right back after you stop dieting. What makes the task even more complicated is the vast array of diet programs and diet books, all promising a quick fix to your weight problem.

Many mildly obese women who sought help at our clinic for their weight problems were disappointed to find that they *weren't fat enough* to be considered for the very-low-calorie diets popularized by talk-show host Oprah Winfrey. Indeed, while these diets (described on the next page) are considered safe and effective for moderately obese people, they can be dangerous when used by mildly overweight people. When calories are severely restricted, mildly overweight people tend to lose more muscle than do the severely obese. Large losses of muscle can have disastrous consequences, including disturbances of heart function and damage to other organs. Losing muscle may also decrease your resting metabolic rate, making it more difficult to maintain a desirable weight after the diet's over. (To get around some of these problems, Kathryn Parker, R.D., our clinic's registered dietitian, developed "Slim-Trim," an adaptation of the very-low-calorie diets that can be used by women with just a little weight to lose, also described on the next page.)

If you're committed to making changes in your eating and exercise habits, however, your chances of successfully taking the weight off and keeping it off are pretty good.

It's best to work with your physician and a dietitian any time you plan to lose weight—even if you want to lose just a few pounds. Your doctor can make sure you're in good physical health. A dietitian can counsel you on the most effective ways to lose weight.

If you can't see a dietitian and are wondering how to make sense of the hundreds of diet programs and diet books available to you, keep the following guidelines in mind:

• **Don't cut calories too severely.** Most adults can safely lose weight on a diet of one thousand to twelve hundred calories a day (if you have a large body frame or are physically active, you may need fifteen hundred to eighteen hundred calories a day). *Diets providing fewer than one thousand calories a day can be dangerous and should not be attempted without medical supervision.*

• **Choose foods high in nutrients and low in calories and fat.** Ideal choices are raw vegetables, some fruits, and complex carbohydrates (rice, pasta, whole-grain breads, and cereals).

• **Take a multivitamin supplement.** It's almost impossible to get all the nutrients you need on a diet providing fewer than twelve hundred calories a day.

• **Beware of diet programs promising a weight loss of more than one to two pounds a week.** Most of the weight you lose will probably be water, which you'll gain right back after the diet's over. Most experts agree that a healthy rate of weight loss is one to two pounds a week.

• **Eat the majority of your calories early in the day.** This way, the calories you eat are more likely to be used for energy than stored as fat.

• **Be prepared to change your eating and exercise habits—permanently.** Guidelines can be found on page 299.

"Slim-Trim"
When an increasing number of mildly obese women came to our clinic anxious to see quick weight-loss results, Kathryn Parker developed a weight-loss program just for them. We call it "Slim-Trim." The program, a modification of the very-low-calorie diets used by more obese women (described below), involves drinking three high-protein shakes per day and eating one seven-hundred-calorie meal plus a snack. We recommend that you eat your meal at lunchtime. This way, you'll burn off some of the calories as energy during the day and will avoid the "triglyceride bulge" (described on page 58).

Over the course of the six-week program, the number of shakes is reduced and the amount of food increased. Throughout the program, patients learn how to break old eating habits and learn new ones.

Rather than using just the scales to measure their progress, patients rely on girth measurements and other means of determining body composition. This helps ensure that they're losing *fat* rather than muscle.

Patients who exercise while they're dieting have the best results, losing an average of two to three pounds (of fat) per week. Sedentary patients lose less rapidly, roughly one to two pounds per week.

If You Are Moderately Overweight

If you're more than 30 percent over your ideal weight (or more than twenty-five pounds overweight), you may be a candidate for a very-low-calorie diet. These diets—which are really modified fasts containing enough protein and nutrients to keep you healthy—provide the quickest way to lose weight without losing vital muscle mass. Today's very-low-calorie (VLC) diets are much safer than the high-protein diets developed in the mid- to late 1970s, which were associated with at least fifty-eight deaths. But they're not for everybody. And they're not without risks.

Very-low-calorie diets aren't safe for people who are mildly overweight. The diets also won't work for people who aren't ready to change their diet and exercise habits permanently. In fact, losing weight is often the easy part; keeping the weight off is the real challenge.

The greatest potential risk occurs in people who undertake these diets without medical supervision—particularly the low-caloric diets that can be bought over the counter. Some people might restrict their consumption of conventional foods to fewer than the recommended eight hundred calories per day. Or they may rely on the commercially available powdered diets as their sole source of nutrition rather than eating one sensible meal per day, as the makers of these products advise.

As a result, these people may suffer such short-term complications as dehydration, electrolyte imbalance, postural hypotension (low blood pressure when you stand up), and increased uric-acid concentrations, which could lead to gout. These complications—as well as other common complaints, including fatigue, dizziness, muscle cramping, headache, gastrointestinal problems, and cold intolerance—can be quickly identified and readily managed by your physician.

A doctor's supervision is particularly important during "refeeding," since too much food after severe calorie restriction can lead to cardiac arrhythmias. Many of the fifty-eight deaths associated with liquid protein diets of the mid- to late 1970s occurred during early refeeding, within the two-week period when the dieters discontinued their consumption of liquid protein and returned to conventional foods.

For the diet to be most effective, your program should include a trained physician, who can monitor your weight loss and ensure that the diet isn't endangering your health; a dietitian, who can help educate you about healthful food choices once you begin eating again; and a behavioral psychologist, who can help you change the eating habits that may have helped contribute to your weight problem in the first place. This will improve your odds of keeping the weight off once you go off the diet.

The long-term effectiveness of these diets is still being debated. Generally speaking, women who learn new eating habits as they lose weight do better than those who diet alone. However, many women *do* regain some of the weight they lost after the diet is over. Remember that even if you regain some weight, the risks to your health will still be substantially lower than if you never lost weight at all.

What to Expect
You should undergo a medical examination and electrocardiogram before beginning the diet. If you've recently had a heart attack or stroke, suffer from arrhythmias (abnormal heart rhythms), or have had kidney or liver disease, cancer, insulin-dependent diabetes, or serious psychiatric problems, this diet is not recommended.

After a complete physical, including an electrocardiogram, your doctor may recommend that you spend two to four weeks on a twelve-hundred-calorie balance diet. This allows you to adjust to a lower calorie intake. The gradual loss of water weight in these few weeks will also help prevent the rapid sodium loss that occurs if you abruptly started the VLC diet. Generally speaking, if you do well on this diet, you will probably do well on the VLC diet—and in sustaining weight loss after the diet is over.

Most very-low-calorie diets involve drinking three to five high-protein shakes per day, equalling four hundred to eight hundred calories. During the diet, you will eat no food at all. Another version of the VLC diet is a protein-sparing modified fast (PSMF), in which you eat three or four meals a day consisting of only lean meat, fish, or fowl. No carbohydrates are permitted and fat is restricted to what's in the meat you eat.

During both diets, you must drink at least two quarts of water a day to prevent dehydration. The diet usually continues for twelve to sixteen weeks. During this time, you'll undergo blood tests at least every other week to monitor electrolytes and other critical variables. After every twenty-four pounds of weight you lose (or every month on the diet), you should undergo an electrocardiogram, as well.

It's not unusual to feel fatigue and experience mild postural hypotension. If you become constipated, your doctor may allow you to take mild laxatives or eat fiber-rich, low-calorie vegetables.

You can expect to lose within four to eight pounds during the first week of the diet, much of which will be water weight. After the first week, you will lose an average of two to three pounds per week. Heavier people may experience even greater losses.

When you've reached your desired weight (or after three months on the diet), you'll gradually be reintroduced to foods: Milk and milk products will be allowed first, followed by vegetables, cereals, and fruits. Carbohydrates, particularly simple sugars, must be reintroduced slowly to avoid an abrupt gain of fluid weight.

This period of refeeding is crucial in helping you learn new eating habits to help keep the weight off. We recommend that you meet with a registered dietitian, who can help you come up with ways to solve the problems and overcome any obstacles that may be keeping you from reaching your goal.

Just as important is increased physical activity, which will be discussed later in this chapter.

If You Are Severely Overweight

For severely overweight people who've failed repeatedly using VLC diets and other methods, "stomach stapling" and other types of surgery may be an option. But surgery should be considered only as a last resort for people who are one hundred pounds or more overweight and who have a life-threatening complication of obesity that has been proven to benefit from weight loss, such as non-insulin-dependent diabetes, hypertension, congestive heart failure, sleep apnea (periodic stoppage of breathing during sleep), or problems affecting the weight-bearing joints, such as arthritis.

The advantages of such a drastic approach to weight loss are many: Most people with non-insulin-dependent diabetes will experience almost a total cure of the disease. Blood pressure and blood-cholesterol levels drop to much safer levels, and problems with sleep apnea are usually resolved after the surgery.

Several different methods of surgically treating obesity have been used over the years, but only two procedures are considered safe and effective today. Each has several advantages and disadvantages.

• **Gastric bypass:** The stomach is separated into two compartments, each closed by four rows of staples. The upper (and much smaller) compartment has a capacity of less than two ounces. A new outlet is created in this small portion of the stomach and connected to the lower part of the small intestine. Food entering the new "small stomach" causes a sensation of fullness, then slowly empties into the intestine through the new outlet. This rerouting causes food to bypass the lower part of the stomach. Digestive juices from the lower stomach combine with food in the lower part of the small intestine, thus permitting digestion of the food.

One advantage of this procedure is that food enters the small intestine directly after leaving the stomach pouch. As a result, most patients who have had gastric bypass experience unpleasant feelings of shakiness, sweating, and palpitations (what's known as the "dumping syndrome") when they eat sweet foods, such as refined sugars, ice cream, and soft drinks. This can be so unpleasant that the patient will never want to try these foods again. In effect, the operation provides a built-in reminder to stay away from such fattening foods. The procedure also cures heartburn caused by a hiatus hernia. Heartburn is caused by stomach acid refluxing up into the esophagus. Since most stomach acid is made in the part of the stomach below the staple line, acid can no longer reflux up the esophagus after gastric bypass.

On the other hand, some patients will develop anemia and a calcium deficiency after a number of years because of reduced absorption of iron, vitamin B_{12}, and calcium. Because of this, lifelong multivitamin and mineral supplements are essential for all patients who have had gastric bypass surgery.

• **Vertical-banded gastroplasty:** This is a newer and much more successful modification of gastric bypass. In this procedure, four staple rows are placed vertically in the upper part of the stomach. The lower end of the pouch created by the staple rows becomes the outlet of the "new stomach" and is encircled by a fine silicone ring, which effectively prevents the opening from ever enlarging.

Because the operation doesn't bypass part of the small intestine, you're not as likely to develop anemia or other nutrient deficiencies years later. However, because this operation doesn't cause "dumping," it may be easier for patients to resume poor dietary habits once the initial weight loss has been achieved.

Of course, any surgery carries risks, including such anesthesia-related complications as pulmonary embolism (blood clot in the lungs) thrombophlebitis, cardiac complications, and wound-healing problems. These risks are significantly greater among the obese than in patients of normal weight. In addition, the procedures themselves involve certain risks. These include injury to the spleen, requiring surgical removal of the spleen, and perforations of the stomach and leakage within the first ten days of surgery, which requires immediate reoperation. Some patients (about 2 percent) develop a peptic ulcer either in the stomach, duodenum (upper part of the small intestine), or, more commonly, at the new stomach outlet. The ulcer can usually be healed with medication. Rarely is surgery required.

You should be aware, too, that the surgery doesn't always permanently solve your weight problems. Usually, you will reach your lowest weight between eighteen and twenty-four months after the surgery. While many regain some of the weight over the next four or five years, most people will keep off about one-third of their preoperative weight.

Exercise: The Energy Connection

Many dieters never consider the *other* way to tip the energy-balance equation in their favor: exercise. However, our clinical experience and a growing body of research now show that no weight-loss program is complete without it. Exercise helps burn calories and *fat*, while helping you to retain vital muscle mass. Some studies suggest that exercise raises your metabolism for several hours after strenuous physical activity. And while other studies have shown the change in postexercise metabolism is negligible, we do know that dieters who exercise are less likely to experience the slowdown in their metabolism that appears to be a natural response to dieting. Adding exercise to your weight-loss program may also increase compliance with your diet, since you won't have to cut calories as severely as when you diet alone, and since exercise actually acts as an appetite suppressant for some people. Finally, exercise counteracts many of the increased health risks associated with obesity, including heart disease, hypertension, and diabetes.

Some women find that increasing their physical activity alone may be all they need to lose weight. However, the weight comes off much more slowly this way; for those who want to lose weight quickly, dieting combined with exercise is probably the most efficient and effective way to shed pounds. Women who exercise while dieting lose weight more rapidly than sedentary dieters. What's more, those who continue to exercise after the diet is over are more likely to keep the weight off than nonexercisers.

Incorporating Exercise into Your Weight-Loss Program

If you want to get the weight off and keep it off, you'll need to participate in a regular program of physical activity. Not just any activity will do: While muscle-strengthening exercises help build vital muscle mass, they don't do much to reduce body fat. On the other hand, low-impact aerobic activities—walking, bicycling, and swimming—burn fat. For this reason, these types of activities should be the major component of your weight-loss program.

Keep in mind that the rules are a little different when you're exercising to reduce your weight. While a twenty-minute aerobic workout is enough to increase your cardiovascular fitness, you'll have to work out a little longer—at least forty-five minutes per session—to lose weight. During the first thirty minutes of exercise, your body relies mainly on glycogen—stored sugars in the muscles—for energy. Only after glycogen stores are depleted does your body start drawing on fat reserves for energy. For this reason, you should choose low-impact activities that can be sustained for longer periods of time. Brisk walking and bicycling (including the use of a stationary bicycle) are ideal.

These low-impact activities are well suited to the overweight for another reason: High-impact activities, such as jogging and running, can place unnecessary strain on the knees, hips, ankles, and joints, thus increasing your risk of musculoskeletal injuries.

What about spot reducing? Exercising only those areas of your body with the most fat makes sense in theory: It is believed that, in some way, disuse of a muscle group causes a disproportionate storage of fat in that area. However, studies comparing the fat content of the right and left forearms of high-caliber tennis players show that the amount of fat in both the dominant playing arm and the nondominant arm was essentially the same. So doing one hundred situps a day probably won't be sufficient to melt away the fat around your abdomen and waist.

Exercise Guidelines for the Overweight

For the most part, being overweight—even up to 130 percent over your ideal body weight—poses no greater medical risk to participating in regular aerobic exercise than that of normal-weight people, provided you have no risks of major coronary heart disease (elevated cholesterol levels, hypertension, cigarette smoking, or an abnormal ECG). Nevertheless, you should undergo a physical examination by your doctor before embarking on an exercise program, particularly if you have any of the risk factors for heart disease we just mentioned. If you're over forty-five, you should have a graded exercise stress test, as well.

If you're one hundred pounds or more overweight, however, you're considered to be at risk for both cardiovascular and musculoskeletal problems, and you should proceed with caution. Begin an exercise program *only* under your doctor's supervision. The same basic guidelines for beginning an exercise program apply whether you're normal weight or overweight—start out slowly, warm up before exercising, and cool down afterward. These guidelines are especially important if you're overweight.

1. Start slowly. Overweight people have a considerably lower tolerance for physical activity than people of normal weight. So the first part of your exercise program should simply get you accustomed to the increased physical activity. If you're walking, start out with a few three- to five-minute walks per day, gradually working your way up to longer periods of continuous walking. It may take eight to twelve weeks of this kind of progressive training before you can continuously walk two miles.

2. Warm up. It's a good idea to stretch your muscles and limber up for several minutes before beginning the conditioning phase of exercise. However, excess body weight may make it uncomfortable for you to do certain stretches and calisthenics for long periods of time. If an activity (such as touching your toes) feels uncomfortable to you, avoid doing it until you've lost a little weight.

Many experts recommend a cardiovascular warm-up in addition to flexibility exercises before engaging in strenuous physical activity. This probably won't be necessary if you plan to engage in such low-intensity activities as walking and bicycling.

3. Cool down. You should allow five to ten minutes of progressively more mild exercise at the end of your session to allow your heart rate and breathing to return to normal levels, particularly if you have been exercising strenuously. Cooling down also helps prevent blood from pooling in the legs, a problem that may be exacerbated in the overweight.

4. Choose your exercise environment carefully. If you're overweight, you may tend to become overheated easily, particularly when you're just starting out. To prevent overheating, drink plenty of fluids before and during your exercise session. If you're working out indoors, make sure the room temperature is cool. If you're using a stationary bicycle, set up a fan near the bicycle to keep you cool. (Some bicycles now come equipped with a fan.) If exercising outdoors, avoid working out in the heat of the day.

Wear lightweight and loose-fitting clothing so that air can circulate between your skin and clothes, helping to cool you. Cottons and linens are better at wicking away moisture from the skin (and keeping you cooler) than clothing containing plastic or rubber (Spandex).

Weight Control: A Way of Life

By far the most difficult part of losing weight is keeping it off for good. Essentially, this means changing your eating and exercise habits not just for a few weeks but for the rest of your life—a tall order even for the most diligent among us.

This is where behavior modification comes in—techniques that help you change the lifestyle habits that may have contributed to your weight problem. Of more than one hundred controlled studies testing behavioral approaches to weight control, many have shown greater and more sustained weight losses among people who received some kind of professional counseling or training in changing their lifestyle habits. Most diet programs, including Weight Watchers, NutriSystem, Medifast, and even fad diets now emphasize the importance of behavioral changes as a key to taking weight off and keeping it off.

Again, if you're losing weight under the guidance of your doctor, a dietitian, or one of the structured weight-loss programs (such as Weight Watchers), these professionals can offer individual or group counseling to help you identify and change some of the habits that may have made you fat in the first place. You may be able to recognize and change some of these habits yourself, too.

Start by becoming aware of your eating habits and activity patterns. Before beginning a diet, keep a record for at least two weeks of what you eat, when and where you eat, what you are doing and how you feel when you're eating. After about two weeks, you'll probably see some patterns emerging. For instance, you may find that you tend to eat snacks while watching television. Or perhaps you turn to ice cream for solace after an argument. These circumstances may trigger an eating response, and your goal is to stop this from happening by creating new associations to replace your previously established patterns of behavior.

Once you understand some of your key eating behaviors, you can begin to substitute different ones. For example, instead of eating snacks in front of the television, try sewing, painting, or writing letters while watching TV. Better yet, set up a stationary bicycle in front of the TV and exercise while watching television. Or try doing ten jumping jacks or taking a brisk walk after an argument instead of eating ice cream.

You can take the same approach to changing your level of physical activity. Keep a record of all your daily activities—including such minimal activities as sleeping and eating—for seven days. Then look for ways to replace your sedentary habits with physical activity. For instance, if you drive to work, park your car a half mile away and walk the remaining distance. Instead of going to a restaurant for lunch, take a thirty- to forty-five-minute walk.

A good reinforcement for dieters: At the start of your diet, wear clothing that fits and feels snug. As soon as these clothes begin to fit comfortably, get rid of the larger sizes you were wearing and start wearing the outfits in your closet that still feel tight.

A Final Word

Losing weight may be one of the toughest challenges you face. But by setting reasonable goals, dieting sensibly, working with your physician, and—perhaps most important of all—keeping physically active, you can do it. Your reward will be better health and an improved sense of well-being, which is well worth your efforts when you consider the toll that obesity can take on your health.

Suggested Reading

Bailey, Covert. *Fit or Fat?* Boston: Houghton Mifflin Co., 1984.
Mirkin, Gabe, M.D. *Getting Thin: All About Fat.* New York: Little, Brown and Company, 1983.

Resources and Support

Weight Watchers International, Jericho Atrium, 500 North Broadway, Jericho, NY 11753-2196. This organization hosts group meetings that offer a nutritionally sound weight-loss program as well as plenty of emotional support for people who need to lose weight. Look in the phone book for a local affiliate or contact Weight Watchers International at the address here for more information.

Taking Off Pounds Sensibly (TOPS) Club, 4575 South Fifth Street, P.O. Box 07360, Milwaukee, WI 53207. Phone: (414) 482-4620. This organization provides group therapy for people who want to lose weight. Members are required to use physician-approved individual eating plans and physician-set weight loss goals. Check your phone directory for a local chapter or write to the national office at the above address.

Overeaters Anonymous, P.O. Box 92870, Los Angeles, CA 90009. Phone: (213) 542-8363. This support group for compulsive overeaters is based on the 12-Step Program of Alcoholics Anonymous. Check your phone directory for a support group near you or contact the national headquarters for more information.

Chapter 16

Cardiovascular Disease

People tend to think of heart disease as a "man's" illness. But cardiovascular disease is the leading cause of death for women, too. Because women are "protected" by estrogen before menopause, the prevalence of cardiovascular disease lags behind that of men by about a decade. However, by about age seventy, the rate in men and women is about the same. In terms of its absolute effect on women's health, cardiovascular disease is a primary concern: *Almost 50 percent of all deaths among women in the United States is due to cardiovascular disease.*

Too often, even the medical profession doesn't take women's heart problems seriously. Two recent studies have shown that physicians generally are less aggressive in their management of coronary disease in women than in men, despite the fact that coronary disease is often more serious and more disabling for women than for men.

We take your heart problems *very* seriously. You should, too—especially since there's a tremendous amount you can do to reduce your risk of cardiovascular disease. The sooner you begin, the better off you'll be. High blood pressure, or hypertension, a major risk factor for heart attacks and strokes, can often be brought under control by losing a few pounds, exercising regularly, and watching your salt intake. We're now discovering that another major form of cardiovascular disease, *atherosclerosis* (progressive narrowing of the arteries—particularly the coronary arteries that nourish the heart muscle), can be slowed and even reversed with such lifestyle changes as a low-fat diet, regular exercise, and stress management.

Cardiovascular disease is a broad term describing many different problems with the heart and circulatory system. The most worrisome for women in midlife are high blood pressure (hypertension), coronary heart disease, and stroke. The program for prevention of cardiovascular disease described in the pages that follow will help protect you from these potential killers.

Hypertension

If there's one type of heart disease that's an equal-opportunity killer, it's hypertension, or high blood pressure. Half of the 58 million Americans with hypertension are women. And while we're not sure why, *after menopause your chances of having high blood pressure are greater than a man's.*

Simply put, blood pressure is the force of blood on the artery walls as it is pumped from the heart. When you have high blood pressure, the arteries that help maintain blood pressure by dilating and contracting as needed remain constricted. As a result, your heart and arteries must strain to pump blood through your body. The heart may eventually enlarge and the arteries may become scarred, hardened, and less elastic. The reduced blood flow means that other organs don't get the nutrients and oxygen they need. Your heart, brain, and kidneys are particularly susceptible to damage by high blood pressure. If left untreated, hypertension can lead to heart failure, stroke, kidney damage, and more.

Making a Diagnosis

Hypertension is often called a "silent" killer because it is virtually symptomless. Many people have high blood pressure for years without knowing it. That's why it's paramount to have your blood pressure checked periodically. Most physicians now regularly check your blood pressure every time you visit.

A blood pressure reading consists of two numbers written as a fraction: The top number (*systolic* pressure) represents the force of blood on the arteries as the heart contracts; the bottom number (*diastolic* pressure) is blood pressure when the heart is at rest. A reading of 120/80 is about normal for most people.

If your doctor finds that your blood pressure is elevated during a routine office visit, it doesn't necessarily mean you have high blood pressure. Your blood pressure varies widely over time, depending on many variables. Blood pressure often rises when you are nervous or excited, for example, but normally it goes down again almost immediately. Indeed, some 15 percent of people with mildly elevated blood pressure may suffer from what's called "white-coat hypertension," in which their blood pressure is elevated only at the doctor's office. If your blood pressure is above 140/90, your physician will want to measure it again on at least two subsequent visits before making a diagnosis of hypertension.

Most people with elevated blood pressure have what is known as *essential* or *primary* hypertension, which has no known cause. However, about 5 percent of people with high blood pressure have *secondary hypertension*—high blood pressure that is a symptom of an underlying medical problem, which, when treated, causes blood pressure to return to normal. If your blood pressure doesn't fall after drug therapy, or if your blood pressure suddenly worsens, your physician may look for an underlying cause.

Can your blood pressure be *too low*? Some women, particularly the elderly, do have a problem with *postural hypotension,* a sudden drop in blood pressure when they stand up too quickly or get out of bed in the morning. What happens when you stand or sit up from a lying position is that gravity pulls the blood to your extremities and your brain is temporarily left without an adequate blood supply. The problem may be compounded in older women by the decline in cerebral blood flow that naturally occurs with age, by illness, and by certain medications (see pages 304–305). The danger is dizziness, which could cause you to lose your balance and lead to a fall. Some women may actually faint. Older women and those at high risk of osteoporosis should have their blood pressure checked while seated and again while standing to see whether this is a problem for them. A drop in systolic blood pressure greater than or equal to twenty points and a ten-point drop in diastolic pressure means you have postural hypotension. Otherwise, low blood pressure is generally not a problem. (For tips on coping with postural hypotension, see page 304.)

A Lifestyle for Lowering Blood Pressure

Fortunately, most cases of high blood pressure respond well to a few sensible lifestyle changes. If you have mild to moderate hypertension, your physician will probably recommend that you start with these strategies for lowering your blood pressure:

1. **Shake the salt habit.** From one-third to one-half of all people with hypertension are salt-sensitive; that is, their blood pressure rises when on a high-sodium diet and falls on a low-sodium one. You may find that lowering your sodium intake to about 1 teaspoon per day (2,000 milligrams) is all you need to do to control your blood pressure. (For tips on reducing the sodium in your diet, see page 74.)

2. **Keep up your calcium intake.** Several population studies have associated a low calcium intake with high blood pressure. Moreover, calcium supplements totalling 1,500 milligrams per day have been shown to lower blood pressure in hypertensive men. Although more evidence is needed before we can start prescribing calcium supplements to help control blood pressure, it can't hurt to make sure you're getting plenty of calcium in your diet. (See Chapter 4 for ways to increase the calcium content of your diet.)

3. **Lose weight.** Overweight women are two to three times more likely to develop high blood pressure than normal-weight women. Usually when your weight drops, your blood pressure falls to a more healthy level, too. (For hints on losing weight, see Chapter 15.)

4. **Exercise.** Regular moderate exercise has been shown to be *as effective as medication* for lowering mildly to moderately elevated blood pressure. Even if you take drugs to lower your blood pressure, you can often reduce the amount you take by exercising regularly.

If you have high blood pressure and want to begin an exercise program, you should do so *only* after you've had a complete medical evaluation by your physician, and only under your doctor's supervision. (See Chapter 5 for instructions on beginning an exercise program.)

5. **Cut back on alcohol.** You've probably heard that alcohol helps protect against cardiovascular disease. This is not necessarily so when it comes to hypertension. Consuming three or more drinks per day is associated with

•   Get up slowly after sitting or lying down to reduce dizziness and the risk of falling. Ideally, you should rise slowly from a lying to sitting position and wait a few minutes before standing. You should stand *only* when there is support available to prevent you from falling.

•   Wear elasticized support hose to help keep blood from pooling in the legs and to help circulate blood back up toward the brain when you stand.

•   Avoid alcohol, which can aggravate postural hypotension.

•   Don't stay in bed because you feel dizzy—this will only perpetuate the problem. Rather, try the following prestanding exercises before getting out of bed in the morning.

1. Sit up in bed, letting your feet hang over the side of the bed. Flex your feet up toward you five or six times. This exercise prevents blood from pooling in your feet by stimulating the veins in your calves to pump blood back up toward your heart.
2. Tense and relax your abdominal muscles several times. This exercise also helps encourage blood flow from the lower extremities back toward the upper body.
3. Tense the muscles in your hands and arms several times by making a fist. Or squeeze tennis balls with your hands. These isometric exercises are some of the most potent stimulators of blood pressure.

•   If hot baths, steam baths, saunas, and whirlpools make you feel dizzy, avoid them. Heat dilates the blood vessels in the skin and lowers your blood pressure.

•   Drink plenty of fluids, particularly when flying on airlines, in hot weather, and when you have a diarrheal illness or the flu. These conditions can cause you to lose fluids and become dehydrated, which will make the problem worse.

•   Try elevating the head of your bed by stacking books or two-inch by six-inch blocks under the legs of the bed.

•   If you take one of the medications listed here that's associated with postural hypotension, ask your physician if you can switch to another medication that doesn't have this side effect.

If you take . . .	*Ask about switching to . . .*
Antihypertensive medications	
Diuretics; clonidine (Catapress); guanabenz (Wytensin); methyldopa (Aldomet); prazosin (Minipress); terazosin (Hytrin)	Calcium channel blockers; ACE inhibitors; beta-blockers; hydralazine (Apresazide, Apresoline, Hydra-Zide, Resorpine, Ser-Ap-Es)

• Your physician may also recommend that you take salt tablets (take these only under the supervision of your doctor, since excessive sodium can *increase* blood pressure in some susceptible people) or other medications that may help improve postural hypotension.

an *increased* incidence of hypertension. One study found that women who consumed more than three drinks per day increased their risk of developing hypertension by 90 percent. For this reason, if you have high blood pressure, you should limit your alcohol intake to *no more than two drinks per day* (one drink equals one ounce of hard liquor, four ounces of wine, or twelve ounces of beer). Better yet, cut out alcohol from your lifestyle altogether (tips for sensible social drinking—and stopping altogether—can be found in Chapter 7).

6. **Control stress.** Many people think of high blood pressure as a "stress" disease, caused by overworking and other modern-day pressures. Some studies *have* suggested that chronic stress can lead to permanent increases in heart rate and blood pressure. That's not to say that stress *causes* hypertension. As we mentioned earlier, we don't know yet what causes high blood pressure. But stress can contribute to the problem.

On the other hand, relaxation techniques, such as deep breathing, progressive muscular relaxation, yoga, meditation, and biofeedback can help undo the effects of stress on your body. Relaxation techniques have been found to reduce blood pressure by several points when used in the treatment of hypertension— the higher the blood pressure to begin with, the greater the drop that occurs.

More long-term studies are needed before relaxation therapy can be recommended for the treatment of hypertension. But if you have mild hypertension, you may want to try some of these techniques (for details, see Chapter 6) in conjunction with other nondrug therapies. They can't hurt, and they just might help.

Common Antihypertensive Medications

If your diastolic blood pressure is higher than 95, or if lifestyle measures fail to lower even mildly elevated blood pressure, your physician may recommend one of several types of antihypertensive drugs to help bring down your blood pressure, including thiazide diuretics, beta-blockers, ACE inhibitors, and calcium channel blockers. Beta-blockers, ACE inhibitors, and another class of drugs occasionally used to treat hypertension, known as *central alpha agonists*, may also reduce the likelihood of *left ventricle hypertrophy*, a condition in which the heart wall thickens and that can lead to congestive heart failure. The only antihypertensive drugs that *don't* have this protective effect are diuretics. For this reason, your physician may prescribe a small amount of diuretics along with other antihypertensive medications.

Estrogen has also been found to lower blood pressure in postmenopausal women. In a study we conducted on the effects of estrogen therapy and exercise on blood pressure, women who took oral estrogen alone experienced nearly a 4 percent decline in systolic blood pressure. (The estrogen patch also lowered blood pressure—but by only 1.5 percent.) The combination of estrogen and exercise really packed a one-two punch: These women experienced a 6 percent decline in blood pressure. Still, our findings are preliminary, and while it's probably safe for women with hypertension to take estrogen to help ease menopausal symptoms and protect their bones, more research needs to be conducted before estrogen is *routinely* prescribed to help lower blood pressure.

You may have to visit your doctor as often as once a week when you first start taking your blood pressure medication to ensure that the drug is working properly and that you're not suffering any adverse side effects. If you have mild hypertension that has been kept in check with drug therapy for at least a year, your physician may gradually reduce the amount of medication you take, particularly if you also have been using nondrug methods (diet, exercise, weight loss) to help control your blood pressure. However, regular medical checkups are a must, since blood pressure can rise again to hypertensive levels, even after years without therapy.

Coronary Heart Disease

Although coronary heart disease affects more men than women, it's still the leading cause of death for women in the United States today. Coronary heart disease occurs when the arteries that supply oxygen and nutrients to the heart muscle become narrowed or blocked.

How do the arteries become constricted? Some thickening and hardening of the arteries is a part of normal aging, a process called *arteriosclerosis*. Far more insidious, however, is *atherosclerosis,* a type of arteriosclerosis in which deposits of fatty substances, cholesterol, cellular waste products, calcium, and fibrin (the tough fibers of a blood clot) build up on the inner lining of the artery, forming a hard *plaque*. As plaques grow larger, they reduce the flow of blood through the arteries (see Figure 16.1).

When blood flow to the heart muscle is restricted, chest pain (*angina pectoris*) may result, particularly during strenuous activity. This is the heart's way of saying it isn't getting enough oxygen. Angina often subsides when you rest, since a resting heart doesn't need as much oxygen as a working heart.

A *heart attack* occurs when blood flow through a coronary artery (see Figure 16.2) becomes completely blocked, either through progressive narrowing (*stenosis*) of a coronary artery, when a blood clot (*thrombosis*) forms in a coronary artery, or when a spasm occurs in the artery. With no oxygen and nutrients, the heart tissue supplied by the blocked artery begins to die.

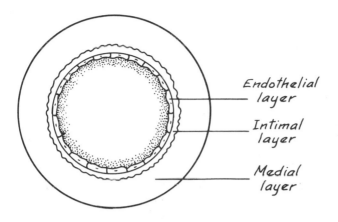

Endothelial
layer

Intimal
layer

Medial
layer

Normal artery

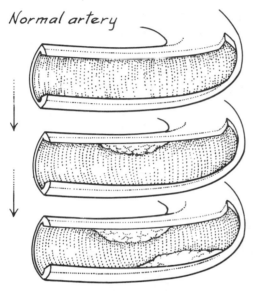

Artery with atherosclerotic
plaque

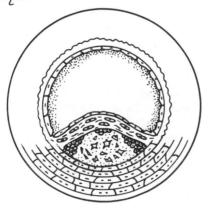

**Figure 16.1
How Plaque Forms
on Artery Walls**

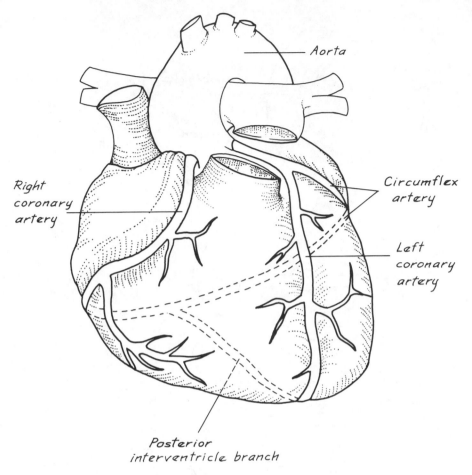

Figure 16.2   The Heart and Coronary Arteries

(Narrowing of the arteries that supply the brain with blood can increase the risk of stroke, too. For more on stroke, see page 331.)

Atherosclerosis doesn't just happen overnight—or immediately after menopause, for that matter. Rather, it's a gradual process that takes years—possibly half a lifetime or more—to develop. Researchers studying the risk of heart disease among children in the town of Bogalusa, Louisiana, found that *children as young as age ten have fatty streaks in their arteries that are believed to develop later into artery-clogging plaques.*

You've undoubtedly heard that cholesterol, the fatty substance that circulates in your bloodstream, is a major contributor to coronary heart disease. Indeed, with all the hype about cholesterol in recent years, you may have been led to believe it was the *only* cause. But cholesterol is just one of many contributing factors. More recently, researchers have begun focusing on the role of your body's ability to make (and dissolve) blood clots, and the role of insulin. And, of course, there's estrogen, which is now known to *protect* women from coronary heart disease in the premenopausal years. A family history of premature heart disease and such lifestyle factors as cigarette smoking, lack of exercise, poorly controlled diabetes, unchecked hypertension, and stress also play a part.

Cholesterol's Role in Coronary Heart Disease

We've known for some time that the development of plaques is strongly associated with high levels of cholesterol circulating in your blood. Cholesterol is a fatty substance found in meat, eggs, and dairy products and in every cell in your body, where it is used to form cell membranes that help carry out the cell's basic functions. Cholesterol also helps manufacture certain hormones, notably estrogen and vitamin D. Indeed, cholesterol is so essential to your survival that *your liver manufactures virtually all the cholesterol you need.*

But there's much more to the cholesterol story than the "good" high-density lipoproteins and "bad" low-density lipoproteins you may be familiar with. When we talk about cholesterol, we're actually referring to several different types of fat and cholesterol, collectively known as *blood lipids.* Since fat and water don't mix, the liver pairs up fat and cholesterol with protein carriers called *apolipoproteins* so they can be transported in the bloodstream and deposited into cells. The resulting particles are known as *lipoproteins.* Each has a role in your body's processing and handling of fat and cholesterol—and many are involved in the development of atherosclerosis.

• **Triglycerides:** Essentially, triglycerides are a form of fat your body can use. The liver makes some of the triglycerides circulating in your bloodstream. Fats in the foods you eat are also broken down in the small intestine and converted to triglycerides, to be used for energy or stored as fat.

It's still not clear what role triglycerides play in the development of heart disease. However, researchers associated with the Framingham Heart Study report that elevated triglycerides are a powerful predictor of coronary heart disease in women over age fifty. This is particularly true when high triglycerides (above 300 mg/dl) are combined with low levels of HDL cholesterol (below 40 mg/dl).

Triglyceride levels are determined partly by the amount of fat in the foods you eat (most of the fat in your diet is triglyceride) and partly by your genes. Triglycerides also rise with age. Being overweight can raise triglyceride levels, too, as can oral contraceptives and oral postmenopausal estrogens.

• **Very-low-density lipoproteins:** These fat particles, manufactured by the liver, are laden with triglycerides. They also contain some cholesterol. Their chief role is to carry triglycerides to the muscles for energy and to fat tissues for storage. Again, we don't know the precise role of VLDL in the development of heart disease, but animal studies have shown that an unusual form of VLDL, known as *beta-VLDL, is* involved in the development of artery-clogging plaques.

• **Low-density lipoproteins:** After their cargo has been delivered, the VLDL break up into smaller particles containing mostly cholesterol. These are known as *low-density lipoproteins* (LDL), and their chief role is to transport cholesterol to your cells. Some of the LDL is also returned to the liver, where it can be broken down and cleared from the body.

LDL cholesterol truly does live up to its reputation as the "bad" cholesterol. High levels of LDL cholesterol appear to cause white blood cells called *monocytes* to penetrate the innermost lining of the artery wall (the *endothelium*) and take up residence just beneath the surface. These white blood cells are transformed into scavenger cells, or *macrophages*. The scavenger cells attract LDL cholesterol and become heavily loaded with fat droplets, forming *foam cells*. The accumulation of foam cells leads to the development of a *fatty streak*, believed to be a precursor of plaque.

New research shows that LDL cholesterol must somehow become "damaged" before it is taken up by monocytes and converted into foam cells. Many researchers now are convinced that *oxidation* caused by *oxygen free radicals* is one of the main culprits. Free radicals are highly charged particles that are missing one electron. They're naturally occurring by-products of metabolism in your body, and are also formed by certain drugs, cigarette smoking, excessive sun exposure, and some substances in foods. Essentially, free radicals bombard the fat particle, thus adding an oxygen molecule to the chain of molecules that make up LDL cholesterol.

There are also several subtypes of LDL cholesterol believed to be more or less atherogenic. For instance, studies have shown that high levels of a small, densely packed cholesterol molecule, known as *small-molecule LDL* cholesterol, are associated with a threefold increased risk of heart attack. Another type of low-density lipoprotein known as lipoprotein (a), or Lp(a), is so closely associated with coronary heart disease that it is now considered to be an independent risk factor for heart disease. Elevated levels of Lp(a) even in people with normal cholesterol levels signal an increased risk. Researchers are now developing more practical ways of measuring Lp(a) in the blood that will make future lipid tests even more accurate than those currently available at predicting your risk of heart disease.

One reason that postmenopausal women appear to be more vulnerable to heart disease is that LDL cholesterol levels rise after menopause.

• **High-density lipoproteins:** High-density lipoproteins, which are manufactured in the small intestine and the liver, are believed to haul cholesterol back to the liver for processing and disposal. HDL cholesterol may even help remove cholesterol deposits from the artery walls, which is why it is often referred to as the "good" cholesterol. There are two main types of HDL cholesterol: HDL_2 and HDL_3. HDL_3 is believed to be a precursor of HDL_2. High levels of HDL cholesterol are believed to help protect against heart disease.

As with the other lipids circulating in your bloodstream, levels of HDL cholesterol are determined partly by your genes and partly by such lifestyle factors as your weight, how much you exercise, the amount of alcohol you consume, and whether you smoke cigarettes. Women generally have higher levels of HDL cholesterol than men, which may help explain the lower incidence of heart disease among women—at least until after menopause. Ironically, it appears that you may need *some* fat in your diet for your body to manufacture HDL cholesterol. A study by British researchers found that while exercise raised levels of HDL cholesterol, the effects of exercise on HDL cholesterol levels were greater when study participants ate a diet moderately high in fat.

• **Apolipoproteins:** Several different types of apolipoproteins have been identified, and all are receiving increased scrutiny for their role in the development of (or protection from) coronary heart disease. Apolipoprotein A is the protein carrier of HDL cholesterol. Apolipoprotein B carries LDL cholesterol through the bloodstream.

Of particular interest in recent years is a newly discovered particle called apolipoprotein (a). Researchers have found that high blood levels of apolipoprotein (a) are associated with an increased risk of heart attacks among people with a genetic predisposition to dangerously high blood-cholesterol levels, a condition known as *familial hypercholesterolemia.*

Guarding Against High Cholesterol

Clearly, a major goal of any preventive program is to keep your blood cholesterol at "safe" levels. It's becoming increasingly apparent that you should also protect against the oxidation of LDL cholesterol circulating in your bloodstream.

The first step, of course, is to find out what your cholesterol levels are and how your menopause is affecting them. Eventually, a cardiovascular evaluation will include blood tests for apolipoproteins, small-molecule LDL cholesterol, and other subgroups of cholesterol that will allow us to gauge your risk more accurately. For now, however, these tests are too complicated and too costly to be of any practical value.

Typically, the first step is to undergo a blood-screening test that measures your total cholesterol levels. (Total blood-cholesterol levels over 200 are now considered "borderline high" and levels exceeding 240 milligrams per deciliter (mg/dl) are considered "high.") However, this test simply isn't comprehensive enough to evaluate your risk of heart disease after menopause. For a more accurate assessment of your risk, it is essential that you undergo a complete lipid profile, which will give you not only your total cholesterol levels but levels of triglycerides, HDL cholesterol, LDL cholesterol, and the ratio of HDL to total cholesterol. Because the test results (mainly triglycerides) can be influenced by what you eat, you should have the test done after an overnight fast. The lipid profile is important because it can often help uncover possible causes of high blood cholesterol, which will influence the type of treatment you receive. Some lipid profiles—high triglycerides and normal levels of LDL cholesterol, for example—suggest the cause may be genetic and you may need to take cholesterol-lowering drugs under the care of a cardiologist or lipid specialist. If your cholesterol levels rise only after menopause, the problem is probably menopause-related, and hormone therapy may be appropriate.

We recommend that all women have a lipid profile at least once before menopause. If your blood-cholesterol levels are normal (see Cholesterol Tests: What the Results Mean on page 312), you should repeat the test once every five years until menopause. After menopause, you should have a lipid profile every one to two years to monitor any menopause-related changes.

If your cholesterol levels are elevated to begin with, your physician will probably want to test you more frequently—even as often as every six months—to see how well various lipid-lowering therapies (including diet and exercise) are working.

Cholesterol Tests: What the Results Mean	
Total cholesterol	
Below 200 mg/dl	Desirable
200 to 239 mg/dl	Borderline high risk
240 mg/dl or above	High risk
Low-density lipoproteins	
Below 130 mg/dl	Desirable
130 to 159 mg/dl	Borderline high risk
160 mg/dl or above	High risk
High-density lipoproteins	
Below 35 mg/dl	Increased risk
35 to 50 mg/dl	Good
50 mg/dl or above	Better
Triglycerides	
20 to 140 mg/dl	Normal
140 to 190 mg/dl	Above normal—monitor
Above 190 mg/dl	High
Ratios:	
Total cholesterol/HDL cholesterol	
Below 4.5	Increased risk
Above 4.5	Desirable

If you have high blood cholesterol, a family history of heart disease, or if you are already experiencing signs of coronary artery disease (such as chest pains), you may also be advised to undergo an exercise stress test. This is essentially an electrocardiogram (ECG) that monitors your heart rate and rhythm while you exercise on a treadmill (you'll find a complete description of the various types of exercise stress tests in Chapter 5).

Nutritional Strategies for Lowering Blood Cholesterol

As you can see, how much cholesterol you have circulating in your bloodstream is determined by many different factors working together, including your gender (women generally have higher levels of protective HDL cholesterol than men), your age (cholesterol levels naturally rise with age), and even your genes. Regardless of your age, your gender, or your genes, however, your blood-cholesterol levels are also affected by what you eat. And even people with a genetic predisposition to high blood cholesterol can usually lower it to safer levels by making a few key changes in their diets.

• **Reduce the amount of total and saturated fat and cholesterol in your diet.** Population studies show that rates of coronary heart disease are relatively low among cultures that consume low-fat diets. In Japan, where coronary heart disease rarely develops, the average diet is just 10 to 20 percent total fat, and average blood-cholesterol levels are between 125 and 166 mg/dl. On the other hand, the average American diet is about 38 percent fat, and average blood cholesterol levels are 205 mg/dl. Most experts recommend that you limit the total amount of fat in your diet to *no more than 30 percent of your total calories.*

A Prudent Diet for the Prevention of Heart Disease

- Reduce the amount of total and saturated fat and cholesterol in your diet.

- Eat foods high in soluble fiber (up to 35 grams) every day to help keep LDL cholesterol levels in check.

- Eat foods high in beta carotene and other antioxidants.

- Drink coffee in moderation (no more than three cups per day)—particularly decaffeinated coffee.

- Limit the amount of sodium in your diet to about one teaspoon (2,000 milligrams) per day to help control your blood pressure.

- Eat plenty of calcium-rich foods.

- Eat fish at least twice a week.

- Drink alcohol only in moderation (no more than two drinks per day).

- Eat several small meals throughout the day instead of three large meals.

One type of dietary fat that's particularly important to cut back on is *saturated fat,* found mostly in meat and dairy products but also in some vegetable fats. Many people confuse cholesterol and saturated fat, thinking they're one and the same; they aren't. Remember, saturated fat is a type of fatty acid that's generally solid at room temperature. Cholesterol is a fatty substance found in all animal products—meats, milk, eggs, cheeses, and seafood. *Both* saturated fat and cholesterol in foods can raise your blood-cholesterol level. But saturated fat is particularly adept at it.

The problem is that some vegetable fats, such as chocolate, hydrogenated vegetable shortenings, palm oil, and coconut oil, are high in saturated fat but free of cholesterol. Some shellfish, such as shrimp, crab, and lobster, are high in cholesterol but very low in saturated fat. Confounding matters even further are products on your supermarket shelf whose labels boast "low cholesterol" or "no cholesterol." Many of these same products are quite high in saturated fat and can still raise your blood-cholesterol level.

To help resolve this dilemma and help you make wise food choices, researchers Sonja L. Connor, R.D., and William E. Connor, M.D., at the Oregon Health Sciences University in Portland developed the Cholesterol–Saturated Fat Index (CSI). They assigned a CSI value to various types of food—

TABLE 16.1   *The Cholesterol–Saturated Fat Index of Some Common Foods*

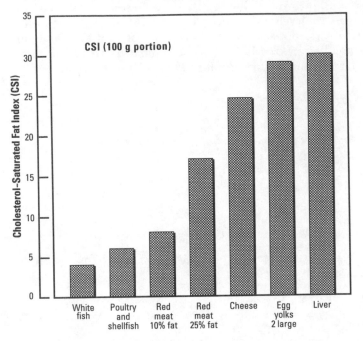

Note: Table reprinted from S. L. Connor, et al., "The Cholesterol Saturated Fat Index: An Indication of the Hypercholester-olaemic and Atherogenic Potential of Food," *Lancet* i: (May 31, 1986) 1229–1232. Copyright © 1986 by The Lancet Ltd.

the higher the CSI, the more atherogenic the food (See Table 16.1). For instance, a 3.5-ounce portion of cooked fish contains 66 mg of cholesterol and .20 grams of saturated fat, compared with 96 mg of cholesterol and 8.1 grams of saturated fat in 3.5 ounces of 20 percent–fat cooked beef. The CSI for the fish is 4; the CSI for the beef is 13.

The Connors' Cholesterol–Saturated Fat Index is fully described in their book, *The New American Diet System* (New York: Simon & Schuster, 1991), which also includes hundreds of recipes and tips for eating out. You'll find more tips for cutting back on saturated fat on pages 60–66.

• **Use monounsaturated oils instead of saturated fats.** The incidence of fatal heart attacks among Greeks and Italians is roughly half that of Americans, and many experts have pointed to the traditional Mediterranean diet—a diet low in saturated fats and rich in complex carbohydrates and monounsaturated olive oil—as an explanation. Several studies now show that monounsaturated oils are as effective as polyunsaturated fats in lowering LDL cholesterol. And a recent study of nearly five thousand Italian men and women showed that those whose diets were high in monounsaturated oils (olive and peanut oils) had lower blood-cholesterol and blood-sugar levels and lower blood pressure than those whose diets were high in saturated fats such as butter. Monounsaturated fatty acids may help protect in another way: They're much more resistant to damage from oxygen free radicals, possibly protecting against oxidation of LDL cholesterol. Polyunsaturated fatty acids are much more readily oxidized.

314

Based on this evidence, most experts recommend that 10 to 15 percent of the total fat in your diet should consist of monounsaturated oils. Increasing your intake of monounsaturated fats is easy. If a recipe (or salad) calls for cooking oil, use olive and peanut oils instead of vegetable oils.

• **Eat foods high in soluble fiber, such as oat bran.** Several studies have suggested that oat bran and other foods high in *water-soluble fiber* can lower blood-cholesterol levels. Although one highly publicized study refuted these findings, it's been criticized for its small numbers and poor design. More recent studies support the original findings that oat bran does, in fact, help lower blood-cholesterol levels.

Remember that oat bran should be used *in addition* to a low-fat diet, not as a substitute for it. In particular, watch out for some of the new oat-bran products, including cookies, snack crackers, and chips, which contain enough fat to undo any cholesterol-lowering effects of oat bran. Check the label for the fat content of these foods before you buy them.

Keep in mind that several foods besides oat bran are also high in soluble fiber. Barley and dried peas and beans (including black and kidney beans, lentils, split peas, and chick peas) contain the soluble fiber *beta glucan,* also found in oat bran. Rice bran (found in some breakfast cereals) and psyllium seed, the active ingredient in the bulk fiber laxative Metamucil, are also high in soluble fiber. These foods are also naturally low in fat, making them doubly good choices for your heart. (See our list of high-fiber foods on page 70 and our guide to heart-healthy foods on pages 316–317.)

• **Eat foods high in beta carotene and other antioxidants.** If damage from oxygen free radicals can increase your risk of atherosclerosis, can antioxidants help protect against heart disease? Preliminary evidence suggests the answer is a hearty yes. Researchers have found, for instance, that when antioxidants such as vitamin E or the food preservative BHT (butylated hydroxytoluene) are added to LDL cholesterol cells in a laboratory dish, they are completely prevented from becoming oxidized.

Several animal studies—most involving rabbits afflicted with a genetic predisposition to high levels of LDL cholesterol—are even more encouraging. Scientists treating the rabbits with the cholesterol-lowering drug *probucol,* which also happens to be a powerful antioxidant, found that the rabbits developed atherosclerotic lesions much more slowly than untreated rabbits. (Unfortunately, probucol also lowers protective HDL cholesterol among people who take it.)

Even more convincing evidence comes from a six-year study of 333 male physicians with heart disease, those who took a 50 mg beta carotene supplement every other day had a 50 percent lower rate of heart attack and stroke than those who didn't take beta carotene. The researchers suspect that beta carotene may neutralize the damaging effects of oxidized LDL cholesterol on the artery wall. Another study by British researchers found a lower incidence of angina among men whose blood levels of vitamins C, E, and carotene were high. The apparent protective effects of vitamin E remained even after the researchers included cigarette smoking, a major risk factor for heart disease, in their data.

While it's too early to make any specific recommendations (particularly

To make low-fat, low-cholesterol eating easier, use this food guide from the National Heart, Lung, and Blood Institute.

	Choose	Go Easy On	Decrease
Meat, Poultry, Fish and Shellfish (up to 6 ounces a day)	Lean cuts of meat with fat trimmed, like: • beef: round, sirloin, chuck, loin • lamb: leg, arm, loin, rib • pork: tenderloin, leg (fresh), shoulder (arm or picnic) • veal: all trimmed cuts except ground poultry without skin fish shellfish		Prime grade Fatty cuts of meat such as: • beef corned beef brisket, regular ground, short ribs • pork spareribs, blade roll • fresh goose, domestic duck • organ meats • sausage, bacon • regular luncheon meats • frankfurters • caviar, roe
Dairy Products (2 servings a day; 3 servings for women who are pregnant or breast-feeding; one serving equals 8 ounces of milk or 1 ounce of cheese or ⅔ cup of cottage cheese)	Skim milk, 1% milk, low-fat buttermilk, low-fat evaporated or nonfat milk Low-fat yogurt Low-fat soft cheeses, like cottage, farmer, pot Cheeses labeled no more than 2 to 6 grams of fat an ounce	2% milk Yogurt Part-skim ricotta Part-skim or imitation hard cheeses, like part-skim mozzarella "Light" cream cheese "Light" sour cream	Whole milk, like regular, evaporated, condensed Cream, half and half, most nondairy creamers, imitation milk products, whipped cream Custard-style yogurt Whole-milk ricotta Neufchâtel Brie Hard cheeses, like Swiss, American, mozzarella, feta, cheddar, Muenster Cream cheese Sour cream
Eggs (no more than 3 egg yolks a week)	Egg whites Cholesterol-free egg substitutes		Egg yolks

	Choose	Go Easy On	Decrease
Fats and Oils (up to 6 to 8 teaspoons a day)	Unsaturated vegetable oils: corn, olive, peanut, rapeseed (canola oil), safflower, sesame, soybean Liquid or tub margarine made from unsaturated fats listed above; or shortening made from unsaturated fats listed above; liquid, tub, stick, diet stick margarine or shortening made from unsaturated vegetable oils	Nuts and seeds Avocados and olives	Butter, coconut oil, palm oil, palm-kernel oil, lard, bacon fat Margarine or shortening made from saturated fats listed above
Breads, Cereals, Pasta, Rice, Dried Peas and Beans (6 to 11 servings a day; one serving equals 1 slice of bread or ½ cup cooked pasta or ½ cup dry grains or cereal)	Breads, like white, whole-wheat, pumpernickel, and rye; pita; bagel; English muffin; sandwich buns; dinner rolls; rice cakes Low-fat crackers, like matzo, bread sticks, Ry-Krisps, saltines, zwieback Hot cereals, most dry cereals Pasta, like plain noodles, spaghetti, macaroni Any grain rice Dried peas and beans, like split peas, black-eyed peas, chick-peas, kidney beans, navy beans, lentils, soybeans	Store-bought pancakes, waffles, biscuits, muffins, corn bread	Croissant, butter rolls, sweet rolls, Danish pastry, doughnuts Most snack crackers, like cheese crackers, butter crackers, those made with saturated oils Granola-type cereals made with saturated oils Pasta and rice prepared with cream, butter, or cheese sauces; egg noodles, soybean curd (tofu)
Fruits and Vegetables (2 to 4 servings of fruit and 3 to 5 servings of vegetables a day; one serving fruit equals ½ cup cut up or 1 piece whole fruit—apples, oranges, pears, plums, etc.—or 6 ounces juice; one serving vegetable equals ½ cup cooked)	Fresh, frozen, canned, or dried fruits and vegetables		Vegetables prepared in butter, cream, or sauce

Heart-Healthy Foods (cont.)

	Choose	Go Easy On	Decrease
Sweets and Snacks (avoid too many sweets)	Low-fat frozen desserts, like sherbet, sorbet, Italian ice, frozen yogurt, Popsicles Low-fat cakes, like angel food Low-fat cookies, like fig bars, gingersnaps Low-fat candy, like jelly beans, hard candy Low-fat snacks, like plain popcorn, pretzels Nonfat beverages, like carbonated drinks, juices, tea, coffee	Frozen desserts, like ice milk Homemade cakes, cookies, and pies using unsaturated oils sparingly Fruit crisps and cobblers	High-fat frozen desserts, like ice cream, frozen tofu High-fat cakes, like most store-bought, pound, and frosted cakes Store-bought pies Most store-bought cookies Most candy, like chocolate bars High-fat snacks, like chips, buttered popcorn High-fat beverages, like frappes, milk shakes, floats, and eggnogs

Note: Chart adapted from *Eating to Lower Your High Blood Cholesterol*, NIH Publication No. 87-2920, U.S. Department of Health and Human Services, Public Health Service, National Institutes of Health.

about taking vitamin supplements), it certainly can't hurt to eat plenty of foods high in vitamins E and C and beta carotene. A word of caution about supplements: Megadoses (more than ten times the recommended dietary allowance), particularly large doses of oil-soluble vitamins such as vitamin A, can cause toxicity and interfere with your body's use of other vitamins and minerals. Too much vitamin A can stimulate bone loss, too, so don't overdo it. You only need 4,000 IU each day.

• **Drink coffee in moderation.** Some studies have suggested that regular caffeinated coffee raises blood-cholesterol levels and may contribute to your risk of heart disease in other ways. Newer studies now show that regular drip-brewed coffee (the kind most Americans drink) *does not* affect cholesterol levels. (Coffee prepared the Scandinavian way—by boiling either whole or coarsely ground beans in water—may raise your cholesterol levels, however.) According to a Harvard University study—the largest and best-designed to date—even three or four cups a day of typical American coffee are safe for virtually everyone, even people with heart disease.

Decaffeinated coffee may be another story, however. Preliminary data from the Harvard study and a Stanford University study have found an *increased* risk of heart disease among heavy drinkers (four or more cups per day) of decaffeinated coffee. Until we know more, drink decaffeinated coffee in moderation (no more than three cups per day). Don't overdo it with caffeinated coffee, either. Remember, too much coffee can jangle your nerves. And more than five cups per day can cause you to excrete excess calcium.

• **Avoid the "triglyceride bulge."** Don't forget that it's not just *what* you eat but *when* you eat that may influence the development of atherosclerosis. Blood-triglyceride levels peak about four hours after eating a fatty meal. If you eat your heaviest meal of the day in the evening, your blood-lipid levels will peak while you're sleeping and may be more likely to be stored in your fat tissues than used for energy. Likewise, cholesterol in the food you eat might be more readily deposited in your arteries.

We recommend that you eat the majority of your calories *before* 5:00 P.M. This way, the fat in the foods you eat is more likely to be used by your body as energy rather than stored as fat. We call this the PPP Principle: Essentially, you eat like a potentate for breakfast, a princess for lunch, and a pauper for dinner.

If you don't see a measurable difference in your blood-lipid levels after cutting back on fat and cholesterol in your diet, you may want to consult with a registered dietitian. Some people find that by doing so they can lower their cholesterol through dietary changes even after their own efforts have failed. (To find a qualified dietitian, see page 93.)

Commonly Used Drugs

If diet, exercise, and other lifestyle changes aren't effective in lowering your cholesterol, your physician may prescribe certain cholesterol-lowering drugs, including *cholestyramine* (Cholybar, Questran), *colestipol* (Colestid, Cholesta-byl), a prescription form of the B-vitamin *niacin, lovastatin* (Mevacor), *simvastatin* (Zocor), *gemfibrozil* (Lopid), or *psyllium seed,* found in over-the-counter bulk fiber laxatives, such as Metamucil.

Remember, too, that cholesterol is just one of many factors contributing to heart disease. Read on to see how you can further reduce your risk.

The Role of Blood Clots

The formation of blood clots in the arteries plays such a critical role in cardio-vascular disease that the condition might be more appropriately named *ather-othrombosis* (a thrombosis is a blood clot that lodges in a major artery). Blood clots and bleeding in the body are controlled by a sophisticated system of *hemostasis.* Your body's ability to form blood clots keeps you from bleeding to death when you're injured. On the other hand, when a blood clot forms in a vital artery, it can trigger a life-threatening heart attack or stroke.

Hemostasis is a complex process, involving the blood vessel itself, specialized molecules that circulate in the bloodstream, known as *platelets,* and dozens of *coagulation factors* and *anticoagulation factors* in the blood.

When a blood vessel is injured or broken, platelets begin sticking to the exposed collagen in the blood-vessel wall. The collagen triggers a number of biochemical changes in the platelets that ultimately lead to the formation of a clot. The platelets begin churning out *thromboxane A$_2$,* a compound that increases their "stickiness" and constricts the blood vessel to help prevent excessive blood loss. Other biochemical changes in the platelets trigger a chain reaction among several blood-coagulation factors, ultimately resulting in the activation of *thrombin*. This powerful blood coagulant converts the coagulation factor *fibrinogen* into tough *fibrin* strands that hold the platelets together.

The blood-vessel wall itself secretes compounds called *endothelins,* some of the most powerful blood-vessel constrictors known. We still don't know much about the exact role of endothelins in the regulation of blood flow and the formation of blood clots. But blood levels of endothelins are elevated after a heart attack.

For every action, there is an equal and opposite reaction. *Anticoagulants* help ensure that your blood circulation isn't threatened by the formation of blood clots. The cells lining the blood-vessel wall manufacture *prostacyclin,* a prostaglandin that keeps platelets from sticking together. Prostacyclin is also a powerful vasodilator, widening the blood vessel to maintain blood circulation. This anticoagulant works in direct opposition to thromboxane A_2 and endothelins.

The blood vessel's ability to manufacture prostacyclin decreases with age and among people with diabetes or atherosclerosis. This means there may be a direct link between the production of prostacyclin in blood-vessel walls and its vulnerability to the development of blood clots or atherosclerosis.

More recently, scientists have discovered that the blood-vessel wall also secretes *endothelium-derived relaxing factor* (EDRF), the body's own version of the widely used heart medication *nitroglycerin.* Nitroglycerin has been prescribed since the nineteenth century to widen the coronary arteries and relieve bouts of angina. Apparently, EDRF acts together with prostacyclin to inhibit platelet aggregation and keep blood vessels open.

Antithrombin III is one of several substances manufactured by the liver that neutralizes the action of thrombin and thus limits blood coagulation. Blood levels of antithrombin III are a good gauge as to whether you're likely to develop blood clots.

Plasminogen is a precursor of plasmin, an enzyme that dissolves the tough fibrin strands that hold a blood clot together. It's produced in the liver and also in the blood-vessel wall.

We now know that there is a link between cholesterol metabolism and the body's blood-clotting system: As it turns out, apolipoprotein (a), the protein carrier for lipoprotein (a), is closely related to plasminogen and may be a genetic mutation. We suspect that apolipoprotein (a) somehow competes with plasminogen after a clot begins forming in a blood-vessel wall, short-circuiting the blood vessel's natural ability to dissolve the clot.

As you can see, blood coagulation plays a key role in the development of heart attacks and strokes. Fortunately, there are ways to influence your body's system of hemostasis and further reduce your risk of cardiovascular disease.

Preventing Blood Clots

There are no mass screening tests to determine whether you are at risk of developing a blood clot. However, there are some things you can do to protect yourself from blood clots. (Keep in mind that *anything* you do to try to alter your body's delicate system of hemostasis should be done *only* with your doctor's permission and under his or her supervision. Otherwise, there's a danger of excessive bleeding.)

•   **Eat fish at least twice a week.** Fish oils appear to protect against heart disease in several ways but probably *not* in the way you think. Many people are under the impression that fish oils lower blood cholesterol. In fact, fish oils may even *raise* your cholesterol levels. Rather, omega-3 fatty acids in fish and fish-oil supplements are believed to interfere with the normal metabolism of blood platelets, making them less likely to stick together. Fish oils may also alter the function of monocytes so that they're not as likely to take up residence in the artery wall and develop into foam cells. Some studies have found that omega-3 fatty acids lower triglycerides, which may also reduce your risk of heart disease.

What about fish-oil supplements? It's probably better to eat fish rather than pop fish-oil supplements. Many of the studies on the benefits of fish oils are still preliminary. Plus, the supplements have side effects, including loose stools, gas, abdominal distension, and a possible increased need for vitamin E. Supplements containing cod-liver oil also contain high levels of vitamins A and D, which can be toxic at high doses. Until we know more, stick with fish—two to three times a week.

•   **Ask your physician about taking aspirin.** One way of reducing your risk of a life-threatening blood clot is as close as your medicine cabinet. Aspirin is a powerful anticoagulant that works by tipping the balance between the anticoagulant prostacyclin and the blood coagulant thromboxane so that blood-thinning prostacyclin gets the upper hand. When you take aspirin, it suppresses the production of both prostacyclin in the blood-vessel wall and thromboxane, manufactured by blood platelets. But aspirin's effects on prostacyclin last for only six hours, while the drug suppresses thromboxane for three days. As a result, when you take aspirin regularly, your blood becomes more resistant to forming a clot.

A few major studies—all involving men—suggest that taking aspirin reduces the risk of heart attacks and strokes caused by blood clots (thrombosis). However, those in the studies who took aspirin suffered more strokes from cerebral hemorrhage than those who took a placebo.

A recent study involving women also found aspirin to have beneficial effects. Women who took between one and six aspirin a week experienced a 25 percent reduction in the risk of having a heart attack. Women over fifty and those at high risk of developing coronary heart disease had the greatest reduction in risk. Women who took seven or more aspirin per week, however, didn't enjoy any greater protection, and those who took fifteen or more aspirin per week were at a greater risk of suffering a cerebral hemorrhage.

Should you regularly take aspirin to prevent a heart attack or stroke? Don't do so without first discussing it with your doctor. Although aspirin is readily available over the counter, it's not safe for everybody. If you have liver or kidney disease, a peptic ulcer, gastrointestinal bleeding, or other bleeding problems, you may not be able to take aspirin at all, or you may need to adjust the amount you take. Since aspirin prolongs bleeding, you should notify your physician that you're taking aspirin if you're scheduled for any kind of surgery. Also, if you have uncontrolled hypertension or any condition that might increase the risk of a stroke, you should not take aspirin routinely without first checking with your physician. When we prescribe aspirin to patients in our clinic, we recommend taking a junior aspirin (60 milligrams) every three days.

The Role of Insulin

It's probably no coincidence that people with diabetes also have high blood-cholesterol levels, often suffer from hypertension, and are at an increased risk of cardiovascular disease. Indeed, we're just beginning to recognize the importance of insulin in the development of hypertension and atherosclerosis, a condition referred to as *syndrome X.*

How can elevated insulin levels contribute to high blood pressure? The link appears to be the *sympathetic nervous system,* which regulates your heart rate, blood pressure, blood flow, metabolism, and other involuntary body functions. Fasting suppresses the sympathetic nervous system and helps you conserve energy. Overeating, on the other hand, stimulates the sympathetic nervous system. This may be your body's way of burning off some of the excess calories you eat and protecting you from getting too fat. Overeating also triggers insulin production from the pancreas, and high levels of insulin appear to stimulate the sympathetic nervous system into action. This, in turn, raises blood pressure.

Insulin has also been implicated in aiding and abetting the development of atherosclerosis. High blood-sugar levels are believed to damage or alter the lining of the artery wall somehow, allowing insulin to interact with the underlying tissues and making them more sensitive to the development of foam cells, fatty streaks, and, ultimately, artery-narrowing plaques. To add insult to injury, insulin is also associated with lower levels of protective HDL cholesterol.

Protecting Against High Insulin Levels

Have a fasting blood-glucose test as part of your cardiovascular work-up. If glucose levels are high, there are a number of ways you can help keep insulin levels from peaking.

• **Eat several small meals throughout the day instead of three large meals.** Nibbling nutritious foods throughout the day instead of gorging on a few large meals helps keep insulin levels at a more even keel.

• **Eat a diet low in fat and high in complex carbohydrates.** Once again, soluble fiber, found in dried peas and beans, oat bran, and oatmeal, has been shown to help stabilize insulin levels among diabetics. (See page 70 for a list of foods high in soluble fiber.)

• **Exercise.** Regular physical activity helps your body use insulin more efficiently. We showed that women who exercise regularly experienced increased sensitivity to insulin, thus helping to offset the natural age-related increase in insulin resistance that can lead to adult-onset diabetes. More recently, exercise has been shown actually to help *prevent* the development of diabetes in men. The more active the men were in a fourteen-year study by researchers at the University of California at Berkeley, the less likely they were to develop diabetes. Moreover, the men at highest risk—those who were overweight, those who had had high blood pressure, and those with a family history of diabetes— enjoyed the greatest protection. Among the nearly six thousand men who participated in the study, there was a 6 percent reduction in risk for each five-hundred-calorie-per-week increase in activity level.

•   **Control your weight.** Insulin resistance increases with obesity, resulting in elevated insulin levels. Losing weight usually increases insulin sensitivity and brings insulin levels down again.

•   **If you have diabetes, work closely with your physician to control it.** The above guidelines often suffice to keep Type II diabetes under control. If your blood-sugar levels are still high, your physician may prescribe oral hypoglycemic agents. If these drugs don't work, you may have to take insulin injections.

The Role of Estrogens

Premenopausal women seem to enjoy a built-in biological protection from cardiovascular disease. And the protective mechanism appears to be the reproductive hormone estrogen. Indeed, postmenopausal women who take oral estrogen for ten years or more have *50 percent less coronary heart disease than women who don't.*

How does estrogen protect? We know that estrogen has a powerful effect on blood lipids and lipoproteins. Our studies and those of other researchers have shown that blood-cholesterol levels rise sharply after menopause—an average of twenty-five points. This translates roughly into a 50 percent increase in your risk of developing heart disease. Moreover, women who take postmenopausal oral estrogen experience a decline in total and LDL cholesterol and a rise in protective HDL_2 cholesterol. The change in blood lipids depends on the amount of estrogen you take: The higher the dose, the greater the change. On the average, women who take the higher dose of oral conjugated estrogen (1.25 mg of Premarin) per day experience a rise in HDL cholesterol of 14 to 17 percent, while LDL cholesterol falls an average of 8 percent. In our study of the effects of oral estrogens on blood lipids, women taking 1.25 mg of estropipate (Ogen) daily experienced an increase of nearly 10 percent in HDL cholesterol after 12 months, a drop of 8 percent in LDL cholesterol, and a marked improvement in the ratios of HDL cholesterol to total cholesterol.

Postmenopausal estrogen appears to protect your heart in other ways, as well. Contrary to popular belief, postmenopausal estrogens *don't* raise blood pressure. In fact, several studies have found that oral estrogen can actually *decrease* blood pressure. As you may recall, we found that estrogen alone decreased blood pressure by an average of 3.8 percent.

Another common misconception about postmenopausal estrogens is that they increase your risk of developing a blood clot. While oral estrogen *does* increase the liver's production of several different coagulation factors, these factors are not biologically active until they're exposed to an injured blood vessel. Plus, "normal" levels for many of these coagulation factors vary widely, and it's impossible to predict who is at higher risk of developing blood clots by measuring levels of these enzymes.

On the other hand, we found that estrogen *doesn't have any effect at all* on anticoagulants, particularly antithrombin III, which is a good marker for predicting whether you will develop a blood clot. In addition, we've found that menopause itself raises levels of potential anticlotting factors, such as plasminogen, possibly providing some natural protection against the formation of blood clots. This may help explain why postmenopausal estrogen therapy appears less likely to cause blood clots in older women. Indeed, *there is no study showing a cause-and-effect relationship between taking estrogen therapy and the development of blood clots.* Estrogen's poor reputation comes from studies on the use of older, high-dose oral contraceptives among older women who smoked. As for insulin, estrogen *decreases* fasting blood-sugar levels, possibly because it prevents the breakdown of insulin. This may provide added protection against heart disease.

Estrogen may protect in other ways, as well: For instance, estrogen improves blood flow. The hormone also appears somehow to protect the innermost lining of the blood vessel wall, where artery-narrowing plaques form. At least three studies have shown that women who take estrogen are less likely to have occluded arteries. Angiograms, in which a dye is injected into the bloodstream and an X ray is taken as the dye passes through the coronary arteries, showed that estrogen users had significantly less stenosis (narrowing) than nonusers, even when other risk factors, including hypertension, diabetes, cigarette smoking, and obesity, were taken into account. Indeed, estrogen appeared to reduce the risk of severe coronary artery disease by a striking 56 to 63 percent. Estrogen also protects against spasms of the coronary arteries, which can trigger a heart attack. And animal studies suggest that estrogen somehow protects against atherosclerosis.

The picture grows a little more complicated when progestogen (a synthetic form of the reproductive hormone progesterone) is added. You may have heard reports that progestogen, which is often prescribed along with postmenopausal estrogen to protect against endometrial cancer, may cancel out estrogen's protective effect and possibly even *raise* your risk of heart disease. Long-term studies are now under way to determine the exact role of postmenopausal progestogen in the development of heart disease. However, preliminary results suggest the fear of heart disease associated with progestogen use may be exaggerated. An eight-year study of the use of oral contraceptives among 119,061 women by Dr. Meir Stampfer found no increased risk of cardiovascular disease among women who had used oral contraceptives in the past. Indeed, the relative risk of major coronary disease for users was 20 percent *lower* than the risk for nonusers.

Progestogen does appear to somewhat dampen the effects of estrogen on blood lipids. However, the cyclic use of progestogen with intermediate doses of oral estrogen (.625 mg per day of conjugated equine estrogens or the equivalent) still results in a meaningful *overall increase in cardioprotective factors,* such as an increase in HDL cholesterol. One study showed that the combination of progestogen and oral estrogen lowered LDL cholesterol and raised protective HDL cholesterol, although the increase in HDL—6 percent—was about half that of women receiving estrogen alone.

In the near future, new types of progestogen and different ways of administering the hormone may make the whole issue of progestogen's effects on blood lipids obsolete. Preliminary evidence suggests that a new class of synthetic progestogens, including *gestodene, desogestrel,* and *norgestimate,* as well as oral micronized progesterone, will have little effect on HDL cholesterol in women taking estrogen. A transdermal skin patch containing both progestogen and estrogen may also reduce the negative effects of progestogen on blood lipids because the skin patch allows the hormones to enter the bloodstream without first passing through the liver.

Contrary to popular belief, the low levels of progestogens used in today's oral contraceptives have no adverse effect on blood pressure. Again, the idea that progestogen raises blood pressure was based on studies involving the older oral contraceptives, which contained large doses of progestogen.

As for blood clots, progestogen may even help protect against them. We found that postmenopausal progestogens *increase* the activity of the anticoagulant plasminogen by 16 to 20 percent. Although we don't yet know what effect these changes have in the body, it's possible that they have a protective effect. This effect of progestogen on plasminogen may be particularly important in the prevention of heart disease. It's possible that the higher levels of plasminogen among women taking progestogen may help guard against the ill effects of apolipoprotein (a) on the artery wall. Remember, apolipoprotein (a) is genetically similar to plasminogen and high levels of apolipoprotein (a) may raise your risk of developing a blood clot.

Progestogen *does* increase insulin resistance somewhat, which may be a problem for some women, particularly diabetics. These women may need to be more closely monitored.

Animal studies have also suggested that progestogen may *reduce* blood flow, and this may dampen the positive effects that estrogen has on blood flow, particularly through the coronary arteries. Overall, however, it appears that progestogen doesn't totally cancel out the good that estrogen does for your heart. Indeed progestogen may add some protective measures of its own.

Should You Take Hormones to Protect Against Heart Disease?

Yes—particularly if you have:

- a family history of premature heart disease
- high blood-cholesterol levels
- high blood pressure
- premature menopause (before age forty)

However, you will have to work with your physician to determine which type of hormone therapy is best for you. Different types and amounts of estrogen may affect you in different ways. For instance, oral estrogens raise blood-triglyceride levels and may not be appropriate for women with high triglycerides. On the other hand, the estrogen patch doesn't seem to have as great a cardioprotective effect as oral estrogen as far as HDL cholesterol is concerned. (We'll discuss these differences in more detail and give you general guidelines for taking hormones to protect against heart disease in Chapter 21.)

Your blood-cholesterol levels should be monitored periodically (every two years if cholesterol levels are normal; once every six months if they're elevated, and once a year if you are taking estrogen *and* a progestogen) after beginning hormone therapy to ensure that the therapy is effective. Again, we recommend you undergo a complete lipid profile rather than just have your total cholesterol levels measured. The lipid profile gives a better idea of how well the hormone therapy is working. You should also keep in mind that hormone therapy works best when used in conjunction with other preventive measures, such as a low-fat diet and exercise.

The Role of Iron

As a woman, you're probably used to worrying about getting enough iron to ward off iron-deficiency anemia. In fact, throughout your childbearing years, you lose iron every time you menstruate, which tends to keep your body's iron stores (the backup supply of iron tucked away in muscle and other tissues) low. Once you stop menstruating, however, your body's iron stores rise quickly (see Table 3.2 on page 35). According to a 1992 report from Finnish researchers, therein lies the problem. The Finnish scientists found that the level of stored iron in men is a strong risk factor for heart disease—possibly stronger than the risk factors of elevated blood cholesterol, high blood pressure, or diabetes. In the five-year study involving 1,931 men, even "normal" levels of stored iron were strongly associated with an increased risk of heart attack, and every 1 percent increase in serum ferritin (storage iron) was associated with a more than 4 percent increase in the risk of heart attack. A high ferritin level—200 micrograms or more per liter of blood—more than doubled the relative risk of a heart attack. If further research confirms these results, the iron theory could help explain why women appear to be safe from heart attacks until after menopause, when iron stores accumulate quite rapidly.

How can high levels of storage iron contribute to heart disease? The researchers point out that the release of iron from ferritin molecules may contribute to the formation of oxygen free radicals, which could help transform LDL cholesterol into an oxidized form that more readily adheres to and clogs artery walls. The ferritin molecules are also capable of releasing iron at injury sites, which could cause the injury to the heart muscle that follows a heart attack. Some animal experiments have suggested that iron depletion may inhibit both the clogging of the arteries that leads to a heart attack and the injury to the heart muscle after a heart attack. The iron theory could also help explain the protective effects of aspirin, fish oils, and a cholesterol-lowering drug called cholestyramine. Aspirin and fish oils increase bleeding times, which may increase chronic blood loss and therefore lower iron stores in the body. Cholestyramine, which passes through the body without being absorbed, has been used to make animals iron-deficient.

The researchers say that donating blood three times a year is enough to reduce a postmenopausal woman's iron stores to those of a menstruating woman. However, no research has yet been conducted on regular blood donors to see whether their lower levels of stored iron actually reduce their risk of heart disease. It's still not clear what effect low iron stores will have on your overall health, either. Low body-iron stores is a frequent cause of fatigue in women. And low storage iron is just a step away from iron-deficiency anemia, a medical condition that causes fatigue, dizziness, heart palpitations, and reduced resistance to infection. An iron supplement is usually required to correct iron-deficiency anemia. So before you become a regular blood donor to protect against heart disease, wait for more definitive studies. If you already regularly donate blood, you should periodically have your blood tested to ensure that you have an adequate iron supply—particularly if fatigue and lack of energy are problems for you. Another way you can protect yourself is to eat foods high in vitamins A, E, and C. These foods have antioxidant properties that help protect against damage from oxygen free radicals.

Other Essential Protective Measures

Coronary heart disease is the result of many different factors working together. Your program of prevention should also include the following measures:

• **Quit smoking.** Nearly three times more smokers die of heart disease than lung cancer. The risk of stroke—both from blood clots and cerebral hemorrhage—is doubled among women who smoke; heavy smokers (more than twenty-five cigarettes per day) have six times the risk of suffering a stroke than nonsmokers.

Carbon monoxide in cigarette smoke reduces the blood's oxygen-carrying ability, so there's less oxygen available to your heart and other organs. Cigarette smoking raises levels of LDL cholesterol and decreases HDL cholesterol. Smoking also damages the lining of the coronary arteries, setting the stage for the development of coronary lesions.

Cigarette smoking adversely affects blood coagulation, too, increasing the likelihood that blood clots will form and cause a heart attack.

By speeding up the activity of the sympathetic nervous system, which controls heart rate and other bodily functions, cigarette smoking may trigger coronary spasms, which could lead to a heart attack. Cigarette smoke may also interfere with the electrical activity of the heart, leading to irregular heart rhythms (*arrhythmias*) and increasing the likelihood of sudden death. What's more, women who smoke experience menopause an average of two to three years earlier than nonsmokers. The earlier menopause puts you at an earlier increased risk of heart disease.

No matter how long you've smoked, when you quit your risk of heart disease begins to decline. *Within two years of quitting, your chances of having a heart attack will be cut in half. Ten years after quitting, your risk of dying from a heart attack will be almost the same as if you'd never smoked.* Your risk of suffering a stroke declines, as well. So do your heart a big favor and quit. (For tips on quitting, see Chapter 7.)

• **Exercise.** Sedentary living is now considered a major risk factor for heart disease, along with high blood pressure, high blood cholesterol, and cigarette smoking. Conversely, regular physical activity appears to be a powerful deterrent against heart disease.

Exercise lowers your blood pressure and heart rate; burns body fat, which helps counter obesity, a serious risk factor for heart disease; promotes more efficient use of insulin, which may reduce your risk of developing adult-onset diabetes (and syndrome X); raises levels of protective HDL cholesterol and lowers detrimental LDL cholesterol; may even help prevent blood clots; and reduces stress, which may contribute to an increased risk of heart disease.

For protection against heart disease, we recommend aerobic activities—those that involve increasing your heart rate and breathing and using the large muscles of your body. Brisk walking, bicycling, and swimming are ideal for women in midlife. (Keep in mind that nonaerobic activities, such as weight lifting and stretching, are important, too. While these activities do little to increase the efficiency of your heart, they do increase your muscle strength and flexibility, which improves your ability to do aerobics and decreases your risk of injury.)

You'll find everything you need to know to start an exercise program for cardiovascular protection in Chapter 5.

• **Drink alcohol in moderation.** Several population studies have suggested that *moderate* amounts of alcohol (one or two drinks per day) may help prevent heart disease, particularly among women. Alcohol appears to protect against coronary heart disease by raising levels of HDL cholesterol. Moderate alcohol consumption is also associated with several changes in blood coagulation, which could also explain its possible protective effect. Alcohol apparently decreases the stickiness of blood platelets, and increases the anticoagulant prostacyclin, keeping it dominant over the blood coagulant thromboxane. Alcohol also interacts with aspirin to prolong the time it takes blood to clot. (It's *not* a good idea to take aspirin and drink alcohol at the same time, however; doing so may accelerate the rate at which alcohol enters your bloodstream.) European researchers have identified a substance in red wine that they believe may be responsible for conferring protection against heart disease in the French, whose diet is fairly high in fat and cholesterol but who enjoy a low incidence of heart disease. The substance is *phenol,* an antioxidant. Finally, alcohol lowers the levels of fibrinogen, a potent risk factor for coronary heart disease.

Before you raise a glass or two, however, keep in mind that the studies are by no means conclusive. Dr. Meir Stampfer and his colleagues at Harvard Medical School found that moderate alcohol consumption among middle-aged women *did* decrease the risk of coronary heart disease and stroke. But in this study, moderate drinkers also had a higher risk of suffering a cerebral hemorrhage (a stroke caused by bleeding in the brain).

Keep in mind, too, that *heavy drinking* (more than three drinks per day) can damage the heart muscle, trigger disturbances in the heart's rhythm, and reduce blood flow from the heart. Even three or four drinks per day can raise blood pressure. Heavy drinking also raises blood-triglyceride levels.

Until we know more about the possible protective effects of alcohol on heart disease, limit yourself to no more than two drinks per day. If you have more than two drinks a day, try to curb your alcohol consumption. If you find you can't cut back by yourself, this may be a sign that you have a drinking problem and should consider seeking professional help. (See Chapter 7 for tips on cutting back and help in recognizing and treating an alcohol dependency.)

• **Keep your blood pressure in check.** Elevated blood pressure is one of the most powerful contributors to cardiovascular disease. Even mildly elevated blood pressure leads to a greater incidence of premature atherosclerosis, heart attacks, and strokes. The greater your blood pressure, the greater the risk. For tips on lowering your blood pressure, see page 303.

• **Control your weight.** JoAnn Manson, M.D., and her colleagues at Harvard University's School of Medicine in Boston found that even mildly overweight women (those with a body-mass index of 25 to 29) are up to forty times more likely to develop coronary heart disease than normal-weight women. (To determine your body-mass index, see page 29.) And women who gain weight *during the middle years* have double the risk of developing coronary heart disease than women who have been overweight all their lives. Women who tend to put on weight around the waist and abdomen ("apple" shapes) are more likely to have lower levels of HDL cholesterol, elevated LDL cholesterol, triglycerides, and insulin, and are more likely to develop hypertension and adult-onset diabetes.

Dr. Manson estimates that *as much as 40 percent of coronary disease in women could be prevented by weight loss alone.* Losing weight is often enough to lower elevated blood cholesterol and blood pressure and to keep adult-onset diabetes in check without drugs and their sometimes serious side effects. If you have a weight problem, simply cutting back on fat in your diet and increasing your physical activity may solve it. If these measures don't work, see Chapter 15 for ways to bring down your weight.

• **Keep tabs on diabetes.** Diabetes mellitus is particularly hard on women. Several studies have confirmed that the condition somehow completely wipes out the biological protection against heart disease that healthy women enjoy.

High blood cholesterol is more common in diabetics, and HDL cholesterol is lower in people with uncontrolled diabetes. Remember, too, that high blood-sugar levels may damage the lining of the artery walls, increasing their susceptibility to the formation of plaques. Uncontrolled diabetes may cause blood platelets to stick together more readily, allowing blood to clot more easily. These and other characteristics of people with diabetes substantially raise their risk of developing cardiovascular disease. Indeed, cardiovascular disease is the major cause of death in people who have diabetes.

Heart disease is just one of several major complications associated with diabetes, including kidney failure, amputations due to infection, and blindness. Better control of diabetes is associated with fewer complications. And the majority of women with non-insulin-dependent diabetes can control it with dietary changes alone. But don't attempt to treat this serious metabolic disorder by yourself. Rather, plan to work closely with your physician (and possibly a registered dietitian), who will develop a diet plan to control your diabetes and prescribe blood-sugar lowering medications, if necessary.

• **Control stress.** Events you find emotionally taxing—getting stuck in a traffic jam on the way to the airport, for example—can trigger a physiological response in the body called the "fight or flight" response, in which your body releases a flood of chemicals from the adrenal glands, notably *epinephrine* and *norepinephrine.* These hormones accelerate your breathing and heart rate, raise your blood pressure and blood-sugar levels, and release high-energy fats into the bloodstream for quick energy—essentially preparing you for a fight with or a quick flight away from a physical threat. The hormones also increase the stickiness of blood platelets, which make blood clot more easily (in case you're wounded in the ensuing battle). *Cortisol,* another hormone released from the adrenal glands when your body is chronically stressed, raises blood-cholesterol levels.

Several studies have suggested that the constant firing of the "fight or flight" response from living in a stressful environment (particularly one in which you have a lot of responsibility but little control) may lead to permanent increases in heart rate and blood pressure. Blood-cholesterol levels may also be grossly elevated by stress. Other studies have found a correlation between a cluster of personality traits, including competitiveness, aggression, hostility, impatience, and time urgency, and an increased risk of heart attacks. One landmark study by Meyer Friedman, M.D., and Ray H. Rosenman, M.D., authors of the 1974 best-seller *Type A Behavior and Your Heart* (New York: Knopf), found that men who exhibited these personality traits—what they called *Type A behavior*—were 2.2 times more likely to develop coronary heart disease than the more relaxed Type B's. Other researchers have found no significant correlation between Type A behavior and increased risk of heart disease. Few studies have been conducted on women, so the issue remains controversial.

Although many questions remain unanswered about the role of stress and heart disease, it makes sense to take stock of the stresses in your life and reduce stress whenever possible. Exercising regularly is an ideal place to start, since it also helps protect against heart disease and high blood pressure. Relaxation techniques, such as deep breathing, progressive muscular relaxation, yoga, meditation, and biofeedback can also undo the effects of stress on your body. You'll find other practical ways to manage stress in Chapter 6.

Warning Signs of a Heart Attack

Prevention is the best medicine, and making lifestyle changes now can significantly reduce your odds of having a heart attack later. However, preventive measures can't guarantee that you won't develop heart problems.

Fortunately, lifestyle changes and treatment advances in the last ten to fifteen years have vastly improved the outlook for people who suffer a heart attack: Of the estimated 1.5 million Americans who have a heart attack today, *roughly two-thirds will survive.* One key to survival is to *seek medical help at the first signs of heart trouble.* Here are a few symptoms to watch out for:

•   **Angina pectoris:** Discomfort in the chest, often described as a feeling of pressure or tightness. Attacks of angina pectoris usually last several minutes and are often triggered by physical exertion, exposure to cold, or stress.

If you have an angina attack, notify your physician as soon as possible. Your physician may also want to perform a few diagnostic tests, such as an electrocardiogram, an exercise stress test, or a coronary angiogram. He or she may also prescribe drugs, such as nitroglycerine, calcium channel blockers, or beta-blockers, to see whether the angina can be controlled.

•   **Heart attack:** If you're at increased risk of developing coronary heart disease, it is imperative that you know the warning signs of a heart attack. According to the American Heart Association, *you should immediately call for emergency help if you experience*:

- an uncomfortable pressure, fullness, squeezing, or pain in the center of the chest that does not go away in a few minutes
- severe chest pain
- pain spreading to the shoulders, neck, or arms

330

- light-headedness and palpitations
- fainting
- sweating associated with chest discomfort
- nausea associated with chest discomfort
- difficulty breathing

Prompt medical attention may reduce the damage to your heart; the more quickly you receive medical care, the greater are your chances of surviving the attack.

Stroke

Stroke is another major cause of disability and death among women in the middle and later years that can often be prevented. A stroke occurs when the blood supply to the brain is disrupted, either by a blood clot or excessive bleeding from a ruptured artery. There are four main types of stroke: *cerebral thrombosis*, the most common, occurs when a blood clot (thrombus) forms and blocks blood flow in an artery supplying blood to part of the brain (see Figure 16.3); *cerebral embolism* occurs when a wandering clot (embolus) or some other particle forms in a blood vessel away from the brain (usually in the heart) and is carried by the bloodstream until it lodges in an artery leading to or in the brain (see Figure 16.3); *cerebral hemorrhage* occurs when an artery in the brain bursts, flooding the surrounding tissue with blood (see Figure 16.4); *subarachnoid hemorrhage* occurs when a blood vessel on the surface of the brain ruptures and bleeds into the space between the brain and the skull—but not into the brain itself (see Figure 16.4).

When nerve cells in the affected area of the brain don't get the oxygen and nutrients they need, they begin to die within minutes. Therefore, the part of the body controlled by these cells can't function, either. This tissue damage may result in severe losses in mental and bodily functions—sometimes even death.

The best way to prevent a stroke from occurring is to reduce the risk factors for stroke. Some risk factors can't be changed. These include your age (the incidence of stroke more than doubles in each successive decade after age fifty-five), your sex (women are 30 percent less likely to have a stroke than men), your race (stroke is more prevalent among blacks), and whether you have a personal or family history of stroke. People with diabetes, particularly women, are more susceptible to stroke regardless of whether the diabetes is kept under control. If you have an *asymptomatic carotid bruit* (an abnormal sound when a stethoscope is placed over the carotid artery in the neck), you are also at an increased risk of stroke.

However, four risk factors are at least partly within your control:

• **Hypertension:** This is the most important risk factor for stroke. In fact, the risk of stroke rises as blood pressure rises, and women with hypertension are just as susceptible as men. On the other hand, studies now show that reducing blood pressure *definitely* reduces the risk of stroke. For this reason, it is essential that you have your blood pressure checked regularly and that

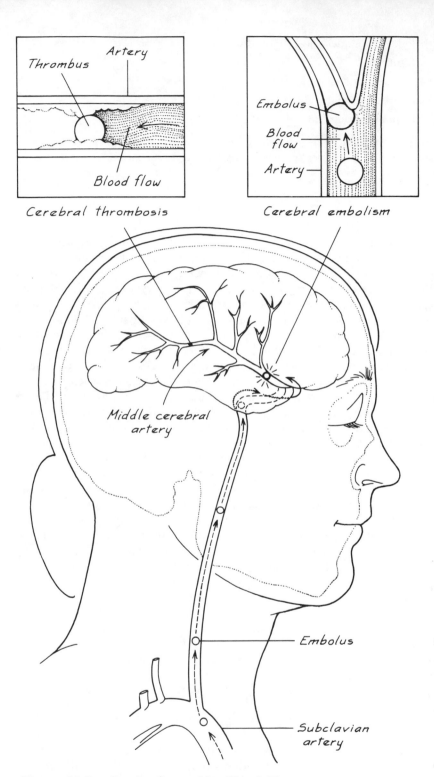

Figure 16.3   Stroke Caused by Blood Clots

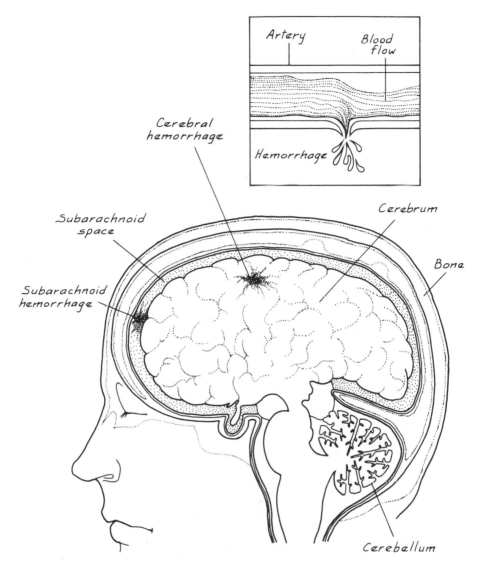

Figure 16.4   Stroke Caused by Bleeding (Hemorrhage)

you keep high blood pressure under control. (For ways to control blood pressure, see page 303.)

•   **Heart disease:** People with heart problems have more than twice the risk of stroke than people with normally functioning hearts. So by preventing heart disease by following the guidelines in this chapter, you are also lowering your risk of suffering a stroke.

•   **High red blood cell count:** A marked or even moderate increase in the red blood cell count is a risk factor for stroke. We don't know exactly why this is so. One theory has it that the sheer number of red blood cells may cause blood flow to become more sluggish, particularly in the smaller capillaries, which may increase the likelihood of developing clots. If you have a high red blood cell count, your physician may recommend that you take aspirin to help prevent the formation of a clot (see page 321).

• **Transient ischemic attacks (TIAs):** About 10 percent of strokes are preceded by "little strokes," or transient ischemic attacks. TIAs occur when a blood clot temporarily clogs an artery and part of the brain doesn't get the blood it needs. Symptoms include temporary weakness, clumsiness, or loss of feeling in an arm, leg, or the side of the face, temporary loss of vision in one eye, temporary loss of speech or difficulty speaking, and sometimes dizziness, double vision, and staggering. Symptoms generally don't last long. More than 75 percent of TIAs last less than five minutes. However, TIAs can last up to twenty-four hours (although this is very unusual). Unlike stroke, when a TIA is over, people return to normal. If you suffer any of these symptoms, it is essential that you see your physician. Your doctor can help determine whether you've experienced a TIA or whether the symptoms arose from another condition.

Warning Signs of a Stroke

Prompt medical attention is essential for minimizing the damage of a stroke. According to the American Heart Association, *you should immediately call for emergency help if you experience*:

- sudden weakness or numbness of the face, arm, and leg on one side of the body
- loss of speech, or trouble talking or understanding speech
- dimness or loss of vision, particularly in only one eye
- unexplained dizziness, unsteadiness, or sudden falls

Your physician can determine whether you have suffered a TIA or a stroke, or whether the symptoms are caused by another medical problem, such as seizure, fainting, or migraine. Prompt medical or surgical attention to these symptoms could prevent a fatal or disabling stroke from occurring.

Other Cardiovascular Problems

Arrhythmias

You've undoubtedly experienced it at some point in your life: a pounding sensation in your chest or a feeling that your heart is racing. Or perhaps you've felt occasionally that your heart skipped a beat. These are known as *arrhythmias*, irregularities in the heart's rate or rhythm. Generally speaking, arrhythmias occur when the heart's natural pacemaker develops an abnormal rate or rhythm, when the normal conduction pathway is interrupted, or when another part of the heart takes over as pacemaker.

The occasional "skipped beat" or a racing heart, particularly just before or after an anxiety-producing situation or after one too many cups of coffee, is usually harmless and nothing to worry about. If you suffer from menopausal hot flashes, you may experience a pounding or racing heart with every hot flash. Again, while the feeling can be uncomfortable, it is rarely life-threatening. That's not to say that *all* heartbeat irregularities are to be tossed off as harmless. Some, in fact, can be life-threatening and require immediate medical attention.

How can you tell harmless arrhythmias from life-threatening ones? *Any* recurring or persistent heartbeat irregularities or abnormal heart rhythms accompanied by chest discomfort or dizziness should be brought to the attention of your doctor, even if you think they're harmless. Your physician can properly evaluate your condition and recommend appropriate treatment.

Mitral-Valve Prolapse

Mitral-valve prolapse (MVP) occurs when one or both leaflets that make up the mitral valve (see Figure 16.5) billow up into the heart's atrial chamber,

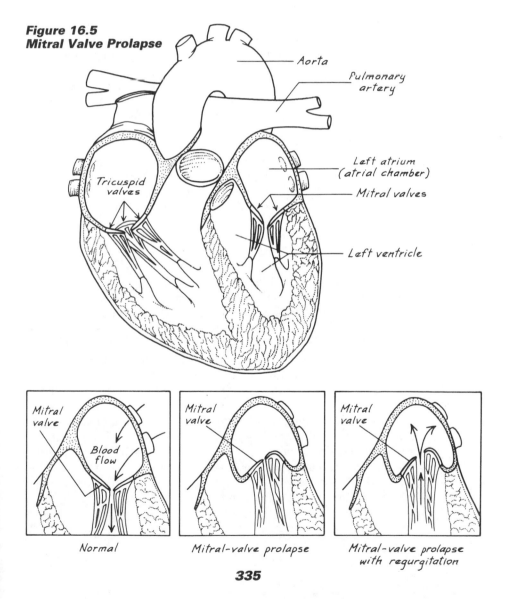

**Figure 16.5
Mitral Valve Prolapse**

Aorta

Pulmonary artery

Tricuspid valves

Left atrium (atrial chamber)

Mitral valves

Left ventricle

Mitral valve — Blood flow

Normal

Mitral valve

Mitral-valve prolapse

Mitral valve

Mitral-valve prolapse with regurgitation

often resulting in a clicking sound, or heart murmur. The condition sometimes causes blood to be regurgitated or spilled back into the atrium.

For reasons unknown, mitral-valve prolapse is more common in women than men, affecting about 5 to 6 percent of women, compared with 2 to 3 percent of men. There are two types. Patients with Type I MVP have no other heart abnormalities, only slight thickening of the mitral valve and mild regurgitation. Those with Type II MVP, the more serious form, often develop abnormalities of the valve itself, severe thickening, and increased regurgitation of blood.

Chest pain is the most frequent symptom, occurring in as many as 50 to 60 percent of women with MVP. Palpitations, chronic fatigue, and a feeling of anxiety are common, too. Some women experience shortness of breath and/ or dizzy spells. Only rarely, however, does MVP lead to more serious heart problems.

Your physician may be able to diagnose MVP simply by listening for the characteristic heart murmur that accompanies the condition. Your doctor can determine the severity of the condition with the help of an echocardiogram, in which sound waves are used to view the mitral valve in motion.

While symptoms may be bothersome, most women—particularly those with Type I MVP—won't require any treatment at all. (Keep in mind that chest pain and palpitations may be aggravated by nicotine, caffeine, and alcohol. If these symptoms are a problem, try to avoid these substances altogether.) Some women with Type II MVP may be advised to take a large dose of antibiotics an hour before having extensive dental work or surgery and again six hours later. This precaution is meant to help protect against *bacterial endocarditis,* an infection of the heart muscle caused by bacteria circulating in the blood-stream that may become attached to the prolapsed mitral valve.

A Final Word

There's no cure for cardiovascular disease—at least not yet. So a far better strategy is to reduce your risk of developing heart disease in the first place. This means adopting a heart-healthy lifestyle early on—preferably before the increased risks of heart disease associated with menopause kick in. A low-fat, low-cholesterol, low-sodium diet and regular exercise are cornerstones to a program of heart-disease prevention. If you smoke, quitting may be one of the kindest things you can do for your heart. You should limit your consumption of alcohol, too.

You will also need to regularly see your physician, who can monitor your cholesterol levels to determine how effective your efforts are. Your doctor can also diagnose and help you control hypertension and diabetes, two other risk factors for heart disease. If additional measures are needed, such as cholesterol-lowering medications, postmenopausal estrogen, or even over-the-counter aspirin, your physician can provide advice and a prescription.

·····································
Suggested Reading
·····································

HEART DISEASE PREVENTION

Legato, Marianne J., M.D., and Carol Colman. *The Female Heart: The Truth About Women and Coronary Artery Disease*. New York: Simon & Schuster, 1992.

Ornish, Dean, M.D. *Dr. Dean Ornish's Program for Reversing Heart Disease*. New York: Ballantine Books, 1990.

COOKBOOKS

The American Heart Association Cookbook, 5th ed. New York: Ballantine Books, 1991.

Connor, Sonja L., and William E. Connor. *The New American Diet System*. New York: Simon & Schuster, 1991.

Cooley, Denton A., M.D., and Carolyn E. Moore, Ph.D., R.D. *Eat Smart for a Healthy Heart Cookbook*. Woodbury, NY: Barron's, 1987.

Starke, Rodman D., M.D., and Mary Winston, Ed.D., R.D. *The American Heart Association Low-Salt Cookbook*. New York: Random House, 1990.

·····································
Resources and Support
·····································

American Heart Association, National Center, 7272 Greenville Avenue, Dallas, TX 75231. (800)AHA-USA-1 (800-242-8721). The AHA has a wealth of information on heart disease, hypertension, and stroke, including pamphlets and booklets on low-fat, low-sodium eating, smoking cessation, and other ways to reduce your risk of heart disease. Contact the national headquarters or your local office.

National Cholesterol Education Program (NCEP), National Heart, Lung and Blood Institute Information Center, Suite 530, 4733 Bethesda Avenue, Bethesda, MD 20814-4820. Phone: (301) 951-3260. This government agency provides free pamphlets, fact sheets, and other publications related to blood cholesterol, high blood pressure, cigarette smoking, and risk factors for cardiovascular disease. Call or write for information.

Chapter 17

....

Osteoporosis: What You Can Do to Prevent It, Plus New Techniques for Managing the Disease

Sixty-eight-year-old Helen Young isn't sure what startled her out of a sound sleep one night a couple of years ago. But when she sat up in bed, she heard a crunching noise and felt an excruciating pain in her back. She learned from a bone specialist a few days later that the noise she had heard was the collapse of several vertebrae in her spine. Helen has *osteoporosis,* a condition marked by severe or prolonged bone loss that makes bones less likely to withstand the physical stresses of everyday living.

Helen Young's story is not unusual. In fact, it's all too common. According to the National Osteoporosis Foundation, one-third of all women over sixty-five will suffer one or more vertebral fractures as a result of osteoporosis. Another 300,000 women each year will suffer a hip fracture. Indeed, one out of every six women will suffer a hip fracture in her lifetime— a risk *equal to the combined risks of developing breast, uterine, and ovarian cancer.*

The cost to individuals and society is enormous: About $10 billion is spent each year on acute care associated with hip fractures alone. This does not include hired nursing care, nursing-home stays, or costs attributable to changes in lifestyle as a result of disability from a fracture.

There's no cure for osteoporosis, but it can be prevented. A key is knowing how much bone you have to start with and having your bone mass monitored through the critical menopausal years, when the rate of bone loss accelerates. This is now possible thanks to the development of various reliable and fairly inexpensive bone-density tests. These tests can help determine whether you have experienced an excessive amount of bone loss for your age, which puts you at a greater risk of suffering a fracture, a condition known as *osteopenia,* or whether you have experienced such a profound loss of bone mass that microscopic or obvious fractures have already occurred, the technical definition of *osteoporosis.*

Knowing whether you have low bone mass is important, since further loss of bone mass can often be slowed or stopped—and possibly even reversed—with appropriate lifestyle measures and medication. And while it's not possible to "uncollapse" a collapsed vertebra, straighten a dowager's hump, or regain height lost as a result of spinal fractures, there are several ways you can reduce both physical pain and your risk of suffering further fractures if you already have osteoporosis. Nine months after Helen Young first visited our clinic, the pain associated with her vertebral fractures had subsided considerably and the bone mass in her spine had actually *increased*.

Before we talk about how to protect your bones, it helps to know a little bit about them.

Bone Basics

Although you probably don't think much about them, the 206 bones in your body play a vital role in your health and well-being. Your bones give you support, allow you to go about your daily activities, and protect your vital organs. Bone marrow manufactures new blood cells. Your bones are a virtual warehouse for storing calcium, a mineral needed for muscle contraction, blood clotting, blood pressure regulation, and nerve impulse transmission. In fact, ninety-nine percent of the calcium in your body is stored in your bones.

Each of the bones in your body is made up of two types of bone tissue: *trabecular bone* consists of a network of bony plates resembling lattice-work or scaffolding that is lightweight yet extremely strong. Trabecular bone is found mostly in the vertebrae of the spine, the breastbone, the top of the pelvis, and in the ends of the long bones of your body (arms and legs). Surrounding the trabecular bone is a thin sheet of denser *cortical bone*. Cortical bone is also the major type of bone tissue in the arms and legs (see Figure 17.1).

Old Bone, New Bone

Although we tend to think of bone as inert and unchanging, bone is living tissue, and like all living tissue, it is constantly changing—breaking down old bone cells and replacing them with new ones, a process called *bone remodeling*. Bone remodeling replaces old bone damaged by wear and tear and helps maintain a constant level of calcium in the bloodstream.

Two major cells are involved in bone remodeling. *Osteoclasts* are responsible for removing old cells. Once activated, osteoclasts secrete powerful enzymes that dissolve old bone cells, carving out microscopic cavities in the bone. *Osteoblasts* are smaller cells that are somehow attracted to the hollowed out spaces made by osteoclasts. Osteoblasts manufacture the basic building material of bone, known as *osteoid*, or bone matrix, consisting mostly of collagen fibers.

Approximately ten days after the osteoid is laid down, crystals—mostly of calcium and phosphorus—are added to the framework, a process called *bone mineralization*. A number of other minerals are also present in bone, such as fluoride, sodium, potassium, magnesium, and zinc. These minerals act as the "mortar" to hold the "bricks" of calcium and phosphorus crystals together. The calcium crystals give your bones their strength, hardness, and rigidity,

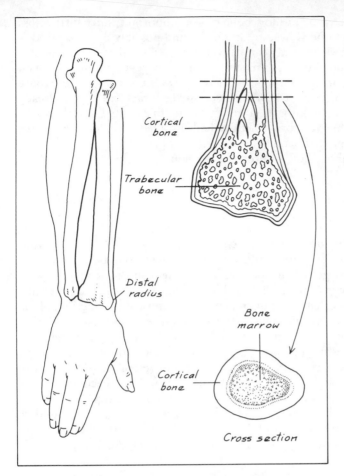

Figure 17.1   Cortical and Trabecular Bone

while the collagen fibers give them their relative capacity for flexibility, or *elasticity*.

At any given time, from 5 to 20 percent of your skeleton is undergoing remodeling. Bone breakdown (*resorption*) and new bone formation takes four to eight weeks to complete. Mineralization requires two to three months more.

About 10 percent of cortical bone is remodeled each year. Because trabecular bone has a larger surface area for osteoclasts to work on, about 40 percent of trabecular bone is remodeled each year. (This may also be why vertebral fractures occur more frequently than fractures of the hip and wrist, which contain more cortical than trabecular bone.)

How Your Body Regulates Bone Mass

Your bone mass—the total amount of bone in your skeleton—is maintained by a delicate balance between the breakdown of old bone and the formation of new bone. Several different mechanisms are involved in the control of this bone-remodeling process.

Calcium and the "Bone Hormones"

Calcium is so vital to the human body that an elaborate system of hormones has evolved to ensure that there is always enough of it in your blood. This "calcium thermostat" is chiefly regulated by three hormones: parathyroid hormone, vitamin D, and calcitonin. The thermostat is influenced by several other hormones, including the reproductive hormones estrogen and progesterone, adrenal hormones, and thyroid hormones.

• **Parathyroid hormone:** If the calcium in your bloodstream falls below critical levels, four tiny glands in your neck, known as parathyroid glands, release *parathyroid hormone*. This hormone signals the kidneys to put calcium back into the bloodstream rather than excrete it through urine. It also stimulates the conversion of vitamin D from an inactive to an active form. (Vitamin D helps the intestines absorb calcium from the food you eat.) Finally, parathyroid hormone stimulates osteoclasts to break down bone, releasing stored calcium into the bloodstream.

• **Vitamin D:** Vitamin D, produced by ultraviolet irradiation of an inactive form of vitamin D in your skin, and derived from certain foods, increases the absorption of calcium in the intestines. It also increases the reabsorption of calcium through the kidneys. Vitamin D is responsible for maintaining a proper level of calcium in the blood. But if levels of vitamin D are high, it can actually withdraw calcium from the bones, leading to bone loss. This is why you should not consume more than 1,000 milligrams of vitamin D per day.

• **Calcitonin:** When calcium levels in the bloodstream rise, this hormone, secreted by the thyroid gland, protects bones by inhibiting the activity of osteoclasts and slowing the bone-remodeling cycle. Levels of calcitonin naturally decline with age. What's more, women have lower levels of calcitonin than men, a difference which is even greater after menopause. These lower levels of calcitonin may contribute to gender-, age-, and menopause-related losses of bone mass.

• **Reproductive hormones (estrogen, progesterone, androgen):** Estrogen receptors have been found in osteoblasts, suggesting that estrogen has a direct effect on bone. Estrogen also interacts with several other hormones and, in this way, indirectly influences the regulation of bone mass. Estrogen blocks the bone-dissolving actions of parathyroid hormone. It also stimulates the activation of vitamin D and the release of calcitonin from the thyroid. Finally, estrogen stimulates the liver to produce a protein that binds to certain adrenal hormones, decreasing their ability to dissolve bone.

Progesterone, the female hormone produced during the second half of the menstrual cycle, appears to help protect bone mass, too. Low levels of progesterone have been associated with loss of bone mass in premenopausal women whose estrogen levels are normal. Progesterone is thought to prevent the bone-dissolving adrenal hormones from attaching to bone-cell receptors, thus offering further protection to bone.

341

Androgens, the "male" sex hormones, which are produced in small amounts by women, also affect bone mass. Androgens apparently stimulate the activity of osteoblasts, helping to build new bone.

• **Adrenal hormones:** Several hormones released from the adrenal glands, known as *glucocorticoids,* act directly on bone by attaching to receptors on the surfaces of bone cells. This causes the bone to respond to the dissolving effects of parathyroid hormone and activated vitamin D.

• **Thyroid hormones:** Overactivity of the thyroid gland stimulates the breakdown of trabecular bone by increasing the number of bone-remodeling sites.

Other Regulators of Bone Mass

The bones themselves also contain powerful regulators of the bone-remodeling cycle.

• **Electrical impulses:** Bones create electrical energy, which is not surprising, since the heart and other bodily functions are driven by electrical currents. These small electrical currents appear to stimulate the formation of new bone somehow.

• **Growth factors:** These proteins are responsible for tissue repair and regeneration throughout the body. Numerous growth factors have been found either to stimulate or inhibit bone formation. Some growth factors are produced by osteoblasts or other bone cells; others come from elsewhere in the body. A number of them are present in bone matrix.

Prostaglandins, fluoride, and phosphates also play a role in the bone-remodeling process.

How Bone Loss Occurs

From the time you are born until you reach early adulthood, you produce more new bone tissue than you lose through bone breakdown. Around age thirty-five, however, you reach skeletal maturity, or *peak bone mass*, and an imbalance in the bone-remodeling system develops, so that old bone removal outpaces replacement with new bone. We're not sure exactly why this is so. It may be that the chemical "switches" that normally signal osteoblasts to lay down new bone are less effective. Calcium absorption declines with age, too. One probable cause is a decrease in your body's manufacture of vitamin D. Another cause is the drop in estrogen after menopause (estrogen enhances the body's ability to absorb calcium). As a result of these changes, blood-calcium levels decline. To bring blood-calcium levels back to normal, the parathyroid gland may secrete more PTH, releasing calcium from the bones and leading to a loss of bone mass. Levels of calcitonin, which, as you may recall, is secreted by the thyroid gland to help stop bone resorption, also appear to decline with age, compounding the problem. Because of these changes, either osteoclasts carve out cavities that are too deep, or osteoblasts don't make enough new bone to fill existing cavities, and you lose bone mass.

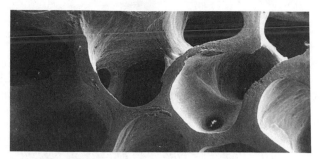

Photo 17.1 **Healthy Bone**

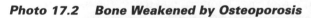

From age thirty-five until menopause, you lose cortical bone at a rate of .3 to .5 percent per year. After menopause and until about age sixty-five, the rate of cortical bone loss increases to about 1 percent per year, slowing down after age sixty-five to 0.18 percent per year. Some experts believe you experience a steady loss of trabecular bone after you reach peak bone mass in your twenties. Others say the bone loss pattern for trabecular bone is similar to that for cortical bone; that is, you lose 0.19 percent per year before menopause, increasing to 1.1 percent thereafter.

The bottom line is that a woman can expect to lose about 35 percent of her cortical bone and 50 percent of her trabecular bone over a lifetime. Men lose only about two-thirds these amounts.

The End Result of Osteoporosis: Fractures

Under severe stress or trauma, *any* bone can break. However, bones weakened by progressive loss of bone mass will break more easily (see photos 17.1 and 17.2). The most vulnerable bones are the vertebrae of the spine, which are

Photo 17.2 **Bone Weakened by Osteoporosis**

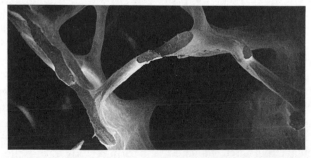

Note: Photographs 17.1 and 17.2 are reprinted with permission from D. W. Dempster, E. Shane, W. Holbert, and R. Lindsay, "A Simple Method for Correlative Light and Scanning Electron Microscopy of Human Iliac Crest Bone Biopsies: Qualitative Observations in Normal and Osteoporotic Subjects," *Journal of Bone Mineral Research* 1 (1986): 15–21.

composed primarily of latticelike trabecular bone. As the vertebrae become more porous and weak over the years, they go through various stages of structural deformity and can actually collapse (see Figure 17.2). Unlike fractures of other bones in the body, which can mend themselves under the proper conditions, the structural damage to the spinal vertebrae cannot be undone.

Hip fractures (actually, fractures of the upper part of the thigh bone, or *femur*)—usually the result of an accident or injury—are by far the most disabling and life-threatening consequence of osteoporosis. *Fewer than one-half of all women who suffer a hip fracture regain normal function. Fifteen percent of women die shortly after their injury, and nearly 30 percent die within one year.* Deaths from hip fractures are not caused by the fracture itself, but from some condition resulting from confinement to a hospital or nursing home bed, such as pneumonia, thrombosis (blood clots), or a fat embolism (bone marrow fat trapped in the lung). So you can see why preventing the bone loss that can lead to fractures is imperative.

Who Will Get Osteoporosis?

Some women are more likely than others to develop osteoporosis. Characteristically, women at risk are described as white (Caucasian) or Asian, blond, petite, with small body frame, and/or a family history of low bone mass (*osteopenia*) or osteoporosis (in either parent). Women are especially at risk if they have had a premature or surgical menopause and have not taken postmenopausal hormone therapy.

Other markers are women who started menstruating after age sixteen; those with a history of irregular menstrual cycles; eating disorders (anorexia or bulimia); athletic amenorrhea; anovulatory cycles (menstrual cycles in which the ovaries did not release an egg); low calcium intake; and scoliosis.

However, while these risk factors can give you and your physician an idea of whether you will develop osteoporosis later, their powers of prediction are limited. By some estimates, using risk factors alone to determine who will develop osteoporosis detects only 30 percent of all women at risk. One patient of ours, sixty-seven-year-old Margaret Lambert, had few of the risk factors for osteoporosis. On the surface, it appeared she would be at *low* risk because she was black; black women generally have greater bone mass than white women and therefore are less likely to develop osteoporosis. However, a bone-density test revealed that Margaret had lost a considerable amount of bone in her spine and was a prime candidate for osteoporosis. Another patient of ours, Pamela Cooley, was overweight, which again would suggest that she was somewhat protected from developing osteoporosis. Yet when she underwent a bone-density screening test, the bone-mineral content of her wrist was found to be just 65 percent of peak bone mass, putting her in a high-risk category for suffering a fracture later on.

Our clinical experience is backed by a formal study at our clinic, in which we compared actual bone-density measurements of 859 women with various risk factors, including height, weight, age of menopause, estrogen use, family history of osteoporosis, vitamin D and calcium intake, physical exercise, alcohol and caffeine consumption, and cigarette smoking. Our objective was to see how well the risk factors could predict which women had low bone mass. We

Figure 17.2   Types of Spinal Fractures

Crush fractures occur when both the front and back sections of a spinal vertebra collapse. *Wedge fractures* occur when the front but not the back section of the vertebra collapses. *Codfishing* describes the beginning of the collapse of two spinal vertebrae, which causes the space between them to take on a fish-shaped appearance. When spinal fractures occur over time, they lead to the stooped posture or "Dowager's Hump" commonly used to describe "little old ladies."

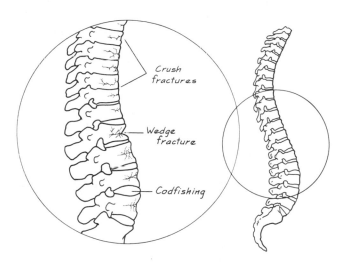

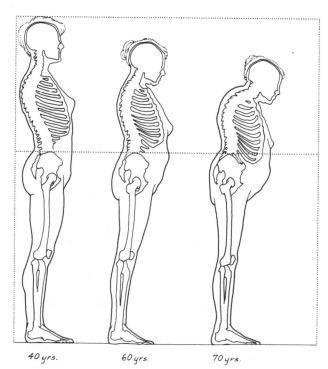

40 yrs.   60 yrs.   70 yrs.

345

found that the most reliable means of determining who had low bone mass was actual bone-density measurements. Our research was buoyed by studies by others, who also found that *the best way to determine whether you're at risk of developing osteoporosis is to have your bone density tested.*

Are You Losing Bone?

Obviously, you don't want to wait until you have a fracture to find out whether you are losing bone. Yet until quite recently, osteoporosis was almost always diagnosed only after a woman had suffered a fracture. By that time, the loss of bone mass was so severe that little could be done to reverse the process.

Now, however, a variety of tests have been developed to help assess the health of your bones. As you have probably gathered by now, your overall bone health depends on a number of different factors, including your *bone-mineral content* (how much mineral—mainly calcium—is in your bones), the activity of your bone-remodeling cycle, the *micro-architecture* of your bones (for instance, the latticework struts that make up trabecular bone), and bone *elasticity* (the ability of bone to bend a little rather than break under stress). A combination of the tests described here can give your doctor a better picture of your bone health and can be used to help design and monitor an individualized prevention or treatment plan for you.

Bone-Density Tests

These tests measure the amount of calcium and other minerals in your bones in relation to the width of the bones.

Screening Tests
Measurements of the hand, arm, or heel can give you and your physician an idea of your overall bone health. We have demonstrated that bone density is lost from the entire skeleton; so, in effect, if you are losing bone in your wrist, you are probably losing bone elsewhere in your skeleton, as well. Essentially, these tests tell you there is a problem somewhere, but further tests are needed to find out where the problem is.

• **Dual-energy X-ray Absorptiometry (DEXA):** This technology for bone density testing consists of a scanner that emits low levels of X-ray radiation and a detector that measures the amount of radiation absorbed by bone—the greater the absorption, the greater the bone density. The procedure is simple. Your wrist is placed under the DEXA scanner and the scanner passes over the bone several times as it measures the bone-mineral content and the width of the bone. The test is painless and exposes you to just a fraction of the radiation of an ordinary arm X ray.

Your bone-density measurement is then compared with the average bone density of younger women (see Table A.2 on page 475). A bone-density measurement that is 20 to 30 percent lower than average indicates that you have osteopenia.

• **Single-photon absorptiometry (SPA):** This test is similar to the DEXA test described above, except that a single beam of radioactive iodine is used to

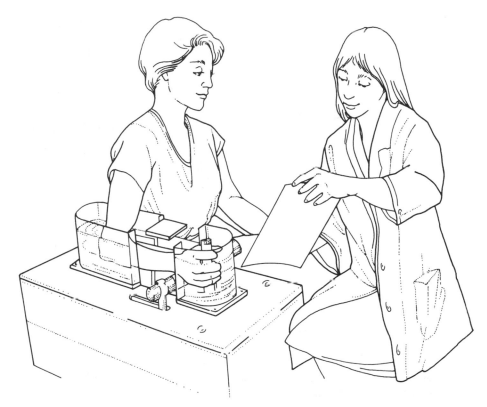

Figure 17.3   Bone Density Testing of the Wrist with Single Photon Absorptiometry (SPA)

determine bone density. In this procedure, your arm or the heel of your foot will be placed in a water bath between the source of gamma rays and the detector (see Figure 17.3); the scanner passes over the bone several times. Again, radiation exposure is just a fraction of that of an arm X ray.

• **Radiographic densitometry:** A routine X ray of the hand can be used to determine bone density, as well. Your hand is placed alongside a standardized aluminum wedge and an X ray is taken. The radiologist can then determine your bone density by comparing the density of your finger with that of the aluminum wedge.

Diagnostic Tests
If a bone-density screening test indicates that you have low bone mass, your physician will want to have you undergo further tests to help pinpoint problem areas. Over the last several years, the technology has been developed that allows measurement of bones located deeper in the body—certain vertebrae in the lower (*lumbar*) spine and the hip, for example—which are more prone to fractures.

• **Dual-energy X-ray absorptiometry:** A DEXA scanner can measure bone density of the hip and spine (areas of the skeleton where osteopenia is usually

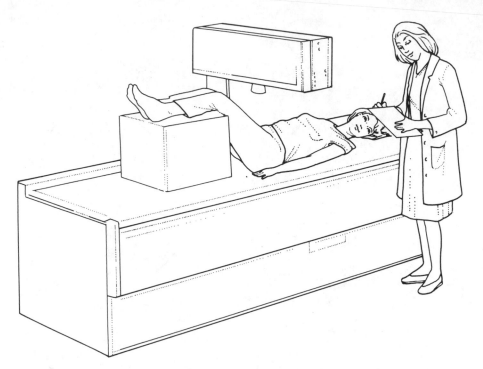

Figure 17.4   Bone Density Testing of the Spine with Dual-Energy X-ray Absorptiometry (DEXA)

the greatest), as well as that of the total body (see Figure 17.4), and is one of the most reliable bone-density screening and diagnostic tests available today. DEXA can detect as little as a 1 percent loss of bone mass from year to year, compared to standard X rays, which can detect low bone mass only after 30 percent or more of bone mass has been lost. Still, the technology is limited in what it can do. DEXA can assess only bone density of the lumbar spine. Most fractures occur in the thoracic (middle) spine. DEXA also includes in its measurements calcium deposits that sometimes form in the body (for instance, around a diseased disk or an arthritic joint or around an old fracture), possibly leading to an *overestimation* of your bone density. Newer models of DEXA that scan from the side of vertebrae may resolve this problem.

In addition, DEXA cannot detect fractures. It measures only the amount of bone mineral you have.

•   **Quantitative computerized tomography:** A CT scan, which creates a three-dimensional view of the body using low-dose X rays and a computerized scanner, is unique in that it can measure purely trabecular bone within the spine, which is where most crush fractures occur. The procedure, in which you lie on an examining table within a cylindrical scanner, takes fifteen to twenty minutes.

However, there are several disadvantages: The procedure exposes you to a relatively high dosage of radiation and can be rather costly. CT scanners also tend to *overestimate* the amount of bone being lost. This is because the scanners also detect fat, which replaces both bone tissue and marrow as trabecular bone ages. For these reasons, CT scanning probably won't be routinely used for bone-density testing.

• **Newer technology:** Ultrasound, involving the use of high-frequency sound waves, is now being evaluated as yet another diagnostic tool for determining bone health. The instruments, which emit sound waves through your body's tissues, measure the collagen content of bone, which may indirectly tell us something about the bone's elasticity. The technology will probably best be used in conjunction with bone-density tests.

Standard X Rays

We still don't have the technology to assess the micro-architecture of bone—particularly the scaffolding structure of trabecular bone, which contributes to

---

Should You Have a Bone-Density Test?

Questions about the accuracy and precision of densitometers and other methods of measuring bone health made bone-density testing controversial in the past. However, further research and technological advances have helped correct some of the early problems with bone-density testing. Now all experts agree that bone-mass measurement is a key to the prevention and treatment of osteoporosis.

The National Osteoporosis Foundation recommends you have your bone density tested:

1. **following a natural menopause,** surgical removal of the ovaries, or prolonged amenorrhea (cessation of menstruation)—regardless of the cause

2. **if you have spinal abnormalities** such as collapsed vertebrae, edging, or "ballooning" of spinal plates

3. **if you take steroids** to control such diseases as rheumatoid arthritis, hepatitis, inflammatory bowel disease, asthma, or chronic obstructive pulmonary disease (steroids can cause rapid bone loss)

4. **if you have hyperparathyroidism** and do not have the parathyroid gland surgically removed, an overactive parathyroid gland can lead to decreased bone mass

Other women who should consider bone-density testing include women with osteopenia or osteoporosis who are taking medication to prevent further bone loss. Bone-density tests can help monitor the efficacy of your treatment.

For more information and referrals to physicians and organizations that perform bone-density testing, contact the National Osteoporosis Foundation, Suite 500, 1150 17th Street, NW, Washington, D.C. 20036.

bone strength. However, regular X rays can help detect fractures and help your physician diagnose osteoporosis.

Generally, in order to diagnose osteoporosis, a regular X ray of the spine is needed—both the thoracic and lumbar spine. Physicians looks for deformities in vertebrae, including codfishing, wedging, and compression fractures. These changes in the spine are irreversible. Two or more nontraumatic fractures indicate that you have osteoporosis.

Spinal X rays can also help determine whether a curvature of the spine is a result of a vertebral fracture or a physical abnormality. For instance, a congenital condition known as *Scheuermann's syndrome* causes marked curvature of the spine, although there are no deformities in the vertebrae.

X rays can be used to diagnose osteopenia, as well. However, this is not the best method, since X rays can't detect bone losses until about 30 percent of your bone mass has been lost (compared to DEXA, which can detect a loss of 1 percent or less).

Bone-Remodeling Cycle Activity

Blood and urine tests can help determine the rate at which you are losing bone mass. Some women lose bone more rapidly than others and may need more aggressive treatment.

Urine Tests

• **Calcium to creatinine ratio:** This is perhaps the most useful marker of the rate of bone-mineral loss. You'll be asked to collect a sample of the second urine that you pass after fasting overnight. The sample is sent to a laboratory and tested for the ratio of calcium to creatinine (a by-product of metabolism). Ratios over 0.16 indicate that the bone-remodeling cycle has been accelerated for some reason. Your calcium intake can influence the result of this test and should not exceed 1,500 milligrams per day.

• **Urinary hydroxyproline:** This test is less frequently used and reflects the breakdown of collagen in bone, which is largely due to the resorption of bone matrix and, as such, goes hand in hand with the calcium-to-creatinine test. Unfortunately, the breakdown of collagen in tissues other than bone is also reflected in the test, so it's not a highly accurate measure of bone resorption. Other disadvantages: The cost of the test, which averages around seventy dollars, you must be on a special gelatin-free diet for at least three days prior to the test.

Promising new markers of bone resorption are urinary levels of certain *collagen cross-links* found in bone and cartilage. Levels of one such cross-link, *pyridinoline* (PYR), are significantly higher after menopause. Hormone therapy returns levels of PYR to premenopausal levels. More research is needed before the test becomes available, however.

Blood Tests

• **Alkaline phosphatase activity:** Blood levels of alkaline phosphatase can reveal whether new bone is forming. Typically, it is used in conjunction with other biochemical markers and in monitoring your response to treatment if you have a medical condition (such as hyperthyroidism) known to increase the rate of bone loss. The test can also be used to monitor the effectiveness of certain drug therapies—notably sodium fluoride, which stimulates the formation of new bone.

Evaluating Secondary Causes of Osteoporosis

A minority of women have low bone mass due to an underlying medical condition that must be treated to prevent further bone loss. Secondary causes include hyperthyroidism, hyperparathyroidism, overactive adrenal glands, malabsorption syndromes (in which the intestines have difficulty absorbing certain nutrients), multiple myeloma (cancer of the bone marrow), other cancers that have spread, and diabetes.

Your physician may look for a secondary cause of osteoporosis if you have symptoms other than low bone mass or when hormone therapy doesn't stop the loss of bone mass. Typically, this entails blood tests of thyroid, parathyroid, and adrenal function. Other tests may be given to determine whether you have a malabsorption syndrome, multiple myeloma (a frequent cause of spontaneous fractures and back pain), or other underlying causes of accelerated bone loss.

Preventing Osteoporosis: Building Bone and Slowing Bone Losses

Remember, the more bone you have to begin with, the more you can afford to lose without impairing your skeleton's strength. That's why it's essential that you start preventive measures early—ideally *before* you reach peak bone mass. But it's never too late to begin. The same measures used to build up bone before you reach peak bone mass can also help slow the loss of bone mass (and possibly even *reverse* it) after menopause.

Our program of prevention consists of a three-pronged approach: exercise to build bone mass, nutrition to ensure adequate bone mineralization, and, for postmenopausal women, estrogen and other nonhormonal means of slowing or stopping the accelerated rate of bone loss after menopause.

Exercise

Bone responds to physical stress in the same way muscles do: by becoming larger and stronger. Mechanical force, muscular activity, and gravity all appear to stimulate bone cells to grow. No one's sure yet how this happens. Exercise may create small electrical currents within the bone, somehow spurring bone growth. Exercise may also stimulate the production of prostaglandins and other bone-growth factors. Whatever the mechanism, exercise is directly associated with increased bone matrix in both trabecular and cortical bone.

Exercise has beneficial effects on the bones both locally and generally. In other words, exercising the legs builds bone mass of the legs, but it also builds bone in the rest of the skeleton, though to a lesser degree.

We know that total inactivity can lead to severe bone loss. For instance, being confined to bed will cause you to lose bone mineral at an alarming rate of 4 percent per month during the first several weeks in bed.

The forces of gravity play a major role: Exercising while lying in bed won't help offset the bone loss associated with bed rest, but standing quietly for three hours a day can help slow it. Four hours of walking prevents bone loss associated with twenty hours of bed rest.

If a little exercise can help maintain bone, how much is needed actually to build bone? Again, we're not certain, but we do know that you must be active on a regular basis. On the other hand, it appears you can exercise *too much*. Repeated and prolonged exercise can cause bone fatigue and microscopic fractures. Stress fractures are common in long-distance runners. (The incidence of stress fractures goes down, however, when bones are allowed sufficient rest between exercise sessions.) What's more, women marathon runners who develop exercise-induced amenorrhea actually *lose* trabecular bone in the spine. (Cortical bone in the runners is normal or only slightly reduced.) The bone loss is believed to be caused by a drop in estrogen associated with decreased body fat, and it may be permanent.

The type of exercise is important, too. Generally speaking, weight-bearing or load-bearing activities—that is, exercises that put stress on the long bones of the body—are best for building bone mass and slowing bone loss. Weight-bearing activities include walking, bicycling, low-impact aerobics, climbing stairs, and racket sports such as tennis. Choose several different activities so that you don't tire of any single one.

Your age is another significant factor: Exercise builds bone mass more readily in "growing" rather than "mature" bone. This is why it's so important to exercise in your premenopausal years, before the predictable postmenopausal bone loss begins to occur.

This is not to say that exercise *won't* benefit older women. Several studies (including our own) have shown that exercise is very effective at slowing the loss of bone mass after menopause. Some studies have even shown that it's possible for postmenopausal women to *gain* bone mass. A study from Washington University School of Medicine in St. Louis found that menopausal women who exercised increased their bone mass by 5.2 percent during the nine-month study, while sedentary women lost an additional 1.2 percent of bone mass. After twenty-two months, the exercisers' bone mass had increased by 6.1 percent, while women who didn't exercise continued to lose bone mass.

Exercise is one of the only preventive (or therapeutic) measures that not only halts bone loss but also *stimulates the formation of new bone*. This is why exercise should be an integral part of any preventive efforts.

Remember, too, that exercise works only for as long as you work out on a regular basis. In the Washington University study, women who stopped exercising once again began to lose bone mass. Thirteen months after the study was over, bone mass of the former exercisers was just 1.1 percent above baseline.

We don't know yet how much exercise is enough. One study of ours suggests that you need to exercise for at least forty-five minutes at a time, three to four times a week, to maintain bone mass after menopause. You'll find step-by-step instructions for beginning an exercise program in Chapter 5.

Nutrition

How well you eat also affects the health of your bones.

• **Calcium:** Calcium is not the only nutrient essential for bone health, but it is the most talked-about one—and possibly the most important. The reason is that bone is roughly two-thirds mineral by weight, and calcium makes up about 40 percent of that mineral.

Clearly, if you don't get enough calcium in your diet throughout your life, your bones will suffer. Several studies have shown that when animals are fed a low-calcium diet, they develop osteoporosis. A link between low calcium intake and an increased risk of fractures has also been found among women. A classic study involved a comparison of bone mass in two groups from different rural areas in Yugoslavia—one group having an average daily calcium intake (940 milligrams) that was more than twice that of the other (441 milligrams). The women in the higher-calcium group definitely had stronger bones at skeletal maturity and a lower incidence of hip fractures later in life than women in the low-calcium group.

These reports on calcium's influence on bone health and other reports showing that women weren't getting enough calcium sparked a "calcium craze" in the 1980s. Sales of calcium supplements skyrocketed. And food manufacturers began adding calcium to all sorts of products—even soda pop! The craze ultimately created more confusion about this mineral than anything else. Adding to the confusion were more recent reports that calcium alone doesn't prevent fractures, nor does calcium by itself slow bone loss as effectively as estrogen.

Actually, this news should come as no surprise, since, as you've already seen, calcium deficiency isn't the *only* cause of osteoporosis. Unfortunately, many women misinterpreted these reports to mean that calcium wasn't all that important in preventing osteoporosis.

New, better-designed studies now show that calcium supplementation may indeed help slow postmenopausal bone loss. A Tufts University study showed that menopausal women whose calcium intake was less than 400 milligrams a day significantly reduced bone loss by increasing their calcium intake to 800 milligrams a day. And a 1993 study by New Zealand scientists reported that even postmenopausal women with higher calcium intakes—750 milligrams a day—could slow bone loss by also taking a 1,000-milligram calcium supplement.

Regardless of whether calcium supplements prevent fractures, your bones need calcium for mineralization. Equally important is the 1 percent of calcium that circulates in your bloodstream, essential for muscle contraction, blood clotting, blood pressure regulation, and nerve-impulse transmission. Remember, if you don't get enough calcium from your diet to maintain adequate levels of calcium in your bloodstream, your body will take calcium from your bones. To find out whether you're getting enough calcium in your diet and how you can increase your calcium intake, see page 75.

• **Vitamin D:** A sufficient amount of vitamin D is essential because it helps to maintain a positive calcium balance, yet too much can have the reverse effect and cause you to lose bone mass unnecessarily.

Getting enough vitamin D doesn't appear to be a problem for premenopausal women. But elderly women and women with osteoporosis have been shown to have a deficiency of the activated form of vitamin D. One recent study of a group of postmenopausal women in Boston showed that one-half of them became vitamin D-deficient during the winter months, when exposure to sunlight was limited. Moreover, women whose daily vitamin D intake was below 220 international units (IU) had higher levels of bone-dissolving parathyroid hormone in their blood in the spring.

The recommended daily allowance for adults is 400 IU, which may be obtained either from your diet or from the sun. While the sun is your primary source of vitamin D, there is no way to measure how much you are getting. Some experts estimate that a Caucasian woman needs from fifteen minutes to one hour of sunshine daily to meet her vitamin D requirement. (Keep in mind that regular use of a sunscreen may limit vitamin D production in your skin; see page 159.)

Vitamin D in the diet is fairly limited: fatty fish, butter, egg yolks, liver, and fortified milk are the best sources. Most multivitamin preparations also contain the 400 units you need each day. But don't overdo it; too much vitamin D can stimulate bone loss. You should avoid amounts in excess of 1,000 units per day.

• **Phosphorus:** The trace mineral phosphorus is a major component of bone. But some evidence suggests that too much phosphorus can lead to bone loss. Early reports suggesting that phosphorus inhibits calcium absorption proved not to be true. However, phosphorus may indirectly affect bone mass by raising levels of bone-dissolving parathyroid hormone in the body. Animals fed high-phosphorus, low-calcium diets develop hyperparathyroidism and, ultimately, osteopenia. A high-phosphorus diet appears to elevate parathyroid hormone in humans, too. In one two-month-long study, fifteen women ages eighteen to twenty-five first ate a balanced diet containing 800 milligrams of calcium and 900 milligrams of phosphorus. Then ten of the women switched to a low-calcium (400 milligrams per day), high-phosphorus (1,700 milligrams per day) diet—a dietary pattern characteristic of teens and young adults. After four weeks on the low-calcium, high-phosphorus diet, the women experienced a 26 to 36 percent increase in levels of parathyroid hormone, while those who continued to eat a more balanced diet experienced no change in levels of parathyroid hormone.

More research needs to be conducted before we know the exact role of phosphorus in bone health. Until that time, it is probably wise to curb your consuption of foods containing excessive amounts of phosphorus. The worst offenders are cola drinks, red meat, and processed foods containing phosphorus additives. (There are plenty of other good reasons to cut back on your intake of these foods, anyway: Soft drinks contain only "empty calories"; red meat is a major source of saturated fat and cholesterol; and processed foods are usually high in sodium, which may raise blood pressure among some women and contributes to excessive calcium excretion in all women.)

• **Magnesium:** Like calcium, this trace mineral is abundant in bone tissue and is important for muscle contraction and nerve-impulse transmission. Because magnesium and calcium have similar functions in the body, an excess of one mineral may cause problems with the other. For instance, excessive amounts of magnesium will inhibit bone mineralization. Too much calcium may inhibit magnesium absorption and trigger a magnesium deficiency. For this reason, experts generally recommend that you balance your intake of both calcium and magnesium. The best calcium-to-magnesium ratio is 2 to 1; that is, that you should take in roughly two times more calcium than magnesium. So if you consume 1, 400 milligrams of calcium per day, this means you should also consume about 700 milligrams of magnesium. (The current RDA for magnesium—280 milligrams for adult women—doesn't take into account the higher recommended calcium intake that most experts now advocate for women in midlife.) Foods high in magnesium include nuts, legumes, cereal grains, dark green vegetables, and seafood.

• **Vitamin K:** This fat-soluble vitamin plays a crucial role in bone mineralization. If you eat plenty of leafy green vegetables, you probably get all the vitamin K you need. (Vitamin K also aids in blood coagulation and clot formation.)

Other Lifestyle Factors

• **Cigarette smoking:** Several studies have associated cigarette smoking with an accelerated loss of bone and a greater risk of osteoporosis. We're still not sure whether smoking actually caused the women in the studies to lose bone mass more rapidly or whether they simply had lower bone mass at skeletal maturity than nonsmoking women.

One important way in which cigarette smoking may affect bone health is that it changes the liver's metabolism of estrogen, making it less biologically active. Cigarette smokers also experience menopause an average of two of three years earlier than nonsmokers, meaning that smokers experience the accelerated rate of bone loss associated with menopause that much earlier than nonsmokers. Also, there's some evidence that cigarette smoking somehow inhibits osteoblasts and new bone formation.

• **Alcohol:** We've known for some time now that alcoholics generally have a lower bone mass than nondrinkers. However, having as few as three drinks per day on a regular basis may contribute to low bone mass. The reasons aren't clear yet: Excessive alcohol consumption is typically associated with poor nutrition, including low intakes of calcium and vitamin D. Alcohol also appears to impair the liver's ability to activate vitamin D. Alcohol inhibits calcium absorption, too.

In terms of calcium and bone loss, we still don't know how much alcohol is too much. Until we know more, limit your alcohol consumption to no more than two drinks per day.

• **Medications:** Some medications can interfere with calcium balance. Aluminum in some antacids binds to and lowers levels of phosphorus, which, in turn, increases calcium excretion. Other antacids contain calcium and can be used both to settle your stomach and as a calcium supplement. Read the label on your antacid. If it contains aluminum, consider switching to a brand that doesn't.

Antacids containing aluminum: AlternaGEL liquid, Amphojel, Basaljel, Maalox, Mylanta, Nephrox, Rolaids, WinGel.

Antacids without aluminum: Alka-Seltzer, baking soda, Citrocarbonate, Milk of Magnesia, Riopan, Tums.

Other medications that cause you to excrete more calcium are *steroids* (often prescribed to reduce the inflammation of asthma, arthritis, and other inflammatory conditions), certain *diuretics* (in particular, *furosemide*, prescribed to relieve water retention associated with congestive heart failure, kidney disease, and cirrhosis of the liver), the antibiotic *tetracycline*, and long-term use of the antituberculosis drug *isoniazid*. If you are taking any of these medications, you may want to discuss with your doctor the possibility of taking alternative types of medications that don't promote bone loss. If substitutions are not possible, you should ask your doctor how you can minimize bone loss. At the very least, you should take a calcium supplement.

Hormone Therapy

Since bone loss accelerates after menopause, it makes sense that giving postmenopausal women estrogen would help slow or even stop this accelerated bone loss. Indeed, estrogen therapy is one of the most effective means of slowing the loss of bone mass after menopause.

• **Estrogen:** No one knows exactly how estrogen works. As we mentioned earlier, estrogen (estradiol) receptors have been found in osteoblasts, which is surprising because all of the clinical evidence we have suggests that estrogen has its main effect on osteoclasts. We now suspect that osteoblasts indirectly affect the behavior of osteoclasts.

Estrogen increases your body's ability to absorb calcium from the intestines. (Some studies have even suggested that women on estrogen therapy can get by with a daily requirement of 1,200 milligrams of calcium, rather than the recommended 1,400 milligrams per day for postmenopausal women.) Estrogen also stimulates the thyroid's production of the bone-sparing hormone calcitonin. In addition, estrogen stimulates the liver's production of cortisol-binding protein and thyroid-binding protein, which helps counteract the bone-dissolving effects of overactive adrenal and thyroid glands.

We know that estrogen increases collagen in other parts of the body (notably the skin), and we suspect it does the same for bone. Remember, collagen in bone forms the bone matrix to which calcium, phosphorus, and other crystals adhere. As a result, estrogen both increases the elasticity of bone and aids in increasing its rigidity.

Estrogen may have an indirect effect as well: By improving your sense of well-being, the hormone may help increase your level of activity. Active women are stronger and more stable than sedentary women, which, in turn, decreases their chances of falling.

Whatever the mechanism of action, estrogen preserves bone mineral, which, in turn, is associated with a decrease in fractures among women who take it. Dr. Bruce Ettinger of Kaiser Permanente in San Francisco determined that the "bone-mineral age" of women taking estrogen was ten to twelve years less than their actual age.

Several long-term studies have shown that the use of estrogen is associated with a *dramatic* decline in fractures of the hip. The actual figures vary from study to study, but the average is about 50 percent. As for fractures of the spine, Robert Lindsay, M.D., of Columbia University in New York has found a *90 percent decrease in spinal deformities* (such as loss of height and dowager's hump) among surgically menopausal women who took estrogen for ten years. In this study, only 4 percent of women taking estrogen suffered spinal vertebral fractures, compared to 38 percent of untreated women.

• **Progestogen:** Although progestogen given by itself isn't as good as a combination of estrogen and progestogen, it does work. One type of progestogen, *megesterol acetate* (Megace), is useful for protecting bone in women who've had breast cancer and can't take estrogen therapy.

• **Combinations:** Estrogen and progestogen help protect bone in different ways; therefore, taking a combination of estrogen and progestogen provides added protection. This is one reason why women who have had a hysterectomy and who have low bone mass (a loss of 30 percent of peak bone mass or more) may want to consider taking combination therapy, even though they don't need progestogen to protect the endometrial lining.

When should you begin? It's never too late to start taking estrogen. Bone-mineral loss is halted whenever estrogen is used—even if you already have osteoporosis. However, the sooner after menopause you begin, the better off you'll be; this way, you can preserve a higher level of bone mass.

Should all postmenopausal women take hormone therapy to protect their bones? No. If your bone density is normal, you probably won't improve it any further by taking estrogen. And remember, hormone therapy, like all drugs, has side effects (see Chapter 20).

The best way to determine whether you should take hormone therapy is to have your bone density tested. Subsequent bone-density tests can help monitor your treatment and tell you how well the treatment is working.

Some premenopausal women may want to consider taking oral contraceptives, particularly women with low bone mass and those who suffer from athletic amenorrhea.

Managing Osteoporosis Once You Have It

If you have osteoporosis, you may have already suffered a certain amount of physical deformity and disability. Nevertheless, there are measures you can take to prevent further bone loss and, in doing so, substantially reduce your chances of more fractures.

Treatment is a bit of a misnomer, since osteoporosis is not a disease that can be treated, cured, and forgotten. *Management* is a better term, since therapy must be continued until there is a natural slowing of bone loss.

When managing osteoporosis, we strive for four goals:

1. slowing or stopping bone loss

2. alleviating pain

3. improving your posture during activities of daily living

4. preventing falls that could lead to more fractures.

Nutrition, exercise, certain medications, and using good common sense all play a role in achieving these goals.

• **Nutrition:** The same nutrition strategies used for prevention are essential ingredients of any management program. You should get at least 1,200 to 1,400 milligrams of calcium and 400 units of vitamin D daily. Also beware of the bone robbers: large amounts of protein, red meat, coffee, salt, and fiber. There's little room in your life for cigarette smoking or alcohol consumption, either, since both of these can adversely affect your bone health; alcohol can also affect your balance, subjecting you to falls.

• **Exercise:** Regular physical activity is a must in managing osteoporosis. Exercise not only helps increase bone mass but also strengthens muscles, which can reduce pain and help prevent falls. An overlooked cause of pain is not so much the fracture itself but muscle spasms resulting from changes in posture caused by the fracture. Moreover, muscle weakness can affect your balance and may increase the likelihood that you will fall.

The trick is to strike a balance between exercise that is beneficial and stimulates new bone formation and overly strenuous exercise that can actually increase your risk of more fractures. Jogging, for example, is inappropriate for women with osteoporosis, as the jarring motions can traumatize the skeleton. Walking is more appropriate for women with osteoporosis because it is a low-impact activity. Although swimming isn't a weight-bearing exercise and can't help build bone mass, it is an ideal activity for women who have already suffered a fracture. According to physical therapist Vibeke Vala, a consultant to the National Osteoporosis Foundation and our clinic, hydrotherapy and water aerobics are particularly effective for strengthening muscles, improving balance, and increasing the range of motion in your joints. Exercising in the water is less stressful on your bones and joints than exercising out of the water. Water assists in lifting your arms and legs while you exercise, so your muscles don't get as tired as when you perform the same exercises outside of the water. On the other hand, the gentle resistance of the water against the force of your movements helps give your muscles a better workout. Most water exercises are performed while standing neck-deep in water. Try the following exercises (see Figures 17.5–17.7), which help strengthen your upper and lower back muscles.

Be careful not to *overdo* it. Because water exercises seem so effortless, some women may overwork their muscles without realizing it, then pay the price in muscle stiffness later on. (Over-the-counter analgesics, such as aspirin, acetaminophen, or ibuprofen, can help relieve sore muscles, as can a warm bath and a day or two of rest.)

If you have recently sustained a spinal fracture, you can still perform a few simple exercises. According to Vibeke Vala, you should concentrate first on activities that involve your abdominal muscles, which help you maintain

Figure 17.5 Underwater Leg Lifts

To strengthen your thighs, stand in the pool with your feet slightly apart, your arms extended out at your sides. Swing your right leg upward about 45 degrees, then slowly return to the starting position. Start with five repetitions, gradually working your way up to ten or fifteen. Then perform the same exercise using the left leg.

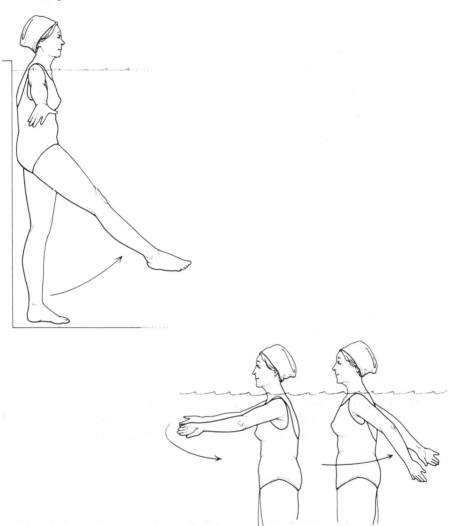

Figure 17.6 The Breast Stroke

To improve upper body strength, extend your arms straight out in front of you with your palms facing outward. Keeping your elbows straight, slowly swing your arms around your body and behind your back in a swimming motion. Bring your arms to your sides and return to the starting position. Start with five repetitions, slowly working your way up to ten or fifteen.

Figure 17.7   Shoulder Pinches

To strengthen the muscles of your upper back (which are needed to help maintain balance), stand with your hands clasped—fingers interlaced—behind your back. Slowly roll your shoulders back as far as they will comfortably go and return to the starting position. Start with five repetitions, gradually working your way up to ten or fifteen. This exercise can be performed in or out of the water.

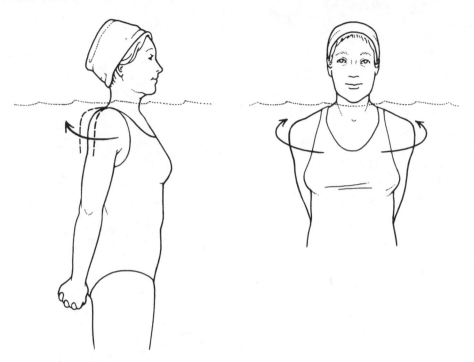

balance. She recommends the following exercises (see figures 17.8-17.9). You may also walk or ride a stationary bicycle if you feel comfortable. You should not, however, engage in any activities that put too much strain on your musculoskeletal system.

Drugs in the Management of Osteoporosis

•   **Estrogen:** This is the most widely studied and accepted method of treating established osteoporosis. Women with osteoporosis who take estrogen are relatively protected from further bone loss, height loss, and fractures.

Remember, if you have an intact uterus, it is imperative that you take a progestogen along with estrogen to protect the uterine lining from overstimulation by estrogen.

•   **Calcitonin** *(Calcimar; Cibacalcin; Miacalcin):* This drug, given by injection (and newly developed nasal sprays), inhibits bone resorption and slows the bone-remodeling process. Several studies have shown that when combined

Figure 17.8   Side-Lying Leg-Lifts

Lie on your side on a carpeted floor or an exercise mat with your legs together and your head resting on your arm, as shown. Keeping your knee straight, toe pointed, slowly lift your leg to about a 45-degree angle, then return to the starting position. Start with five repetitions, gradually working your way up to ten or fifteen. Repeat the exercise with the other leg.

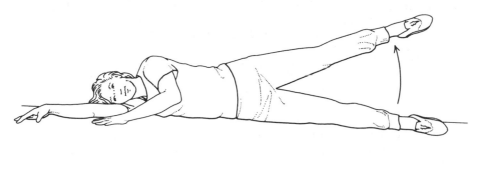

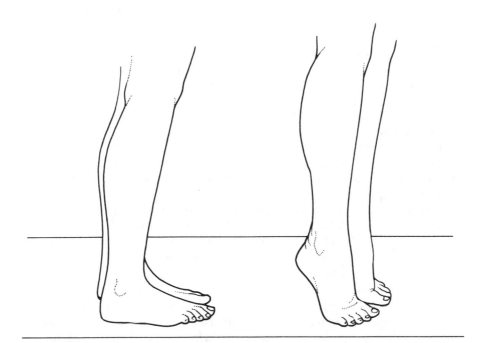

Figure 17.9   Toe Roll-Ups

While barefoot, stand with your feet together, arms at your sides. Slowly lift your heels off the floor so that your weight shifts to the front part of your feet and your toes. Hold for a count of five, then return to the starting position. Repeat the exercise five times, gradually working your way up to ten or fifteen repetitions.

with calcium supplements, calcitonin reduces bone breakdown. A few studies have found that calcitonin may also increase bone density in some women. Calcitonin appears to reduce pain, too.

Side effects include nausea, vomiting, abdominal pain, diarrhea, facial flushing, and tingling of the hands. Side effects are usually mild, and the nasal sprays (which are not yet available in this country) are associated with even fewer side effects. Calcitonin was approved in 1985 by the U.S. Food and Drug Administration for treatment of osteoporosis and is the only other FDA-approved treatment for osteoporosis (besides estrogen).

• **Bisphosphonates** *(Didronel):* This is a group of chemical compounds that have been used to treat various bone diseases over the past twenty years. The most widely tested, etidronate, was previously patented for use as a detergent. To date, none has been approved by the U.S. Food and Drug Administration for the treatment of osteoporosis.

Bisphosphonates, usually given in the form of a pill, adhere to calcium crystals, coating them and somehow decreasing bone resorption. The pills are either given alone in intermittent doses or given along with another drug, phosphate, in a treatment regimen called ADFR (activate, depress, free, repeat). This type of drug therapy attempts to mimic the natural bone-remodeling cycle, helping to stimulate the formation of new bone. In the active phase (A), phosphate is given for several days to increase secretion of parathyroid hormone, which stimulates osteoclasts to begin breaking down old bone. Bisphosphonates are then given to depress (D) bone resorption. This is followed by a free (F), or rest period, in which no drug is given and osteoblasts begin laying down new bone. Then the process is repeated (R).

Two well-designed studies have shown a significant increase in bone-mineral content of the spine and fewer vertebral fractures among women who took etidronate compared with those who took a placebo. Overall, the rate of vertebral fractures was reduced by one-half in women who took etidronate. What's more, women with the lowest bone-mineral density of the spine at the beginning of the study had the lowest subsequent fracture rate. The rate of new vertebral fractures was two-thirds less among these women than that of a control group.

Side effects include stomach upsets among some users. Of greater concern are long-term side effects. If given in sufficiently high doses for long periods of time, some bisphosphonates may slow bone mineralization, resulting in *osteomalacia,* a condition in which newly formed bone fails to become mineralized. More research is needed before these drugs become widely available for treatment of osteoporosis.

• **Vitamin D** *(Calcitriol):* This hormonally active form of vitamin D, taken as a pill, has been shown to increase bone mass among women with osteoporosis. Calcitriol slows down bone resorption and helps the body retain calcium.

Some studies have shown that high doses of calcitriol are associated with such side effects as hypercalcemia (an excess of calcium in the blood) and a deterioration in kidney function. More long-term studies are needed to determine the safety and effectiveness of this drug.

• **Fluoride (sodium fluoride):** This is a naturally occurring mineral found in trace amounts in seafood, vegetables, meats, cereals, fruits, and tea. It is often added to drinking water.

362

It has long been known that fluoride helps prevent cavities. A 1960 study also found a higher incidence of osteoporosis among people with low levels of fluoride in their drinking water. Several other studies showed that without a doubt fluoride actually stimulates the formation of new bone—particularly trabecular bone—although the precise mechanism is unknown.

One problem with fluoride: Some research suggests that bone formed while taking sodium fluoride is not as strong as normal bone. There have been several reports of increased fractures of the hip. However, most of the earlier studies didn't include enough healthy women for comparison. A 1990 study by Lawrence Riggs, M.D., at the Mayo Clinic in Rochester, Minnesota, was the first well-designed study to find an association between fluoride therapy and increased hip fractures. He advised against using fluoride in the treatment of osteoporosis. Dr. Riggs's study was criticized, however, because patients received more than twice the dose of sodium fluoride that's commonly recommended.

Newer, slow-release forms of sodium fluoride are associated with lower blood levels of fluoride and may be associated with fewer fractures. Also, fluoride might work better in combination with other therapies, particularly estrogen therapy. This way, the new bone being formed by fluoride will have enough bone matrix (boosted by estrogen therapy) for calcium crystals to adhere to.

Another problem with fluoride therapy is its side effects. The most common are gastrointestinal problems, such as stomach pains, nausea, vomiting, and diarrhea. Some patients also suffer from foot pain and occasional tenderness around the ankle, knee, or hip. Side effects are minimized by using time-release preparations or coated sodium-fluoride tablets.

Sodium-fluoride tablets are widely available without a prescription at local pharmacies. However, until we know more about the effectiveness of fluoride in the treatment of osteoporosis, you should take fluoride tablets only on your physician's recommendation.

• **Tamoxifen** *(Nolvadex):* This drug is commonly used in treatment of patients with estrogen-dependent breast cancer. Tamoxifen tablets block the action of estrogen by binding to estrogen receptors on cells. Researchers were initially concerned that the antiestrogenic effects of tamoxifen might be harmful to bone. They found, to their surprise, that tamoxifen acts differently in bone tissues. Instead of blocking estrogen in bone, the drug enhances the effects of estrogen on bone, inhibiting bone resorption and preserving bone mass. In women receiving tamoxifen for treatment of breast cancer, bone of the lumbar spine is preserved and even increases.

More research is needed before tamoxifen can be used to treat osteoporosis, but so far the results are encouraging.

• **Thiazide diuretics:** These drugs, which are widely used to treat high blood pressure, decrease the amount of calcium excreted in urine. Not surprisingly, they appear to increase or at least preserve bone density in older women and may even reduce the risk of suffering a hip fracture by up to one-third. There are numerous different types of thiazide diuretics, however, and it's still not clear which are most effective. Researchers with the Framingham Heart Study found that women who took pure thiazides (as opposed to a combination of thiazides and a potassium-sparing drug called *triamterene*) had a significantly lower risk of hip fracture than nonusers. A 1985 study from our clinic, however, found no differences in bone densities or fracture rates between women who took thiazide diuretics and those who did not. Our findings suggest that any bone-conserving effects that thiazide diuretics have may not be enough to compensate for the bone loss associated with low estrogen levels at the time of menopause.

Additional Treatment

•   **Braces:** Should you wear a brace? If you are in acute pain after having suffered a vertebral fracture, you may want to consider wearing a back brace. This helps ease muscle pain often associated with vertebral fractures.

•   **Analgesics and antispasmodics:** If you experience back pain more than twelve weeks after a fractured vertebra has healed, the pain is probably not related to the fracture itself. Rather, persistent pain is usually caused by muscle tension and muscle spasms related to the change in your posture caused by the fracture. Your physician may recommend a narcotic, such as Demerol, to help relieve the acute pain immediately following a fracture. Once the pain has subsided somewhat, he or she may prescribe a milder analgesic, such as Tylenol with Codeine, or Fiorinal.

Antispasmodic drugs may sometimes be prescribed for muscle spasms. However, physical therapy is usually a much more effective and long-lasting treatment for muscle spasms than drugs.

Preventing Falls

While not all falls result in a hip fracture, over 90 percent of hip fractures are the result of a fall. So you can see how important it is to prevent yourself from falling after you've been diagnosed with either severe osteopenia or osteoporosis.

Falls are much more common in women over age sixty-five. This is partly due to such age-related changes as loss of vision and hearing, a slowdown of reflexes, and muscle weakness. A number of illnesses can contribute to a fall, too. Stroke, dementia, Parkinson's disease, arrhythmias, and arthritis all may make you more susceptible to falling. Many drugs can cause dizziness and postural hypotension (a sudden drop in blood pressure when you stand up), thus increasing the risk that you may fall. These include antihypertensive drugs, tricyclic antidepressants, and alcohol.

There are several measures you can take to protect yourself from falling.

•   **Practice good body mechanics.** Essentially, this means adjusting your activities of daily living—standing up, sitting down, lifting, reaching—to accommodate your back. According to physical therapist Vibeke Vala, you should concentrate on maintaining stability in your trunk at all times. She recommends taking a deep breath, tightening your pelvic-floor muscles (the same muscles that control your bladder and bowel—see page 427), and "pulling your belly away from your belt line" when you get up out of bed or move from a sitting to a standing position. This helps keep your trunk in a neutral position. Also, when lifting, be sure to use your *knees*, not your back (see Figure 17.10).

Figure 17.10 **Proper Form for Lifting**
(A) Correct (B) Incorrect

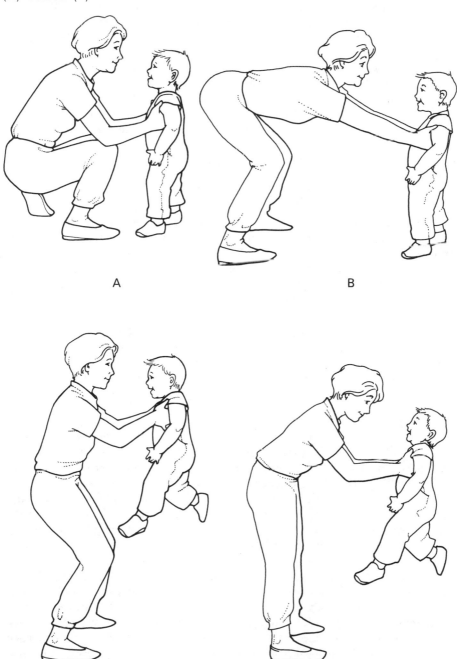

A

B

- **Safeguard your house.**

  Floors: Slippery floors and loose rugs are two major contributors to falls in the home. If finances allow, you may want to consider having wall-to-wall carpeting installed. (Avoid thick pile carpet, however, which can also contribute to falls.) If this is not practical, keep your floors bare. At the very least, try to find scatter rugs with nonskid rubber backing.

  When walking on slippery floors, wear slippers or shoes with nonskid rubber soles. *Don't walk around in your stocking feet.*

  Lighting: Make sure your home is well lighted and that light switches are close to the entrance to every room. Try to avoid groping around in a dark room to find the light switch. You could easily trip and fall over furniture, loose rugs, or other unseen objects on the floor.

  Excessive glare can be almost as dangerous as too little light. Choose "soft" light bulbs and be sure to cover all exposed light bulbs with a lamp shade, globe, or other appropriate covering. (Don't throw a handkerchief or scarf over a bare light bulb; this could be a fire hazard.)

  Stairs: Be sure the stairs in your home (including outside porch stairs) have handrails. Make sure stairwells are well lighted. Have worn stair treads replaced.

  Bathroom: Use nonskid bath mats on bathroom floors to keep the floor dry and prevent falls. Install grab bars in the bathtub and near the toilet. Be sure your bathtub or shower has a nonskid rubber mat or nonskid rubber appliqués to keep you from slipping.

  Bedroom: If your bed is high, consider purchasing an inexpensive metal frame that's lower to the ground. If your bed has wheels, make sure the wheels are in a locked position. Again, the bedroom should be well lighted and you should have easy access to a light switch from the bedroom entrance *and* the bed.

- **Other tips.**

  Have your physician examine your back and musculoskeletal system. He or she can help assess the strength of your back muscles and determine whether you have a disparity in leg length, which could lead to imbalance and a greater risk of falling. Your physician can then recommend exercises to strengthen your muscles or offer other suggestions to help prevent falls. If you are in pain, a simple back examination can often uncover the cause of the pain—and the cure. More often than not, our patients have found symptomatic relief of back pain by learning good body mechanics and undergoing physical therapy rather than by taking any single drug or combination of drugs.

  Avoid postural hypotension. Your physician can help determine whether you are suffering from postural hypotension by taking your blood pressure while seated and again while standing. Some medications can cause postural hypotension. If you can't switch to a medication that doesn't have this side effect, you'll need to take extra precautions to get up slowly from a lying or sitting position. Wearing support hose helps keep blood from pooling in your legs when you stand up, too. (For more tips on coping with postural hypotension, see page 304.)

  Look where you walk. Take a little extra time to get where you're going. Beware of curbs, hard-to-see low steps, and high steps.

Ask your physician about the hip protector. If you have severe osteopenia or osteoporosis, you may want to consider wearing a device called the hip protector. This device, which is strapped around the pelvis, acts as a shock absorber to help diffuse the stress on the hip as a result of a fall.

Don't be vain; use a cane. Although you may have a hard time accepting the fact that you may need a cane or walker to get around, a little hurt pride heals a lot faster than a broken hip. If you're reluctant to use a cane or walker because you feel it takes away from your dignity, try to put your feelings aside and think of your physical well-being.

A Final Word

It's never too early to start preventing bone loss, but it can be too late. So start your program of osteoporosis prevention now by paying attention to good nutrition, getting plenty of exercise, and, if you are postmenopausal, possibly taking hormones to protect your bones from an excessive loss of bone mass.

Suggested Reading

Notelovitz, Morris, M.D., Ph.D., and Marsha Ware. *Stand Tall! The Informed Woman's Guide to Preventing Osteoporosis.* Gainesville, FL.: Triad Publishing, 1982.

Resources and Support

National Osteoporosis Foundation, 1150 17th St., NW, Suite 500, Washington, D.C. 20036. The National Osteoporosis Foundation serves as an information clearinghouse, linking patients and their families with up-to-date information, resources, and services for the prevention, diagnosis, and treatment of osteoporosis. Write for referrals to physicians specializing in the treatment of osteoporosis and for hospitals and/or clinics in your area that offer bone-density testing.

Cancer is one of the most frightening prospects associated with growing older, mostly because our society has been conditioned to think of cancer as a terminal illness that causes painful, lingering deaths, and for which there is no cure. Yet many, many people now are surviving cancer and leading full, productive lives. One of your best means of protection is to learn all you can about the most common types of cancer among women in midlife, the steps you can take to prevent them, and their early warning signs. Undergoing regular cancer screening tests and knowing the early warning signs of cancer may be the two most important things you can do to protect yourself: One of the main reasons why more people are surviving cancer today is that more cancers are being detected in the earliest and most curable stages.

What Is Cancer?

Cancer is not one illness but rather many different diseases with one thing in common: the uncontrolled growth and spread of abnormal cells. Usually, the cells in your body reproduce in an orderly fashion, replacing worn-out tissues, healing injuries, and proceeding with normal growth. Occasionally, however, certain cells undergo abnormal changes, touching off a process of uncontrolled growth and spread. These cells may grow into masses of tissue called *tumors*. Some tumors are *benign* (noncancerous); others are *malignant* (cancerous).

The danger of cancer is that it invades and destroys normal tissue. At first, cancer cells remain at their original site; the cancer is then said to be localized. However, if not treated, cancer cells may *metastasize*, or spread to other parts of the body. This may occur either when the tumor grows so large that it invades neighboring tissues or when cancer cells break away from the original tumor and are carried through the lymph or blood systems to other parts of the body. Eventually, the cancer may spread throughout the body. This condition is known as advanced cancer and usually results in death.

Cancer is usually defined by the stage it has reached. Because cancer becomes more serious with each stage, it is essential to detect cancer as early as possible. When caught in their earliest stages, many cancers can be cured. Many others can be prevented.

How Does Cancer Develop?

No one is sure yet exactly how healthy cells turn into cancer cells. Normally, the cells in your body undergo a natural process of growth, *differentiation* (changes that cause some cells to become skin cells, while others develop into blood cells, for example), maturation, and death. This process is what's known as the *cell cycle*. During the cell cycle, a sophisticated network of mechanisms controls the growth of cells, stimulating cells to grow when existing cells are damaged or worn-out and halting cell growth after the damage has been repaired.

Growth of cancer cells occurs when the network somehow breaks down. This appears to be related to a cascade of events involving a number of controls within the body as well as outside influences. Some possible factors include genetics, the strength of the immune system, and environmental influences.

The Role of Genetics

Some people appear simply to be genetically more susceptible to developing cancer than others. We've known for some time now that having a family history of certain cancers (breast, colon, and ovarian cancers, for example) puts you at an increased risk of developing the cancer yourself. Also, the genes for some noncancerous genetic disorders, such as benign colon polyps, are associated with the increased occurrence of certain cancers.

Research into the theory of *oncogenes*, or "cancer genes," now suggests that each of us harbors a set of genes with the potential to convert healthy cells into cancer cells. Normally, these genes, called *proto-oncogenes*, help control the growth and development of cells in the body. Many do so by manufacturing proteins that help regulate cell growth (either stimulating cells to grow and divide or stopping them from doing so). In people who develop cancer, proto-oncogenes are believed to somehow become damaged and transform into oncogenes. When this happens, some of the normal controls governing the growth of certain cells go haywire.

Researchers have also discovered a category of tumor-suppressor genes, or *anti-oncogenes*, that normally help prevent the formation of tumors. If these become damaged, their tumor-suppressing abilities may become inactivated, allowing tumors to grow.

The exact role of oncogenes is still not known at this time, and activation of oncogenes (or deactivation of anti-oncogenes) in itself may not be sufficient to cause cancer. However, it appears to be a critical step in the formation of tumors.

The Role of the Immune System

Not long ago, experts believed that your body's immune system was your primary defense against cancer. The body was thought to have a built-in immune surveillance system that routinely seeks out and destroys cancer cells. Proponents of this theory point out that some virus-associated cancers in humans and animals do appear to trigger a strong immune response, and certain tumors develop chiefly in people whose immune system is suppressed, such as organ-transplant recipients and those with acquired immune deficiency syndrome (AIDS). Moreover, some types of tumors often regress spontaneously, suggesting that the immune system works to snuff them out.

But the theory remains controversial. One major problem is that there's little direct evidence that cancer cells contain *antigens*, or parts of the cells that the body would recognize as "foreign" and against which the immune system could produce antibodies. However, at least one type of immune cell, natural killer cells, does appear to prevent tumors from taking hold and to stop the spread of cancer cells without the need for antigens.

New research suggests that the immune system deters cancer in a totally unexpected way, as well. Disease-fighting white blood cells (*lymphocytes*) appear to produce molecules capable of influencing the growth and function of other tissue cells. Impairment of the immune system may suppress the lymphocytes' role in the regulation of cell growth, allowing tumors to grow.

The immune system is one of the most complex systems of the body, and it appears to protect against cancer in a variety of different ways. As our understanding of the immune system's role in the development of cancer improves, so will treatment and prevention strategies.

The Role of Environmental Influences

Up to 90 percent of all cancers appear to be related to environmental influences, particularly lifestyle practices. The upshot of this is that prevention of most cancers appears to be largely within your control.

As you are probably already aware, numerous substances in our environment are potential *carcinogens*, or cancer-causing agents. Some of these agents directly damage normal cells in the early stages of cancer development—usually by altering or damaging the cell's DNA (the genetic blueprint within each cell that enables it to make an exact replica of itself when it divides); these are called *cancer initiators*. Others don't cause cancer in and of themselves, but they help to fuel the growth of existing cancer cells—somewhat like fanning a fire that has already been started; these are called *cancer promoters*.

Cigarette smoking is one of the main known carcinogenic hazards. In the United States, smoking contributes to about 30 percent of all cancer in men and women combined. Other known carcinogens include alcohol, solar radiation, ionizing radiation (from X rays), asbestos, radon (an invisible, odorless, radioactive gas that comes from the ground), some medications (such as DES, given to women during pregnancy in the 1950s to help prevent miscarriage, and immunosuppressive drugs given to kidney-transplant recipients). Certain viruses (notably the human papilloma virus, which causes sexually transmitted genital warts—see page 278) are also believed to be potential carcinogens.

The foods you eat may increase or decrease your risk of cancer, as well. Too much fat and too many calories in your diet may predispose you to cancers of the breast and colon. A variety of other dietary factors, including additives and contaminants, have also fallen under suspicion as possible carcinogens. Even the way food is cooked may generate hydrocarbons or other carcinogens at high temperatures.

On the other hand, certain vitamins and trace minerals—particularly vitamin C, beta carotene, and selenium—may protect against some types of cancer. These substances are *antioxidants* and help protect against cell damage from *oxygen free radicals*—highly charged particles that are missing one electron and that bombard and damage healthy cells. (Oxygen free radicals are also believed to play a role in the development of heart disease and the aging process; see pages 310 and 84.)

Obviously, many potential cancer-causing agents aren't harmful unless you are exposed to high doses or unless you are regularly exposed to smaller doses for many years; many have a cumulative effect. The main goal of prevention, then, is to minimize your lifetime exposure to known carcinogens.

Although the various types of cancer share many of the same characteristics, they are different in many ways, and each has its own unique risk factors and preventive strategies. Here's a closer look at the diagnosis, treatment, and prevention of the eight most common cancers of women in the middle and later years.

Lung Cancer

Lung cancer is the leading cause of cancer death among women today, and cigarette smoking is largely responsible. In fact, there is a direct correlation between the number of women who started smoking after World War II and— twenty years later—the rise in deaths from lung cancer.

Other risk factors include chronic exposure to certain industrial substances such as asbestos and exposure to radon in the home—particularly if you smoke cigarettes. Exposure to side-stream smoke (also known as passive smoking) also increases the risk for nonsmokers. Nonsmoking spouses have nearly a twofold risk of developing lung cancer if their spouse smokes compared with those married to nonsmokers.

Some studies have shown a relationship between low levels of certain nutrients and an increased risk of lung cancer. Researchers at Johns Hopkins University in Baltimore found that people with low blood levels of beta carotene (a precursor of vitamin A) had a fourfold greater risk of developing lung cancer, and those with low levels of vitamin E were 2.5 times more likely to develop lung cancer than those with high levels of these nutrients. Beta carotene traps free radicals, and a few studies in animals suggest that it may also reduce the development of tumors. Vitamin E reduces damage to lung tissue in animals exposed to such carcinogens as ozone and cigarette smoke.

One published study has found an increased incidence of lung cancer among men being treated with estrogen for heart disease, leading some researchers to suspect that estrogen may play a role in the development of lung cancer. The lungs contain estrogen receptors, and some experts theorize that estrogen may act like a "Trojan horse," carrying the carcinogens from cigarette smoke into the lung cells and possibly promoting cancer.

There's no cure for lung cancer; it is not easy to detect early and it is difficult to treat: The five-year survival rate for lung cancer averages 13 percent. (Up to 37 percent of people with lung cancer will survive if the cancer is detected when it is still localized, but only 20 percent of lung cancers are discovered this early.) This is why prevention is essential. How can you protect yourself?

• **If you smoke cigarettes, quit.** When you stop, your elevated risk of lung cancer declines, eventually returning to that of a nonsmoker. If you stop smoking at the time of precancerous cell changes, damaged bronchial-lining tissues often return to normal. (See Chapter 7 for help in kicking the habit.)

• **Protect yourself from passive smoking.** The antismoking movement in this country has already made some strides in protecting nonsmokers from side-stream smoke. Most major airlines have banned smoking on domestic flights. Smoking is also prohibited now in most hospitals and certain sections of restaurants, malls, and other public areas. You can further protect yourself by encouraging smokers you know to light up outside of your home or office.

• **Have your home tested for radon.** Radon test kits are widely available and fairly inexpensive. The Environmental Protection Agency provides information on radon testing and guidelines for reducing the amount of radon in your home in its booklet *A Citizen's Guide to Radon: What It Is and What to Do About It*. For a copy of the booklet, call your state radiation office or write to the Environmental Protection Agency, Public Information Center, 401 M. Street, SW, Washington, D.C. 20460.

• **Eat foods high in beta carotene and vitamin E.** Leafy dark green vegetables (broccoli, kale, mustard, and other greens) and orange or yellow fruits and vegetables (sweet potatoes, winter squash, carrots, cantaloupe, peaches) are high in beta carotene. Whole-grain foods, such as whole-wheat bread and wheat germ, are good sources of vitamin E.

Should cigarette smokers take estrogen? At this point, we don't know enough about the effects of estrogen on cigarette smokers' risk of lung cancer, so there's no reason not to. However, we do know that cigarette smoking raises your metabolism of estrogen by one-third, which means you may have to take a higher dose of estrogen than nonsmokers.

Early detection of lung cancer is difficult because symptoms—a persistent cough, sputum streaked with blood, chest pain, and recurring pneumonia or bronchitis—often don't appear until the disease is in the advanced stages. If you do experience these symptoms, your doctor will recommend a chest X ray, sputum analysis, and possibly a fiberoptic examination of bronchial passages.

Treatment depends on the type and stage of the cancer but usually includes surgery, radiation therapy, and chemotherapy.

Breast Cancer

This is the cancer women fear most, partly because it is the most common cancer among women (the incidence is rising; now one in nine women will develop breast cancer in her lifetime). Women also fear breast cancer because the scientific community doesn't know yet how to prevent it, and treatment often involves the loss of a breast, a prospect many women find more frightening than the cancer itself.

In spite of the increased incidence of breast cancer, women who have it are living longer. The five-year survival rate is 91 percent for breast cancer that hasn't spread, thanks mostly to early detection and prompt treatment.

The Normal Breast

Biologically speaking, the sole purpose of the breast is to produce milk. It is composed of milk-producing glands (*mammary glands*), fat, supporting ligaments, and milk ducts that lead up to the nipple (see Figure 18.1). Each mammary gland contains fifteen to twenty sections, known as *lobes*. These are divided into smaller compartments called *lobules* and *acini*. Ducts arise from these lobules, forming larger milk ducts as they pass through the breast tissue to the nipple. The glands and ducts are surrounded by fat and connective tissue. The breast itself contains no muscle, but it does contain erectile tissue, which is made of muscle fiber and lies just beneath the nipple. The areola, the dark pigmented area surrounding the nipple, contains sebaceous glands that secrete oil to protect the nipple against chafing.

Your breasts change over time and in response to hormonal fluctuations, beginning with puberty. As you begin menstruating, estrogen and progesterone stimulate the development of the milk ducts and mammary glands and encourage fat to be deposited within the breast tissues, causing the breasts to grow.

Throughout your childbearing years, fluctuating estrogen and progesterone levels during the menstrual cycle may cause cyclical variations in your breasts: During the second week of the menstrual cycle, the supportive breast tissue and ductal cells increase in size and number. Just before menstruation, the lobules, supporting tissues (or *stroma*), and ducts may become engorged, sometimes causing premenstrual lumps and pain. The pain subsides and the lumps generally recede or disappear within a few days of menstruation, when the ducts shrink and their lining cells are shed. These cyclical changes may worsen in the years before menopause.

During pregnancy, the breasts, fueled by high levels of estrogen and progesterone, enlarge, and by the fifth month of pregnancy they begin producing milk. Milk production involves numerous hormones, including estrogen, progesterone, growth hormone, insulin, and cortisone; chief among them are two pituitary hormones—prolactin and oxytocin. Prolactin initiates milk production in the glands, while oxytocin, secreted in response to a newborn's sucking, stimulates the actual release (the "let down") of milk from the breast.

373

Figure 18.1   The Normal Breast

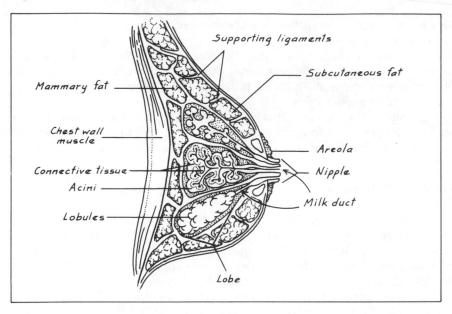

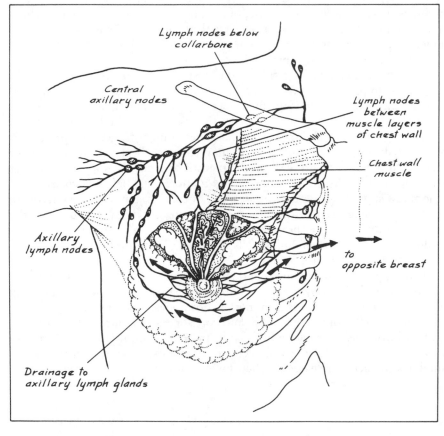

After menopause, decreasing estrogen and progesterone levels cause the mammary glands to shrink. Firm breast tissue is replaced by fat, and the breasts may become soft and saggy.

Common Benign Breast Lumps and Other Changes

It's perfectly normal to have "lumpy" breasts at certain times during the menstrual cycle. During your childbearing years, you may also notice that your nipples occasionally leak fluid. This, too, is normal; throughout your reproductive years, the mammary glands produce secretions that sometimes leak from the nipples. But since breast lumps and nipple discharge are also early warning signs of cancer, these changes can be frightening. Keep in mind that most breast problems are benign. Nevertheless, you should report any changes to your doctor when you first notice them. Only your physician can make a definitive diagnosis. Here are some of the more common—and harmless—breast conditions:

• **Fibrocystic changes (also known as fibrocystic breast disease or fibrocystic breast condition):** This is the most common benign condition of the breast, particularly among premenopausal women. The main symptoms are pain and tenderness, usually in both breasts. These symptoms typically worsen during the second half of the menstrual cycle and subside somewhat after menstruation has begun.

Some women may also develop cysts in the milk ducts. The majority of these cysts are so small that they go unnoticed, but some may grow large (and painful) enough to be felt by hand during breast self-examination, particularly in the years just preceding menopause. Usually, the cysts regress after menstruation begins, but they often return in the next cycle.

The lining of the milk ducts may also thicken, and small, hard plaquelike formations, or *adenoses*, may develop around the smaller milk ducts (acini). Adenosis is more common in women in their thirties and forties and can easily be confused with a palpable early cancer.

Some women with fibrocystic breast changes occasionally develop an *intraductal papilloma*, a benign wartlike growth in the milk duct adjacent to the areola.

• **Fibroadenomas:** These benign tumors that grow in the supporting tissues of the breast are the most common breast lumps in women under age twenty-five. Fibroadenomas usually persist throughout the reproductive years and may occasionally become tender during the menstrual cycle. The tumors regress somewhat after menopause.

If the fibroadenoma is very small and can be seen only with mammography or ultrasound, keeping a watchful eye may be all that's needed. However, if the tumor is palpable, increases in size, or becomes an emotional burden, it should be surgically removed.

• **Nipple discharge:** Only about 3 to 9 percent of women will notice an occasional discharge from one or both nipples. If the discharge occurs after squeezing the breast or the nipple and areola, it's probably benign.

375

Your doctor will first want to perform a series of diagnostic tests to confirm that you have fibrocystic breasts, particularly if you have palpable cysts, adenosis, or an intraductal papilloma. (See Diagnosing Breast Cancer on page 381.)

• **For mild to moderate discomfort, a well-fitted bra** with good support may be all you need. A good support bra is particularly important if you are physically active.

• **For women who need more than a support bra, eliminating methylxan-thines** (chemicals found in coffee, tea, cocoa, caffeine-containing colas and other soft drinks, and chocolate) may be the single most effective means of decreasing pain and tenderness. (You may experience more dramatic results if your consumption of these foods and beverages was excessive to begin with.)

• **Some women find vitamin A and E supplements** to be helpful. Vitamin A is believed to antagonize estrogen production and decreases the plugging of sebaceous ducts. Vitamin E alters hormone production by the body. A daily dose of 1,500 IU of vitamin A for three months is recommended. (Note: Continuing this regimen for more than three months could result in vitamin A toxicity.) Taking 400 IU of vitamin E twice a day may also be beneficial.

• **Taking a mild diuretic** may be helpful for moderate premenstrual breast tenderness. Some women find that thiazide diuretics ease breast pain. This diuretic has the added bonus of helping you to retain calcium.

• **Analgesics** such as ibuprofen, aspirin, or acetaminophen can also be used to relieve breast pain and tenderness.

• **Oral contraceptives** suppress symptoms of fibrocystic changes in 70 to 90 percent of women who take them and may be a good therapeutic choice for women who also need a reliable form of birth control. (For more on oral contraceptives, see Chapter 9.)

• **Other medications** may benefit as well but, because of their side effects, should be used only if other therapies have failed. The drug bromocriptine (Parlodel), normally prescribed for the treatment of endometriosis, may be as effective as oral contraceptives in relieving symptoms.

Likewise, *danazol* (Danocrine) has also been found to be effective. However, it usually takes four to five months for the drug to take effect, and the cost is quite high. In addition, the side effects, including acne, muscle cramps, hot flashes, and menstrual irregularities, are unacceptable to many women. Tamoxifen (Nolvadex), a hormone used to treat women with breast cancer, may be beneficial for reducing fibrocystic symptoms, as well.

• **If you develop a cyst** more than one centimeter in diameter, it should be aspirated, or drained. (For more on this procedure, see Diagnosing Breast Cancer on page 381.)

> • **Having fibrocystic breasts makes it more difficult to examine your breasts**—both for you and your physician. You should practice breast self-examination every week and keep a record of any changes (see the instructions for BSE on page 48 and use the breast diagram there). You should consult with your physician if any change persists for more than one month.

A yellow discharge is usually a result of overstimulation of the breast ducts and glands from estrogen (along with low levels of progesterone), and it may occur in women with fibrocystic breasts.

You may experience a milky discharge for many months following childbirth and breast-feeding, sometimes accompanied by pain (*mastalgia*). Your doctor may prescribe estrogen, androgens, progestogen, or bromocriptine (Parlodel) to stop the release of prolactin causing the discharge.

A thin, translucent, colorless, straw-colored, or green discharge may occur spontaneously during normal menstrual cycles, in early pregnancy, or in women using oral contraceptives. This is a result of excessive stimulation of the lining of the milk ducts by estrogen. If the discharge is accompanied by a single lump just beneath the areola, the cause may be an intraductal papilloma, a benign wartlike growth in the milk ducts. The discharge stops when the growth is surgically removed.

A bloody discharge, which may vary in color from bright red to brown, is a sign of excessive activity of the lining of the milk ducts and is usually caused by estrogen secretion, fibrocystic breast disease, or an intraductal papilloma. However, a bloody discharge may also be a sign of cancer in the breast duct, particularly if it is accompanied by a lump (especially in a postmenopausal woman). While just 7 to 14 percent of all women who have bloody discharges actually have cancer, further diagnostic tests are required of *all* women with a bloody discharge.

The Types of Breast Cancer

Eighty to 90 percent of breast cancers arise from the milk ducts. This type of cancer is known as *ductal carcinoma*. When the cancer is confined to the duct, it is called *intraductal carcinoma in situ* (DCIS). When the cells penetrate the walls of the duct and invade the surrounding tissue, it is called *invasive ductal cancer*. Invasive cancers are capable of spreading to adjacent tissues, the lymph nodes, and other parts of the body. But having invasive cancer doesn't necessarily mean that the cancer has spread.

About 5 percent of breast cancers arise in the lobules, or milk-producing glands. These are known as *lobular carcinomas*, and are classified as either lobular carcinoma in situ or invasive lobular carcinoma.

Some women who receive a negative biopsy or whose mammogram shows an irregularity may be diagnosed as having *hyperplasia*. This simply means that an unusual number of cells have built up in the mammary ducts or lobules. The abnormality is not cancer per se. But if the cells become abnormal—a condition known as *atypia*—a higher than average risk of cancer may exist. These conditions are known as *atypical ductal hyperplasia* and *atypical lobular hyperplasia*, depending on whether they develop in the milk ducts or lobules.

Risk Factors for Breast Cancer

• **Your age:** As a rule, your risk of developing breast cancer rises with age. Until recently, the incidence of breast cancer was higher for women over age fifty. Now, however, for reasons not known, a greater number of women under age fifty are being diagnosed with this cancer. This is why it is essential that you diligently practice breast self-examination and take other measures (including having regular mammograms) to protect yourself from breast cancer *throughout your middle years and beyond*, not just after your fiftieth birthday.

• **Your genes:** Women with a family history of breast cancer (that is, those whose grandmother, mother, or sister have had breast cancer) are two to three times more likely to develop the disease themselves. And women whose mother *and* sister have breast cancer are up to 50 percent more likely to get it than women who have no family history of the disease.

• **Your menstrual and reproductive history:** Women who've never had children, women who had their first child after age thirty, and women who started menstruating early or who experienced a late menopause (after age fifty-five) are also at greater risk of developing breast cancer. Some studies have found that women who never breast-fed are at a higher risk for breast cancer, as well. All of these risk factors suggest that the total number of years you menstruate may somehow play a role in increasing the risk of developing this disease.

One protective factor appears to be surgical removal of the ovaries (bilateral oophorectomy) before age forty. This has been associated with a lifelong reduction in risk of breast cancer of about 50 percent. However, having your ovaries removed solely to prevent breast cancer may not be a very practical prophylactic, since the operation is also associated with an increased risk of osteoporosis and heart disease (see Chapter 13). It's still not clear what effect the estrogen given to surgically menopausal women to prevent these long-term complications has on the risk of developing breast cancer.

• **Your weight:** Being overweight (more than 40 percent over ideal body weight) in your postmenopausal years raises your risk of breast cancer. This may be because excess body fat helps convert postmenopausal androgens into estrogen. Plus, overweight women have lower levels of a liver protein known as *sex hormone–binding globulin*, which binds to estrogen in the bloodstream, making it less biologically active. The result is that heavier women have higher levels of more biologically active estrogen than women of normal weight.

A few studies have also found that "pear"-shaped women—that is, those who tend to accumulate body fat around the abdomen and waist—may also be at a greater risk of breast cancer. (To calculate your waist-to-hip ratio, see page 30.) Gaining weight in adulthood appears to increase the risk of breast cancer, as well. On the other hand, research suggests that *losing* weight in your middle years may have a protective effect.

• **Your diet:** Dietary fat has long been thought to play a role in the development of breast cancer. Most of the evidence comes from population studies showing an increased incidence of breast cancer in countries such as the United States, where the diet is high in fat. More proof: When Japanese women (who eat a low-fat diet and have a low incidence of breast cancer) move to the United

States, their rate of breast cancer rises, presumably along with the increased fat in their diets.

The exact role of dietary fat in the development of breast cancer still isn't clear, however. In the Nurses' Health Study at Harvard University's Brigham and Women's Hospital in Boston, Walter C. Willett, M.D., and his colleagues found that a *moderate* reduction in fat intake (to 30 percent of calories) doesn't result in a substantial reduction of the risk of breast cancer. However, the researchers didn't rule out the possibility that fat intakes of less than 30 percent might reduce the risk. Animal studies have suggested that dietary fat must be cut to less than 20 percent of total calories to reduce the risk of breast cancer. This is about the amount of fat in the diets of Japanese women.

Based on the early reports on breast-cancer prevention, we recommend a diet in which you limit fat to *between 20 and 25 percent of your total daily calories.* (To find out how to cut the fat out of your diet, see Chapter 4.)

Preliminary reports suggest that vitamin D may protect against breast cancer. You may recall (from Chapter 4) that vitamin D is called the "sunshine" vitamin because one of your main sources of vitamin D is exposure to sunlight. Frank Garland, Ph.D., and his colleagues at the University of California at San Diego have now correlated a decreased incidence of breast cancer among women who live in areas that receive more sunlight. Women living in cities with the lowest levels of ultraviolet light (sunlight) also had the highest mortality rates from breast cancer. The lowest mortality rates were in the sunny South and Southwest United States (17 to 19 per 100,000 women), while the highest were in the Northeast (33 per 100,000 women). While the researchers concede that there are many different causes of breast cancer, they suspect that vitamin D may somehow play a protective role.

The current RDA for vitamin D is 200 IU, which you can obtain through exposure to sunlight or through foods (chiefly vitamin D–fortified milk, fish, and egg yolks). (For more information on vitamin D and meeting your RDA, see Chapter 4.)

• **Use of estrogen:** Because certain types of breast cancer are fueled by the hormone estrogen and because a woman's age at menarche, age at first birth, and age at menopause appear to affect her subsequent risk, the hormones in birth-control pills and those used for postmenopausal hormonal therapy have also come under scrutiny. As for birth-control pills, many studies involving hundreds of thousands of women have found no increased risk of breast cancer in the majority of women, regardless of the dose, brand, or type of estrogen or progestogen. Even women with a family history of breast cancer or fibrocystic breast changes aren't at any increased risk from using birth-control pills. Indeed, the only group of women who appear to have a greater risk of breast cancer are women under age forty-five who have used oral contraceptives for relatively long periods of time (eight years or longer) beginning at an early age. The association has been most consistently found for breast cancer diagnosed before age thirty-five, which constitutes only a small proportion of all cases.

What about postmenopausal estrogens? Most current evidence suggests that postmenopausal estrogens either have no effect on the risk of breast cancer or cause a slightly elevated risk with very long-term use (more than fifteen years) or at relatively high doses. No studies have shown an increase in deaths

379

from breast cancer among estrogen users, and some have actually shown an increase in the cure rate of breast cancer among women taking postmenopausal hormones. We don't know yet whether the hormone therapy itself was responsible for the higher cure rate or whether the women taking hormones were screened more diligently, helping to catch their cancers in the early stages, when the cure rate is high. There's some evidence that progestogen may help protect against breast cancer, although most studies have been small.

The story is a little different if you have a family history of breast cancer, however. Studies have shown that among women with a family history of breast cancer, those who had ever used postmenopausal hormones had a twofold greater risk than those who had never taken them. For this reason, many women whose mothers or sisters have been diagnosed with breast cancer are often advised *not* to take estrogen.

More research needs to be conducted before we fully understand what effect, if any, postmenopausal hormone therapy has on a woman's risk of developing breast cancer. At this point, the proven benefits of protection from heart disease and osteoporosis clearly outweigh the possible slightly increased risk of breast cancer for some women. (For more on the benefits and risks of postmenopausal hormone therapy, see Chapter 20.)

• **Alcohol consumption:** In the mid- to late 1980s, several population studies suggested that the amount of alcohol a woman drinks may affect her risk of breast cancer. However, many of these early reports were criticized for not taking into account other risk factors for breast cancer, such as family history and menstrual history. Nevertheless, most investigators did find at least a small increase in risk with increases in alcohol consumption, particularly among premenopausal women and among women who had more than three drinks per day.

Then came a startling report by Dr. Willett and his colleagues at Harvard University, suggesting that as little as one drink per day may raise a woman's risk of breast cancer by 60 percent. Unlike previous studies, this one was well designed; the researchers adjusted their risk estimates for age, menopausal status, age at the birth of the first child, age at menarche, and maternal history of breast cancer, all of which can influence the risk of the disease. And the study involved some ninety thousand female nurses (generally speaking, the larger the number of study participants, the more reliable are the statistics).

At least one subsequent study has found at best a weak association between alcohol consumption and the risk of breast cancer. The researchers suggest that women of higher socioeconomic status are more likely to drink socially, and that it is something about the socioeconomic status of these women (breast cancer *is* more common among women of higher socioeconomic status), not their alcohol consumption, that increases their risk of developing breast cancer.

Compounding the issue is evidence suggesting that moderate amounts of alcohol (one or two drinks per day) may *protect* against heart disease (see page 328), which causes ten times more deaths than breast cancer.

Until we know more, most experts recommend that women who are at especially high risk for breast cancer—those who are obese, who have had few children, who were first pregnant when they were older than thirty, or whose mothers had breast cancer—abstain from drinking altogether, or at least curtail their alcohol consumption. (For tips on cutting back, see Chapter 7.)

• **Exercise:** Regular physical activity may have a protective effect. Studies by Harvard University researcher Rose Frisch, Ph.D., have found that female athletes have about half the incidence of breast cancer (and other cancers of the reproductive organs) as sedentary women. Dr. Frisch says the protective effect may come from healthier lifestyle habits of more active women (including a lifetime of low-fat eating) or a lower percentage of body fat among women who exercise regularly.

• **Silicone breast implants:** Silicone-gel-filled breast implants, used for breast augmentation and breast reconstruction, have not been shown to increase the risk of breast cancer (although at least one study of rats suggests the tiny amounts of silicone that often leak from the implants may be carcinogenic). The major concern is possible delayed treatment of breast cancer due to the difficulty of detecting malignant breast lumps with mammograms. The silicone-gel implants produce a shadow that prevents a significant portion of the breast from being viewed with mammography. Plus, all implants tend to compress breast tissue, making it dense and more difficult for mammograms to detect possible cancerous growths.

For now, the U.S. Food and Drug Administration has asked physicians to stop using the implants with the exception of women who undergo breast reconstruction after mastectomy until more long-term safety data become available. If you are one of the more than 2 million women who have implants already, you should consult a radiologist who is experienced in taking mammograms of augmented breasts. It is usually necessary to take additional X rays of the breast so that all or most of the breast tissue can be seen. If you are considering breast augmentation or reconstructive surgery using silicone implants, you should discuss with your doctor *all* of the pros and cons of the surgery and how it might affect your future risk of breast cancer. (Other surgical options are available for breast reconstruction, although they're not for everybody. Be sure to discuss these with your physician, too. For more on breast reconstruction, see page 387.)

Diagnosing Breast Cancer

Because we still don't have proven ways to prevent breast cancer, early diagnosis is essential. Women whose cancers are diagnosed early live longer and can often undergo conservative surgery—wide excision or lumpectomy (removal of the cancerous breast lump and some of the surrounding tissue) plus local radiation therapy—rather than the more disfiguring mastectomy (removal of the entire breast). And one of the most reliable means of detecting breast cancer early—breast self-examination—is literally in your hands.

• **Breast self-examination:** More than 80 percent of breast lumps are found by patients themselves through breast self-examination. Yet many women refrain from this simple but potentially lifesaving ritual. The reasons are varied and numerous, but two themes seem to predominate: ignorance ("I don't know what I'm feeling for") and fear ("If I don't examine myself, I won't find cancer"). This is perfectly understandable; most women have very little knowledge about the anatomy of their breasts and why it is normal for the breast to feel "lumpy" from time to time. Understanding is the key to overcoming both of these obstacles to breast self-examination.

First, remember that most lumps and nipple discharges are benign. Second, keep in mind that the more you practice BSE, the more familiar you will become with what's normal and what's not. This is one reason we recommend that you perform BSE *once a week* (for instance, "always on Sundays") rather than once a month. You're less likely to forget to examine your breasts if you perform BSE once a week, as well.

A good way to keep track of the "normal" anatomy of your breasts is to use a diagram to chart the changes your breasts undergo each month (see page 48). Keeping a chart also helps notify you of any *abnormal* changes that should be reported to your doctor. If you don't know how to perform BSE, ask your doctor to show you how or follow the instructions for BSE on page 48.

• **Breast exam by your physician:** In addition to BSE, you should have your doctor examine your breasts *at least once a year*. Your physician is highly experienced in examining breasts and may detect an abnormality you may have missed. If you're at high risk of developing breast cancer or if you have fibrocystic breast condition, which can make breast exams more difficult, you should consider having your physician examine your breasts more frequently—every six months or so.

• **Mammography:** Mammography, low-dose X rays of the breast, can be performed both to help diagnose a breast lump found through BSE and to screen for cancers that are too small to be detected by hand. Screening mammography is an integral part of your breast-cancer surveillance program. Indeed, mammography can detect cancers an average of two years before they can be felt by hand. And studies have shown that earlier detection of breast cancers through screening mammography *can* prolong life. *Women whose breast cancers are detected by screening mammography live an average of eight years longer than nonscreened women.* More and more women *are* undergoing this lifesaving procedure. In a 1991 survey by the Jacobs Institute of Women's Health in Washington, D.C., with help from the National Cancer Institute (NCI), 64 percent of the 980 women interviewed reported having at least one mammogram—almost double the number of women in a 1987 survey. Still, only 31 percent of American women are following the guidelines that call for regular mammograms after the age of forty.

Mammography: What to Expect

There are two types of mammograms: *film-screen mammograms,* which yield a black and white picture of the breast, and *xeromammograms,* which produce a blue and white image of the breast. From a layman's perspective, a xeromammogram is essentially the same as a mammogram. The only difference is that the X-ray picture is recorded on paper instead of film and provides a "positive" image of the breast (in contrast to the black and white "negative" image of the mammogram). Some radiologists find the xerographic image easier to interpret.

382

When you are having a mammogram, you first may want to select a mammography facility accredited by the American College of Radiology (ACR). The ACR accredits facilities based on evaluation of equipment, film processing, and the credentials and experience of the technologists who take the mammograms and the radiologists who interpret them. If you have breast implants, be sure to ask the facility whether special mammography techniques are used for women with implants. To find an accredited facility or to get other information on mammography, call the NCI Cancer Information Service toll-free at 800-4-CANCER or a local chapter of the American Cancer Society.

On the day of the exam, don't use any deodorant, perfume, powders, or ointments on your underarms or breasts. They can cloud the X rays. You will have to undress above the waist for the examination, so wear a blouse or sweater and skirt or slacks.

After you have undressed, a lead apron will be placed around your waist to protect the ovaries from X rays. Next, an X-ray technologist will position you at the machine. Depending on the type of equipment being used and the view of the breast to be taken, you will be asked to sit, stand, or lie down (see Figure 18.2). After you are in the right position, a device will be used to compress the breast. This pressure may be somewhat uncomfortable but is essential to achieve high-quality images of the breast.

Usually, pictures of both breasts are taken from at least two angles: top to bottom and side to side. Additional views may be ordered by the radiologist

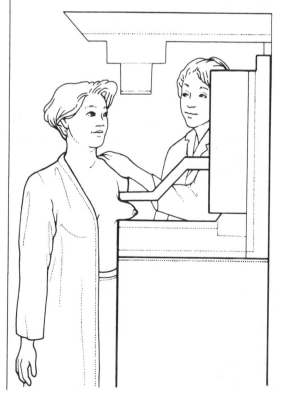

**Figure 18.2   Woman
Having a Mammogram**

to clarify certain indistinct areas or to see areas not shown on original views. This should be no cause for alarm.

After the X-ray film has been developed, a trained radiologist will interpret the results. The radiologist will look for alterations in the density of breast tissue, calcifications, thickening of the skin, fibrous streaks, and nipple changes. Some of these changes may suggest early signs of cancer and warrant further evaluation. Mammography can also aid in identifying fibroadenomas, lymph nodes, or other benign masses. If a suspicious change shows up on a mammogram, more diagnostic tests may be necessary.

•   **Ultrasound (sonogram):** Ultrasound, or the use of sound waves to produce an image of the breast, is typically used as a follow-up when a mass shows up on a mammogram. Ultrasound can usually determine whether the mass is solid or cystic with greater accuracy than mammography. However, since ultrasound cannot identify microcalcifications that are possible signs of early cancer, it should not be used as a substitute for mammography.

During the procedure, the ultrasound technician will apply a lubricating gel to your breast(s), then slide a small ultrasound transducer along the skin.

•   **Needle aspiration:** This procedure is used largely to diagnose and treat benign breast conditions. If you have a palpable cyst, needle aspiration can be used to drain it and test for possible cancerous changes in the fluid. (Only about 0.1 to 1 percent of breast fluid aspirations show signs of malignancy.)

Needle aspiration takes just a few minutes and can be performed right in your doctor's office (see Figure 18.3). Because pain is minimal (it's about the same as a needle stick when blood is drawn from your arm), local anesthesia usually isn't necessary. To aspirate a palpable mass, your physician will immobilize the lump with his or her fingers and insert a needle attached to a syringe through the breast tissue into the cyst. If the mass contains fluid, the fluid will be aspirated into the syringe and the needle withdrawn. If the mass is solid, your doctor may insert the needle into the lump several times to obtain a small amount of fluid or tissue in the syringe. Fluid containing blood or cell samples from a solid mass are then sent to a laboratory for analysis.

You may experience some light bruising or bleeding in the area after the procedure, but major complications are rare.

•   **Biopsy:** A biopsy should be performed if:

fluid from a cyst contains blood

a breast mass fails to disappear completely after fluid has been aspirated

the cyst recurs after one or two needle aspirations

a solid dominant mass exists that is *not* a fibroadenoma

you experience a bloody nipple discharge

you have an ulceration of the nipple or persistent crusting

you have swelling and redness of the skin

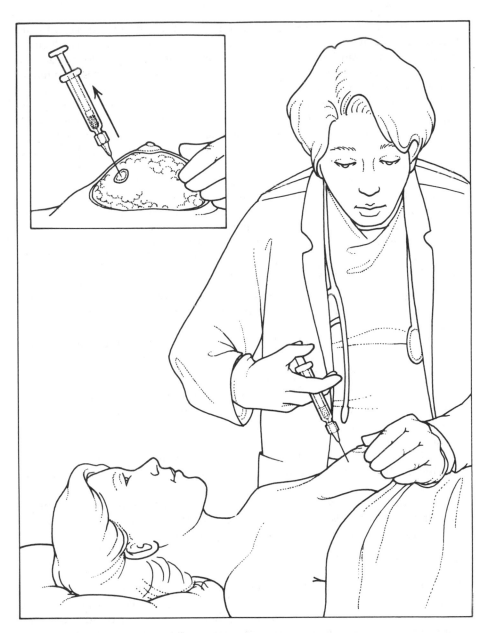

Figure 18.3   Needle Aspiration of the Breast

There are several ways to perform a biopsy. *Needle biopsy* involves the use of a specially designed needle that allows for the removal of a core of tissue. Needle biopsy can be done in your doctor's office under a local anesthetic and is usually used to confirm a diagnosis of cancer made by your physician and/ or as a result of a mammogram. If a needle biopsy is negative, surgical biopsy (see below) is usually recommended.

Some physicians use needle aspiration as a substitute for biopsies of solid breast masses. But this practice is still controversial; if the cell sample is adequate, needle aspiration can identify cancer (although it cannot distinguish intraductal from invasive cancer, or lobular from ductal). However, many times the number of cells taken from a solid breast mass isn't adequate to make a diagnosis.

There are two types of surgical biopsy. *Incisional biopsy* involves removing a portion of a breast lump so it can be inspected under a microscope for any signs of cancer. This may be done in your doctor's office or in the hospital under local or general anesthesia. If the procedure is conducted in the hospital, the results are positive, and you've previously given your consent, your doctor could proceed with surgery. However, many women prefer to wait for the results and consult with their physician about their surgical (or other) options before undergoing further treatment. *Excisional biopsy,* performed when the breast lump is believed to be benign, involves removing the entire mass. It may be done under either local or general anesthesia. (General anesthesia is preferred if the lump is located deep within the breast.) The incision can often be made so that it does not leave a noticeable scar.

• **Prognostic tests:** If biopsy results are positive for cancer, your doctor will perform a few prognostic tests from your biopsy specimen to learn more about the characteristics of the cancer—the tumor's size, how fast it's growing, and whether its growth is stimulated by estrogen, all of which affect the potential for recurrence and the aggressiveness of your treatment.

Estrogen-progesterone receptor test: This test determines whether the cancer contains estrogen or progesterone receptors, which would cause the tumor cells to grow faster when exposed to estrogen or progesterone. "ER-positive" tumors will shrink when exposed to drugs that block estrogen, such as tamoxifen (Nolvadex).

Flow cytometry test: This test determines whether tumor cells have a normal or abnormal amount of DNA and what fraction of the malignant cells are replicating DNA.

Scientists have also found that the number of new blood vessels in breast cancer tumors can also help predict the patient's prognosis: the fewer new blood vessels in the tumor, the better the prognosis.

Treatment of Breast Cancer

• **Surgical treatment:** Whatever the results of the prognostic tests, a positive biopsy usually means surgery. What kind of surgery you have depends on the type and/or number of tumors you have, their size, your breast size, and even your personal preferences. If you are facing surgery for breast cancer, you should learn about all of your options so you can make an informed decision in consultation with your physician.

Lumpectomy (wide excision) followed by local radiation: If the tumor is small and restricted to a single area, you may be a candidate for lumpectomy followed by radiation therapy. During the procedure, which is performed under general anesthesia, the surgeon makes a small incision in the breast and removes the breast lump along with a portion of the surrounding healthy tissue. This type of surgery has been shown to be as safe and effective as modified radical mastectomy, in which the entire breast is removed. Indeed, the overall survival rate for women who undergo lumpectomy followed by radiation therapy is 71 percent—exactly the same as that for women who have a mastectomy. The advantage is that lumpectomy is far less disfiguring than mastectomy.

Women deciding between lumpectomy and mastectomy should get a second and possibly a third opinion. When making a decision, you and your physician should consider your age and whether an experienced radiation oncologist (cancer specialist) is available. Women who *are not* good candidates for this surgery are those whose tumor size is large relative to their breast size and those with more than one tumor or microcalcifications throughout the breast.

Modified radical mastectomy: Most women with breast cancer are treated with modified radical mastectomy, in which the surgeon removes the entire breast, leaving the underlying chest-wall muscles intact. If you have a modified radical mastectomy (by your own choice or because you are not a good candidate for lumpectomy), you should also consider your options for breast reconstruction, since the loss of a breast can be devastating to some women.

• **Postsurgical treatment:** During either lumpectomy or mastectomy, some of the axillary lymph nodes will also be removed to help determine the stage of the disease or the extent of the cancer's spread. This will help determine what follow-up treatment you should consider.

Radiation therapy: All women who have a lumpectomy should receive local radiation therapy, which begins about two weeks after the surgery, or as soon as the incision heals. Radiation therapy is designed to kill any cancer cells that may have been missed during surgery. Generally, you will receive radiation treatments five days a week for up to six weeks.

Chemotherapy: If the cancer is "node-positive" (in other words, cancer cells are found in the lymph nodes), the follow-up treatment is clear: Chemotherapy is recommended for premenopausal women. Chemotherapy may be given in twenty-one-day cycles or twenty-eight-day cycles, as an injection, an intravenous medication, pills, or a combination of intravenous medication and pills. Treatment may last anywhere from three months to one year, depending on the type and severity of the cancer.

Hormone therapy: For postmenopausal women whose cancer involves the lymph nodes, tamoxifen (Nolvadex), a drug that blocks the estrogen receptor on the breast-cancer cell, is a standard treatment. Tamoxifen is given as a pill, which is usually taken twice a day. Studies are now under way to determine whether tamoxifen can *prevent* breast cancer among high-risk women.

Sometimes a progestogen, megesterol acetate (Megace), in the form of a pill may be used to treat estrogen-dependent breast cancers.

Some premenopausal women with estrogen-dependent cancers may have their ovaries removed at the time of surgery to help prevent a recurrence.

Reconstructive Surgery

Many women find the loss of a breast emotionally devastating. However, new techniques now make it possible for a woman to have her breast surgically reconstructed immediately after a mastectomy or at any later time. There are

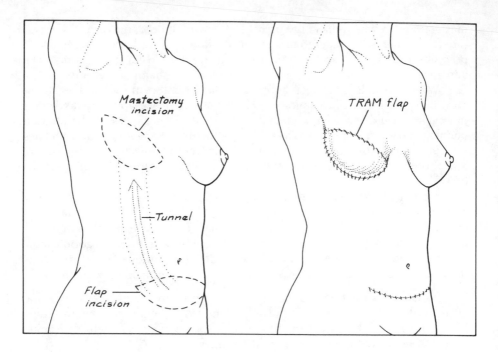

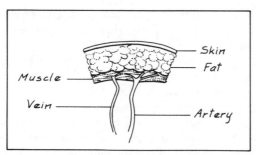

Figure 18.4   TRAM Flap Breast Reconstruction

four major techniques for breast reconstruction. The simplest and most widely used—placing a silicone implant just behind the chest-wall muscles—has come under fire recently because of safety questions involving the use of silicone implants. The silicone-filled implants are still available for use in breast reconstruction, as are saline-filled implants, although the saline-filled implants are not widely used.

Another procedure, known as the TRAM (trans rectus abdominis muscle) flap, involves forming a new breast from the skin, fat, and muscle in the area just below the navel (see Figure 18.4). The abdominal tissue is cut free to form a movable "flap," which remains connected to its artery and vein. The flap is then moved under the skin of the upper abdomen to the chest and brought to the surface through the mastectomy incision, where it is sewn into place.

A third procedure is similar to the TRAM flap surgery, except that a portion of the broad muscle of the back, along with its overlying skin and fat, are used to reconstruct the breast.

Yet another procedure, known as the "gluteus free flap," involves taking tissue from the buttock and reconnecting it to an artery and vein running along the chest wall.

A nipple can be formed for all four types of breast reconstruction, usually by grafting skin from the thigh to the appropriate portion of the breast. Grafted skin tends to become pigmented; if the new nipple isn't dark enough, however, it can be tattooed. (Tattooing is painless, since the relocated skin lacks sensory nerves.)

Reconstructive surgery has improved the quality of life for many women, and should be a consideration for anyone facing the loss of a breast because of cancer.

Colon Cancer

Cancer of the colon and rectum, or *colorectal cancer,* is an equal-opportunity disease, striking as many women as men. It is the third leading cause of cancer death among women, following lung and breast cancer. As with breast cancer, early detection is the key to less disfiguring treatment and better survival. Several reliable screening tests are available for women over forty. There's also evidence that colon cancer can be prevented through dietary measures.

You are at a greater risk of developing colon cancer if you have a personal or family history of cancer or polyps (growths or nodules arising from the mucous membranes) of the colon or rectum. Men and women whose parents have a rare inherited condition known as *polyposis coli* (familial polyposis of the colon) have a 50 percent risk of developing this precancerous disorder, which usually develops into colon cancer at an early age (before age thirty-five). But even individuals in families that aren't affected by polyposis coli are up to 50 percent more likely to develop colon cancer if a parent, brother, or sister has the disease.

Colon cancer also appears to develop more readily in people with inflammatory bowel disease (IBD, also known as *ulcerative colitis*). This is a serious chronic inflammation of the large intestine and rectum. Symptoms include recurrent episodes of abdominal pain, fever, chills, and profuse diarrhea, in which stools often contain blood, pus, and mucus. Inflammatory bowel disease is *not* the same as *irritable bowel syndrome,* a largely stress-related illness that causes abdominal cramping, constipation, diarrhea, or alternating bouts of constipation and diarrhea. Nor is IBD related to *diverticulosis,* a condition characterized by the development of abnormal pouchlike sacs throughout the muscular layers of the colon. Neither irritable bowel syndrome nor diverticulosis is associated with an increased risk of colon cancer.

Some colorectal cancers are believed to arise from a certain type of polyp known as an *adenomatous* polyp. About 30 percent of all men and women in the middle and later years have these polyps, which are usually symptomless and often go undetected. But only a small percentage of these polyps—perhaps 1 percent or less—ever become malignant. Nevertheless, if you are diagnosed with adenomatous polyps, you are considered to be at a higher than average risk of developing colon cancer. For reasons that aren't clear yet, women with a history of breast, endometrial, or ovarian cancer are at a twofold increased risk of developing colon cancer.

By far the greatest risk factors for colon cancer appear to be somewhat within your control: your diet, your weight, and your bowel habits.

• **Your diet:** Population studies have demonstrated a higher incidence of deaths from colon cancer among people who live in countries where meat is a dietary staple. In one of the most convincing studies to date, Dr. Walter C. Willett and his colleagues at Harvard Medical School in Boston found that women who ate beef, pork, or lamb as a main dish on a daily basis had two and a half times the risk of colon cancer as women who ate red meat less than once a month. On the other hand, women who ate chicken (without the skin) and fish had a lower incidence of colon cancer.

In humans and animals, diets high in fat (particularly animal fat) increase the liver's excretion of *bile acids,* which the body uses to break down fats. Animal studies have shown that bile acids act as cancer promoters. Some researchers suggest that eating animal fats leads to an increased number of *anaerobic* organisms in the colon, which may convert normal bile acids into carcinogens. Whatever the mechanism, the message is clear: To help lower your risk of colon cancer, substitute chicken and fish for red meat—or eat no meat at all. (For tips on getting enough protein with a vegetarian diet, see page 72.)

There's also evidence that a high-fiber diet may help *protect* against colon cancer, particularly when the fiber comes from fruits and vegetables (as opposed to cereals and whole grains). In parts of Africa where fiber consumption is high, deaths from colon cancer are low. And in a study by researchers at New York University, men and women who ate more roughage (wheat-bran cereal) had fewer precancerous polyps than those who ate a low-fiber diet.

Dietary fiber is believed to hasten the transit time of food through the intestines—in this way reducing the exposure of colon mucus to potential carcinogens. A high-fiber diet is also thought to dilute potentially carcinogenic bile salts by increasing the bulk of stools. The American Cancer Society recommends that you eat more fiber-rich foods to reduce your risk of colon cancer. (For tips on increasing the fiber in your diet, see page 70.)

Another nutrient receiving increased scrutiny as a possible guard against colon cancer is calcium. Researchers at the University of California at San Diego and the University of Texas in Houston discovered a link between a high intake of calcium and vitamin D (known to help the body absorb calcium) and a lower incidence of colon cancer. Among two thousand men studied, those who consumed more than 1,200 milligrams of calcium in their diets (which also included foods rich in vitamin D) had one-third as much colon cancer as those who ate less than 350 milligrams a day. Calcium supplements have also been found to reduce the growth of colon epithelial cells in family members of people with colon cancer. More research needs to be conducted before any recommendations can be made, but it certainly wouldn't hurt to up your calcium intake, especially since most women in midlife don't get enough, and calcium is also needed to help ward off osteoporosis.

• **Your weight:** Obesity is associated with a 30 percent increase in the risk of colon cancer. Conversely, you can reduce your risk by 30 percent by maintaining normal weight. Lowering your fat intake (see Chapter 4) and exercising (see Chapter 5) are probably the two most effective ways of bringing your weight down. If these measures aren't enough or if you are severely overweight, try the approach to weight control discussed in Chapter 15.

• **Your bowel habits:** Chronic constipation, a condition characterized by small, hard stools, is one of the consequences of eating a low-fiber diet—a risk factor for colon cancer. Although no definitive research has found chronic constipation in itself to be a risk factor for colon cancer, it's reasonable to assume that it could be: If fiber reduces the colon wall's exposure to potential carcinogens by hastening the transit of stool, then constipation must be the antithesis, allowing more time for carcinogens to do damage. At any rate, the problem can easily be remedied and any potential risk eliminated by following a few basic guidelines: Eat foods high in fiber; drink six to eight glasses of water each day; eat a few prunes before bedtime every night; increase your physical activity; avoid using laxatives; and schedule a regular time for a bowel movement every day. (For more on coping with constipation, see page 69.) Practicing good bowel habits will also help you to recognize one of the early warning signs of colon cancer: a change in regularity.

Early warning signs of colon cancer include rectal bleeding, blood in the stool, or a change in bowel habits. But many people with colon cancer have *none* of the early warning signs. (Many people who *do* have these signs don't have cancer.) This is why regular screening is a must. Every woman over age forty should undergo a *digital rectal examination* once a year. This examination allows your doctor to detect any masses in the rectum. You should also have a stool blood test every year after age fifty. This test can detect hidden (occult) blood in the stool. Usually, your physician will provide you with a home test kit, along with instructions on how to obtain a stool sample. In addition to these tests, women over age fifty should undergo *sigmoidoscopy* at least every three to five years. During this examination, your doctor will use a flexible, lighted tube to inspect the upper part of the colon.

If you have symptoms or if screening tests are abnormal, you may have to undergo further tests, including a colonoscopy (examination of the entire colon) or a barium enema, during which a contrast dye is introduced into the colon and your intestines are viewed by X ray.

If cancer is found, surgery, often followed by radiation therapy, is the most effective way of treating it. Chemotherapy and immunotherapy are being investigated, as well. The practice of creating an abdominal opening for elimination of body wastes, or colostomy, is seldom used anymore.

Eighty-eight percent of people whose cancer is detected at an early, localized stage can expect to survive five years or longer. If cancer has spread regionally to involve adjacent organs or lymph nodes, however, the survival rate drops to 58 percent. Survival rates for people with spread of the cancer to distant organs are less than 7 percent, which is why early detection of this cancer is essential.

Endometrial Cancer

Endometrial cancer, cancer of the lining of the uterus (not the uterus itself), is the most common cancer of the reproductive tract in the United States, affecting about one in one thousand women. But when caught in the precancerous

391

stages, it can be treated without radical surgery, and the cure rate is virtually 100 percent.

Endometrial cancer is primarily a disease of postmenopausal women. Less than 25 percent of all cases develop before menopause. The incidence rises steeply among women between the ages of forty-five and fifty-five, reaching a peak among women in their late sixties. In effect, your age is one of the most important risk factors for developing endometrial cancer. Other risk factors include

• **Obesity:** Women who are twenty-one to fifty pounds overweight are three times more likely to develop endometrial cancer than normal-weight women; women weighing more than fifty pounds over ideal weight have a ninefold increased risk. Overweight women with a family history of endometrial, breast, or ovarian cancer are at a particularly greater risk.

• **Estrogen use:** You've probably heard that postmenopausal estrogens increase the risk of developing endometrial cancer. Indeed, early studies showed that postmenopausal women who had not had a hysterectomy (surgical removal of the uterus) and who took estrogen without a progestogen were from two to thirteen times more likely to develop endometrial cancer as nonusers. While the risk may sound high, it must be put into perspective. Essentially, ten to twenty women out of one thousand taking estrogen alone will develop endometrial cancer, compared with one in one thousand nonusers. Indeed, more than 99 percent of postmenopausal estrogen users *do not* develop endometrial cancer. Moreover, taking a progestogen along with estrogen helps prevent overstimulation of the uterine lining by estrogen and wipes out any increased risk associated with estrogen use alone. In fact, progestogen appears to have a protective effect: Postmenopausal women who take progestogen along with estrogen have a lower incidence of endometrial cancer than women who take no postmenopausal hormones whatsoever.

Also, most endometrial cancers associated with estrogen use are less aggressive and are usually caught earlier than those that develop among nonusers, so women with this type of endometrial cancer tend to have a good prognosis.

• **A history of anovulatory menstrual cycles (cycles in which you don't ovulate):** Women who don't ovulate often don't produce the hormone progesterone, needed to protect the uterine lining from overstimulation by estrogen.

• **Diabetes and hypertension:** Women with diabetes are nearly three times more likely to develop endometrial cancer than healthy women. Having high blood pressure is also associated with an increased risk of endometrial cancer, but it doesn't appear to be an independent risk factor.

On the other hand, some women appear to be protected against endometrial cancer. As we mentioned earlier, taking a progestogen along with postmenopausal estrogen has a protective effect. Premenopausal women who take oral contraceptives for as little as twelve months may be protected for up to fifteen years after they stop taking birth-control pills. Regular moderate exercise may help protect against endometrial cancer, as well. The same study by Harvard University researcher Rose Frisch that found a decreased incidence of breast cancer among women athletes also found that women who exercised most of their lives also had less endometrial cancer than sedentary women.

Diagnosing Endometrial Cancer

The single most important early warning sign associated with endometrial cancer is abnormal uterine bleeding. Ninety percent of women with endometrial cancer will experience abnormal bleeding. However, not *all* abnormal bleeding is caused by endometrial cancer. In fact, only about 15 percent of women with abnormal bleeding actually have cancer. Other possible causes of bleeding include use of postmenopausal estrogens, atrophic vaginitis, noncancerous endometrial or cervical polyps, and endometrial hyperplasia. Abnormal bleeding may also occur in women who have cervical cancer, ovarian cancer, or a rare type of uterine cancer known as *uterine sarcoma.* Sometimes, benign fibroid tumors of the uterus cause heavy bleeding, as well.

If you are past menopause and you experience *any* kind of bleeding from the vagina, you should undergo diagnostic tests to rule out endometrial cancer. Postmenopausal women found to have endometrial cells on a Pap smear should be evaluated, as well. Many postmenopausal women who take estrogen are advised to undergo yearly screening tests for endometrial cancer, regardless of whether they have any symptoms. Even pre- and perimenopausal women who experience breakthrough bleeding between periods or increasingly heavy prolonged bleeding should be screened for endometrial cancer, particularly if they have a history of anovulation (failure to ovulate).

Your doctor has several ways of diagnosing abnormal bleeding.

• **Endometrial sampling:** This is a simple and fairly painless procedure that involves removing a sample of endometrial tissue from your uterus so it can be examined under a microscope for possible signs of cancer. The procedure can be performed—usually without anesthesia—right in your doctor's office. First, your doctor will perform a pelvic examination to evaluate the size and position of your uterus. After applying an antiseptic to the cervix and upper vagina, your physician will insert a long, narrow plastic or metal suctioning device through the cervix into the uterus, where a sample of endometrial cells is obtained.

Because endometrial sampling is associated with some cramping and discomfort, you may want to take aspirin or ibuprofen (Advil, Nuprin, Motrin IB) an hour before the procedure. Sometimes, if your cervix has narrowed, or *stenosed*, your doctor may inject a local anesthetic into the cervix to help ease discomfort.

• **Ultrasound:** If your cervical canal is tightly narrowed or if you are extremely sensitive to pain, your physician may instead use ultrasound to measure the thickness of your uterine lining. The test may be performed either abdominally or vaginally. During an abdominal examination, you lie on your back on an examining table and an oil or gel will be spread over your abdomen. The practitioner will move a hand-held ultrasound probe slowly across your abdomen. The probe emits sound waves to project an image of your uterus on a video screen.

Since the abdominal ultrasound requires that you have a full bladder, which can be somewhat uncomfortable, many women prefer a vaginal ultrasound examination. During this procedure, a narrow ultrasound probe is gently placed into the vagina.

An endometrial thickness of less than 5 millimeters is considered normal. If your uterine lining is more than 5 millimeters thick, additional tests, such as hysteroscopy or dilatation and curettage (D&C), may be required to obtain a tissue sample.

• **Color doppler ultrasound:** One drawback to the ultrasound examination is that it doesn't produce a tissue sample that can be examined under a microscope. However, a new color doppler ultrasound technology, now being developed, may be even more accurate than the current method of measuring the uterine thickness.

• **Hysteroscopy:** If there's any question about the results of either endometrial sampling or ultrasonography, your doctor may recommend that you undergo a *hysteroscopy,* in which an endoscope is used to look inside your uterus for possible signs of cancer and possibly to obtain a tissue sample. The procedure may be performed either in the hospital with a general anesthesia or on an outpatient basis with a regional anesthetic or no anesthetic at all.

• **Dilatation and curettage:** If the results of endometrial sampling show some abnormalities, if your uterus is enlarged, or if bleeding remains heavy and persistent, a dilatation and curettage may be recommended. This diagnostic test is performed under local or general anesthesia. During the procedure, the physician first dilates the cervix, then, using a curette (a sharp spoon-shaped instrument), removes the endometrium, or uterine lining. The procedure usually takes less than fifteen minutes to complete.

Classifying Endometrial Cancer

Like most cancers, endometrial cancer is classified by its stage.

• **Hyperplasia:** This is the medical term for overgrowth of endometrial cells. It usually means that your uterine lining has been overstimulated by estrogen. However, having hyperplasia does *not* necessarily mean that you have cancer. Cancer specialists usually distinguish between *hyperplasia without atypia* (that is, without suspicious-looking cells) and *hyperplasia with atypia* (cells that are abnormal in appearance). There's some evidence that hyperplasia with atypia is much more likely to develop into cancer than hyperplasia without atypia. Usually, hyperplasia with atypia doesn't respond to the standard treatment for this condition, hormone therapy (further discussion of treatment of hyperplasia can be found under Treatment of Endometrial Cancer, opposite).

• **Endometrial carcinoma:** When cancer is found, it is generally classified by its stage.

Stage 0: The cancer is localized to the uterine lining and has not spread. Some experts use this stage to describe the most severe form of atypical hyperplasia.

Stage I: The cancer is confined to the uterus. Stage I cancers are further subdivided by the depth of invasion of the cancer into the uterine wall.

Stage II: The cancer has spread to the cervix but not beyond the uterus.

Stage III: The cancer has spread to the vagina and surrounding lymph nodes.

Stage IV: The cancer has spread to the bladder and/or bowel, or to other organs beyond the pelvis.

Treatment of Endometrial Cancer

Treatment depends on whether you have hyperplasia or cancer, and the stage of the cancer. If an endometrial sampling or hysteroscopy shows that you have hyperplasia, your doctor will recommend that you take progestogen for ten days every month for three to six months. After progestogen treatment, your doctor will perform a repeat endometrial biopsy to ensure that the treatment has worked.

If hyperplasia persists after a second trial dose of progestogen therapy or if you have hyperplasia with atypical cells, a hysterectomy (surgical removal of the uterus) is recommended.

For endometrial cancer, an abdominal hysterectomy and bilateral salpingo-oophorectomy (removal of the uterus, Fallopian tubes, and ovaries) is the treatment of choice. Most physicians recommend that your ovaries be removed because women with endometrial cancer are at increased risk of developing ovarian cancer, which is much more difficult to detect in its early stages. A vaginal hysterectomy may be recommended for patients with early (Stage I) endometrial cancer and those who are markedly obese and have other medical problems that place them at high risk for abdominal operations.

Many women, particularly those whose cancer has spread to the lymph nodes or adjacent organs, may require follow-up radiation therapy to prevent recurrence of the cancer in the vagina and lymph nodes.

Overall, the prognosis for women with endometrial cancer is good. Most women with endometrial cancers are diagnosed in the early stages (Stage I), when the survival rate—93 percent—is highest. And virtually 100 percent of women survive when the disease is diagnosed in the precancerous lesion stage.

Cervical Cancer

Cervical cancer is one of the most preventable cancers. If you undergo annual Pap smear testing, you virtually eliminate your chances of developing cervical cancer. On the other hand, the rate of cervical cancer in women who don't have Pap smears is 50 to 60 per 100,000 women ages twenty or older.

Tragically, many older women don't have regular Pap smears. Yet 25 percent of all cervical cancers occur in women ages sixty-five and older. And 40 percent of all deaths from cervical cancer occur in older women.

As with most types of cancer, some women are more likely to develop cervical cancer than others. Women who had their first intercourse at an early age are at a greater risk, as are those with multiple sexual partners. This has led some experts to suspect that perhaps the most important cause of cervical cancer is a sexually transmitted disease. Trichomonas, chlamydia, and herpes all have come under suspicion, but researchers have failed to find a clear connection between these STDs and cervical cancer. Now, several recent studies implicate certain strains of the human papillomavirus (HPV), which causes sexually transmitted genital warts. Studies of cervical-cancer tissue have shown that the genetic material (DNA) for HPV can be found in up to 80 percent of cervical cancers. However, not all strains of HPV are associated with an in-creased risk of cervical cancer; studies have implicated strains 11 and 16 as the most virulent.

Cigarette smokers have double the risk of developing cervical cancer as nonsmokers. Nicotine has been found in vaginal secretions of cigarette smokers at concentrations forty times higher than in their blood. This has led some researchers to suspect that the carcinogens in cigarette smoke play a direct role in triggering cancerous changes of the cervix.

Diagnosing Cervical Cancer

One of the early warning signs of cervical cancer is vaginal bleeding, which usually occurs after intercourse. (Women with more advanced cancer may develop a foul-smelling vaginal discharge.) But one of the most effective ways of catching the cancer in its earliest stages—often before you notice any early warning signs—is to undergo regular annual Pap smears. The test involves having your physician gently remove a sample of cells from your cervix. The cells are then smeared onto a slide, fixed with a solution to keep them intact, then sent to a laboratory for analysis under a microscope. At the laboratory, the cells are classified according to the degree of abnormalities detected.

Class I: a normal smear

Class II: Signs of inflammation were detected.

Class III: Dysplastic cells were detected. This means you have what's known as *cervical intraepithelial neoplasia,* or CIN—small areas of abnormal tissue growth in the outer layer of your cervix that may go on to become cervical cancer if left untreated. Mild or moderate CIN, called CIN 1 or CIN 2, both qualify as a Class III smear.

Class IV: Shows more severe CIN (CIN 3), which may be referred to as carcinoma in situ.

Class V: True cancer cells have invaded the inner layers of the cervix.

Anything other than a Class I Pap smear is considered abnormal and may require further tests to determine the cause of the abnormality. Remember, though, an abnormal Pap smear doesn't necessarily mean you have cancer. Often, the inflammation from a Class II Pap is due to a vaginal infection that can be easily treated with antibiotics or other medication. Your doctor will recommend that you undergo another Pap smear three to six months after the inflammation has cleared to ensure that all cells are normal.

As beneficial as the Pap smear is (the screening test has helped reduce the death rates from cervical cancer by more than 70 percent in the last forty years), it's not perfect. According to the American College of Obstetricians and Gynecologists, between 15 and 40 percent of women who have cancer or precancerous conditions may have a normal Pap smear. Half of the false-negative problem has been attributed to mistakes in taking the sample and the other half to errors by laboratory personnel in reading the sample. But a new cervical-screening test called *cervicography* has been found to improve the accuracy of cervical screening when performed along with your annual Pap smear. During the test, which can be done at the time of your annual examination, your doctor applies a solution of 5 percent acetic acid to your cervix. Then, using a specially designed camera called a *cervixcope,* your physician simply photographs the cervix. The photograph, or *cervogram,* is then sent to a laboratory for analysis. When this test is used along with the Pap smear, more than 90 percent of cervical cancers and precancerous lesions can be detected. (The cervogram is not widely available yet, however.)

If a Pap smear and cervogram both reveal Class III cells, or your cervix looks suspicious, your physician will probably recommend that you undergo a *colposcopy.* This office procedure involves the use of an instrument that magnifies and illuminates the surface of the cervix, allowing your doctor to see the cervix up close. If the colposcopy reveals any abnormal cells, your doctor will perform a cervical biopsy by taking a sample of cells from the cervix. This usually causes only mild cramping and spotting.

Treatment of Cervical Cancer

If the biopsy confirms CIN, your doctor has several ways of removing the abnormal cells, including *cryosurgery* (destroying the abnormal cells by freezing them), laser surgery (in which a laser beam vaporizes the cells), or *electrocoagulation* (in which an intense heat created by an electrical current is used to destroy the cells). These procedures can be performed in your doctor's office without anesthesia, and they enjoy a success rate of about 90 percent.

A new treatment, called *loop electrosurgical excision procedures* (LEEP), may be even better than the standard methods. During this procedure, a low-voltage, high-frequency radio wave running through a thin wire loop is used to remove the cancerous tissue in one piece. The excised tissue can then be examined for evidence of invasive cancer, a rare event, occurring in only one out of one thousand women treated for CIN, but one that can be missed with cryosurgery or laser surgery.

Another advantage of LEEP is that it can be performed right after a colposcopy, making cervical biopsy unnecessary. This way, you are also spared the anxiety of waiting for the upcoming treatment.

LEEP is usually performed under a local anesthetic and takes all of five seconds. The most common side effect—excessive bleeding after the procedure—occurs only about 5 to 6 percent of the time and can be easily treated by having your doctor apply a ferric subsulfate paste to the cervix. For most women, the cervix is completely healed within a month.

The procedure has been used by British gynecologists to treat thousands of patients with CIN over the past several years. It is between 95 to 98 percent successful. More and more American doctors are now being trained to use the technique.

For cervical cancer in situ, a *cone biopsy* may be required. This procedure, performed in the hospital under general anesthesia, involves removing a small "cone" of tissue that includes the entire surface of the cervix and part of the cervical canal. If you are past your childbearing years, your doctor may recommend that you undergo a total hysterectomy (surgical removal of the uterus and cervix).

As we mentioned earlier, cervical cancer is one of the most preventable cancers. Here's how you can reduce your risk:

•   **Have regular Pap smears.** Although some major health organizations recommend that you have a Pap smear every three years, we recommend annual Pap smears, especially since the false-negative rate for Pap smears is fairly high.

•   **If you smoke, quit.** (Advice for quitting can be found on page 150.)

•   **If you're sexually active (particularly with multiple partners), use a condom *in addition to your regular form of birth control.*** Condoms help protect against HPV infection.

•   **Perform a monthly genital self-examination (GSE).** While GSE won't prevent you from getting cervical cancer, it will alert you to possible signs of HPV infection and allow you to seek treatment. (For instructions on how to perform GSE, see page 52.)

If the cancer has spread to the lymph nodes, a radical hysterectomy is often recommended. This involves removing the uterus, cervix, the cuff of the vagina, the supporting tissue around the uterus, and the lymph glands that help drain the pelvis. Postoperative radiation therapy and chemotherapy is usually recommended for women with advanced cervical cancer.

Ovarian Cancer

While ovarian cancer accounts for only 4 percent of all cancers among women, it is a leading cause of cancer death. This is largely because ovarian cancer is a "silent" disease, often causing no symptoms until the cancer has spread. In fact, less than 30 percent of ovarian cancers are confined to the ovaries at the time they are diagnosed. Yet the cure rate for ovarian cancer that hasn't spread may be as high as 90 percent. Improved screening tests hold promise of detecting this cancer earlier and improving the odds of surviving the disease.

The most common type of ovarian cancer is *epithelial ovarian cancer,* the kind we will discuss here. More than 80 percent of these cancers are found in postmenopausal women. Indeed, your age is one of the most significant risk factors for this type of ovarian cancer.

Another telling indicator of whether you are at risk of developing ovarian cancer is a family history. If your mother or sister has had ovarian cancer, your risk increases tenfold. A family history of endometrial or breast cancer appears to double your risk. A history of colon, lung, or prostate cancer in immediate family members increases your risk, as well. Women who have no children are also at greater risk of developing ovarian cancer. The risk appears to decrease with each pregnancy.

On the brighter side, oral contraceptives appear to protect against ovarian cancer, and premenopausal women with a family history of ovarian cancer may want to consider taking oral contraceptive for this reason. Studies have shown that oral contraceptive users are 40 percent less likely to develop ovarian cancer as nonusers. Protection begins in as little as three to six months of oral-contraceptive use and continues for up to fifteen years after you stop taking the birth-control pills.

Early warning signs associated with ovarian cancer are vague and can be easily overlooked. These include enlargement of the abdomen (caused by accumulation of fluid) and vague digestive disturbances, such as stomach discomfort, gas, or distension. If these symptoms persist and can't be explained by any other cause, you should ask your gynecologist to perform a thorough evaluation for ovarian cancer.

Diagnosing Ovarian Cancer

An evaluation usually begins with a pelvic examination to see whether your ovaries are enlarged. If your doctor finds this to be the case, it does not necessarily mean that you have cancer. Often, the cause in premenopausal women may be one of a variety of ovarian cysts. The most common among them—*functional cysts* (also known as cystic ovaries)—are almost always benign. These include *follicular* cysts, which arise from the egg-producing follicles, and *corpus-luteum* cysts, which develop if bleeding occurs in the ruptured follicular sac (known as the corpus luteum) after the release of an egg. These cysts usually regress within a month or two. If not, they often regress after you begin taking oral contraceptives.

Polycystic ovarian cysts, characterized by numerous small cysts that develop in the ovaries along with such symptoms as irregular menstrual bleeding, hirsutism (abnormal hair growth), and obesity, are also considered functional cysts, but do not regress as readily as follicular and corpus-luteum cysts.

Certain ovarian cysts may also be responsible for enlargement of the ovaries in premenopausal women. However, unlike functional cysts, some ovarian cysts, such as *serous-cyst adenomas, mucinous-cyst adenomas,* and *dermoid cysts,* do have the potential to develop into cancer and may require surgical removal.

If you are premenopausal and your physician finds that one of your ovaries is enlarged, but no larger than 3 centimeters in diameter, you may be advised to wait a month or two to see whether it regresses by itself. Premenopausal women whose ovaries are larger than 3 centimeters in diameter, those who have a pelvic mass that *doesn't* regress within three months or after taking birth-control pills, and *all* postmenopausal women whose ovaries can be palpated will be advised to undergo further diagnostic tests.

If your doctor finds a suspicious pelvic mass, he or she may recommend that you have an abdominal or vaginal ultrasound examination. Ultrasound can often distinguish between a large but healthy normal ovary, cystic ovaries (including follicular, corpus-luteum, and polycystic ovarian cysts), and ovarian cysts (such as a dermoid cyst). Ultrasound can also help determine whether the pelvic mass originates in the ovaries or somewhere else (a fibroid tumor of the uterus, for example). However, it is not always reliable in differentiating between benign and malignant ovarian tumors. (Use of a new color doppler ultrasound device may help overcome this problem.)

Certain blood tests have also been found to be helpful in making a diagnosis of cancer. Researchers discovered in 1981 that epithelial ovarian cancers produce a substance known as CA-125, which has become an important "tumor maker" for this type of cancer. If you have a suspicious pelvic mass, your physician may recommend that you undergo a blood test for CA-125. A blood level of CA-125 greater than 34 u/ml is considered positive. You should be aware, however, that other conditions, such as fibroid tumors or endometriosis, can also cause elevated levels of CA-125. If your doctor still has lingering doubts about the nature of the pelvic mass or if test results suggest that you have ovarian cancer, he or she will recommend that you undergo a laparoscopy or an exploratory surgery (laparotomy), in which a biopsy of the ovaries can be obtained. *This is the only definitive way to make a diagnosis of ovarian cancer.*

Treatment of Ovarian Cancer

If cancer is found, treatment involves removal of both ovaries as well as the uterus and Fallopian tubes. Radiation and/or chemotherapy is recommended for women with cancer cells elsewhere in the pelvic cavity. Sometimes a second laparotomy is performed several months later to see whether any cancer cells have been missed (or have recurred).

Cancer of the Vulva

Cancer of the vulva comprises only about 4 percent of all reproductive cancers, but the incidence of precancerous and cancerous diseases of the vulva appears to be rising. Once again, early diagnosis is a key to less disfiguring surgery and longer survival. And as with breast cancer, one of your best means of protection is literally in your hands: genital self-examination.

Ninety percent of vulvar cancer is actually a type of skin cancer, known as *squamous-cell carcinoma.* Vulvar cancer most commonly strikes postmenopausal women. Women who are obese and those with high blood pressure or diabetes also appear to be at somewhat greater risk, as are women who experience an early menopause (before age forty-five). Women with a history of human papillomavirus (the virus responsible for sexually transmitted genital warts, or *condyloma*), herpes simplex Type II, and syphilis may also be at increased risk of developing vulvar cancer.

Cancer of the vulva typically starts with a raised lesion that may be ulcerated, white, or warty in appearance, accompanied by itching or soreness. Some women may experience vulvar bleeding, a discharge, or pain upon urinating. Again, these could be signs of any of a number of benign conditions, such as *lichen sclerosis,* a fungal irritation of the skin, or a sexually transmitted disease, such as condyloma (genital warts) or herpes, so don't panic. If you notice any itching, lumps, sores, discoloration, or inflammation of the vulva, either through genital self-examination (instructions are on page 52) or incidentally, you should report them to your physician right away.

Your doctor can visually inspect the vulva for possible signs of cancer. He or she may also apply a blue dye known as *toluidine blue* on the vulva and wash it off with a dilute vinegar solution. The dye is absorbed by potentially precancerous cells, so any remaining blue coloration of the skin may be a symptom of cancer.

Generally speaking, in postmenopausal women, *any* visible abnormal lesion on the vulva will require a biopsy, which is the most definitive way to determine whether the lesion is cancerous. A biopsy can usually be taken in the doctor's office under local anesthesia.

Surgery is generally required to treat vulvar cancer, but, in the early stages, a wide excision, in which only the cancer and some of the surrounding healthy tissue is removed, is almost always successful. If the disease is more advanced, a radical vulvectomy may be recommended, in which the entire vulva and sometimes the lymph nodes in the groin are removed.

One of your best defenses against such radical surgery is to perform genital self-examination *once a month*. This simple examination takes just a few minutes to perform and is a key to early diagnosis and treatment of vulvar cancer, which is 90 percent curable when caught in its earliest stages.

Skin Cancer

Skin cancer is one of the most common cancers of all. Fortunately, it's also one of the most curable when discovered early. Better yet, most skin cancer can be prevented.

Types of Skin Cancer

• **Basal-cell carcinoma:** Of the three types of skin cancer, this is the most common form, affecting some 500,000 Americans each year. Until recently, basal-cell carcinoma was predominantly a disease of older people, particularly men who worked outdoors. Now, however, basal-cell carcinomas are appearing at earlier ages, and women are getting them almost as often as men.

Basal-cell carcinomas most frequently develop on exposed parts of the body—the face, ears, neck, scalp, shoulders, and back. Because the cancer rarely spreads to vital organs, it is the least dangerous type of cancer. Nevertheless, if left untreated, the tumor can grow, sometimes causing considerable destruction—possibly even the loss of an eye, ear, or nose.

• **Squamous-cell carcinoma:** This is the second-most-common skin cancer, affecting more than 100,000 Americans each year. It arises from the epidermis (outermost layer of skin) and may occur on all areas of the body, including the mucous membranes. Generally speaking, though, squamous-cell cancers most commonly develop in areas exposed to the sun—the face, neck, hands, shoulders, arms, and back. The rim of the ear and the lower lip are especially vulnerable.

Unlike basal-cell carcinomas, untreated squamous-cell carcinomas can penetrate the underlying layers of skin and in a small percentage of cases can spread to other parts of the body. When this happens, the cancer can be fatal.

- **Malignant melanoma:** This type of cancer arises from melanocytes (the skin cells that produce the dark protective pigment called melanin) and is much less common than basal-cell or squamous-cell carcinoma. But it is much more serious because it more readily spreads to other parts of the body (including vital internal organs), where it is much more difficult to treat. On the other hand, the cancer is completely curable when caught in its earliest stages.

Melanoma may suddenly appear on the skin without warning, or it may begin in or near a mole or other pigmented area of the skin. Because the cancer involves melanocytes, it is often black or brown in color, sometimes with red or blue portions. And unlike moles, which usually have regular borders, melanomas have irregular borders.

Perhaps the most significant risk factor for all types of skin cancer is overexposure to the sun. *Anyone* with a history of sun exposure can develop skin cancer. In fact, chronic overexposure to sunlight is the cause of 95 percent of basal-cell and squamous-cell carcinomas. Melanoma appears to occur more often in people who have a history of blistering sunburns in their teens and twenties and who receive intermittent sun exposure as adults.

People with fair skin that burns and freckles easily, light hair, and blue, green, or gray eyes are at the highest risk for all types of skin cancer. People with many moles, certain types of atypical moles, or those with relatives who have had melanoma are more likely to develop it. However, even dark-skinned people can develop skin cancers.

Diagnosing and Treating Skin Cancer

If discovered early enough, all skin cancers—even melanoma—are completely curable. This is why it is essential that you know the size and location of the moles on your body and take note of any other changes that may be early signs of skin cancer. Use the instructions for skin self-examination in Chapter 8 (page 165) to examine your skin *at least once every six months* (once a month if you are at high risk of developing skin cancer). See page 164 for a list of potentially harmful skin changes to watch for.

You should promptly report any suspicious lesions to your physician. After your physician has examined you, a biopsy will be performed to confirm the diagnosis of skin cancer. This involves removing a piece of the affected tissue and examining it under a microscope.

If cancer cells are present, surgery is normally required to remove the tumor. This can usually be performed on an outpatient basis in the physician's office or at a clinic. There are several ways of eradicating skin cancer. The method your doctor chooses—using a scalpel, radiation, a laser, an electrical current, or freezing the cells—depends on the size, location, and type of cancer you have, your age, and your general health.

Preventing Skin Cancer

You can protect yourself from developing skin cancer in the first place by following a few important steps. The most important thing you can do is guard against overexposure to the sun. You should avoid sun exposure between 10:00 A.M. and 3:00 P.M., when the sun's ultraviolet rays are strongest. If you

How can you tell a normal mole from a melanoma? According to the American Cancer Society, a normal mole is an evenly colored brown, tan, or black spot in the skin. It may be either flat or raised, is round or oval in shape, and has sharply defined borders. Moles are generally less than 6 millimeters in diameter (about the size of a pencil eraser) and usually don't change in size, shape, or color for many years. The ABCD rule from the American Cancer Society will help you remember what to look for in a melanoma:

- **A—asymmetry:** One half of a melanoma does not match the other half.

- **B—border irregularity:** The edges are ragged, notched, or blurred.

- **C—color:** The pigmentation is not uniform. Shades of tan, brown, and black are present. Red, white, and blue may add to the mottled appearance.

- **D—diameter greater than 6 millimeters:** Any sudden or continuing increase in size should be of special concern.

Note: Text reprinted with permission from "What You Should Know About Melanoma," prepared by the American Cancer Society.

go out in the sun, wear protective clothing (a wide-brimmed hat, pants, and a long-sleeved shirt if possible). Use a sunscreen with a sun-protection factor (SPF) of 15 or greater. (For more on sunscreens and how to use them, see page 158.)

You should also perform regular skin self-examinations to catch skin cancer in its earliest and most curable stages. Have your doctor examine your skin, as well.

If you have a family or personal history of melanoma, you should *not* take postmenopausal hormone therapy. Estrogen may promote the growth of existing melanomas.

A Lifestyle for Overall Cancer Prevention

Most cancers are related to lifestyle practices within your control. Here are some general guidelines for lowering your overall risk of cancer.

- **Reduce your cancer risk through your diet.** As you've already seen, what you eat may influence your risk of developing a variety of different cancers, including the top three causes of cancer death among women in the middle and later years: lung, colon, and breast cancers. To reduce your overall risk of cancer, follow A Prudent Diet for Cancer Prevention on page 404, based on the American Cancer Society's Guidelines on Diet, Nutrition and Cancer and those of other national health organizations.

• **Maintain a desirable body weight.** Women who are 40 percent above their desirable weight are up to 55 percent more likely to die of cancer than women of normal weight. Obesity is associated with an increased risk of cancer of the uterus, gallbladder, kidney, stomach, colon, and breast. Reducing the fat in your diet (see page 60) and increasing your level of physical activity (see Chapter 5) are ideal ways of keeping your weight down.

• **Eat a variety of fruits and vegetables every day.** People who eat plenty of fruits and vegetables on a daily basis have a lower risk of lung, bladder, esophagus, and stomach cancers. Fruits and vegetables contain vitamins, minerals, fiber, and other substances. These—alone or together—may be responsible for reducing the risk of cancer.

• **Eat plenty of high-fiber foods, such as whole-grain cereals, legumes, fruits, and vegetables.** Some studies have associated a high-fiber diet with a lower risk of colon cancer. Even if fiber is ultimately shown not to have a direct protective effect against cancer, these foods are wholesome low-calorie substitutes for high-calorie fatty foods.

• **Reduce your fat intake.** Excessive fat intake increases the risk of cancers of the breast and colon. You should aim for a daily fat intake of 20 to 25 percent or less of your total calories.

• **Limit your consumption of alcoholic beverages, if you drink at all.** Heavy drinking of all types of alcoholic beverages increases your risk of developing cancers of the oral cavity, larynx, esophagus, and possibly the liver. Some studies suggest that even moderate alcohol consumption may raise your risk of developing breast cancer. If you drink, do so occasionally and sparingly.

• **Limit your consumption of salt-cured, smoked, and nitrite-preserved foods.** Conventionally smoked foods, such as hams, some types of sausage, fish, and so forth, absorb some of the tars that arise from incomplete combustion in the smoking process. These tars contain numerous carcinogens that are chemically similar to the carcinogenic tars in tobacco smoke. This includes foods grilled over charcoal. Some studies suggest that salt-cured or pickled foods may increase the risk of stomach and esophageal cancers. Foods preserved with nitrates and nitrites (such as hot dogs) may enhance the formation of the potential carcinogen *nitrosamine* in foods and in your digestive tract.

• **Eat a varied diet.** Many people worry that such substances as food additives, artificial sweeteners, pesticides, and contaminants that make their way into our food supply may increase the risk of cancer. Rest assured that our food supply is one of the safest in the world. Some experts feel that natural carcinogens in meat, grain, and other food pose a far greater cancer risk than pesticides and food additives. At any rate, your best protection is to limit your exposure to any one potential carcinogen in food (either naturally occurring or man-made) by eating a variety of foods in moderation.

- **Exercise your way to a lower cancer risk.** A landmark study by Harvard University researcher Rose Frisch involving more than five thousand women from twenty-one to eighty years old found that women who participated in organized athletic activity in college had a lower lifetime occurrence of cancers of the reproductive system and breast than their sedentary counterparts. The active women also had significantly fewer benign tumors of the reproductive system and breast. Dr. Frisch and other researchers suggest that active women have less body fat than sedentary women, which may, in turn, reduce their risk of these cancers.

It's still not known whether increasing your activity later in life will help protect against cancer, but it can't hurt: Exercise is an excellent way to help keep your weight in check, and being overweight is another risk factor for cancer.

- **Have regular medical checkups.** Your anticancer strategy should also consist of monthly breast self-examinations (BSE) and regular medical checkups, which help you and your doctor detect cancers in their earliest stages, when they can be easily treated and often cured.

A Final Word

Even if you adopt an anticancer lifestyle, no one can guarantee that you won't get cancer. But by reducing your exposure to certain carcinogens whenever possible, eating a diet rich in nutrients that protect against carcinogens, undergoing regular screening tests that can catch cancers in their earliest, most curable stages, and knowing the early warning signs of cancer, you're bound to improve your odds of living a long cancer-free life.

Resources and Support

American Cancer Society, 1599 Clifton Rd., NE, Atlanta, GA 30329-4251. Phone: (800) ACS-2345. For free information on breast self-examination, how to quit smoking, cancer prevention, breast reconstruction after mastectomy, and more, contact your local branch of the ACS or write to the above address.

National Cancer Institute (NCI), Office of Cancer Communications, National Institutes of Health, Building 31, Room 10A24, 9000 Rockville Pike, Bethesda, MD 20892. Phone: (800) 4-CANCER. Call this toll-free number for confidential answers to your cancer-related questions or to receive information on the early detection, prevention, and treatment of cancer. The staff will provide you with a list of cancer specialists in your area or refer you to an NCI-supported treatment program.

The Skin Cancer Foundation, Suite 2402, 245 Fifth Avenue, New York, NY 10016. Phone: (212) 725-5176. Contact this nonprofit foundation for more information on the world's most prevalent (and most preventable) malignancy: skin cancer.

Suggested Reading

Love, Susan, M.D., with Karen Lindsey. *Dr. Susan Love's Breast Book*. New York: Addison-Wesley, 1990.

Robins, Perry, M.D. *Sun Sense*. New York: The Skin Cancer Foundation, 1990.

Chapter 19

....

*Urinary-Tract
Infections and
Urinary Incontinence:
How to Get an
Accurate Diagnosis
and Treatment*

Bladder problems are some of the most frequent reasons for a visit to the gynecologist, yet two of the most common problems—urinary-tract infections and urinary incontinence (loss of bladder control)—often are not taken seriously enough. Too many women rationalize that "all women get bladder infections, and all you need to do is drink cranberry juice." In fact, no amount of cranberry juice in the world will cure a bacterial infection, and low-grade and undertreated bladder infections can lead to chronic kidney problems.

As for incontinence, your general impression may be, "Well, that's a normal part of aging and there's nothing you can do about it, so you might as well just learn to live with it, right?" Wrong! Most incontinence can be managed, and many cases *can be cured.* But many women don't even bother to seek treatment because they are too embarrassed, they think incontinence is "normal," or they believe that surgery is the only treatment available and they've heard that it is frequently unsuccessful. In one study involving women who were being evaluated for incontinence, 33 percent postponed consulting a physician for one to five years, and 25 percent put off seeking treatment for more than five years. Five years is a long time to put your life on the shelf, which is often what happens to women with incontinence.

While not life-threatening in itself, incontinence can undermine your physical health. The physical inactivity associated with incontinence can have far-reaching effects on the health of your heart, your bones, and your overall sense of well-being.

In this chapter you'll find the information you need to understand and cope with some of the more common bladder and urinary-tract problems you may encounter in the middle and later years.

Urinary-Tract and Bladder Infections

Women are more prone than men to develop *urinary-tract infections,* which are usually caused by some kind of bacteria and may affect the urethra (*urethritis*), bladder (*cystitis*), or bladder and kidneys (*pyelocystitis*). This has to do with simple anatomy. Your urethra (the tube leading from the bladder to the outside of the body) is much shorter than a man's and is situated close to the vagina and rectum (see Figure 19.1). Bacteria from the vagina may work its way into the urethra during intercourse. Or if you clean yourself from back to front after a bowel movement, instead of from front to back, you may inadvertently spread bacteria from the rectum to the urethra. Indeed, the most common bacterial culprit is *E. coli,* found in the colon. Many infections remain localized in the lower urethra, but many, if left untreated, can travel to the bladder and up the ureters to the kidneys.

Having a new sexual partner may increase the risk of infection, as does the use of a diaphragm. Women with diabetes, those with a kidney obstruction or suppressed immune system, and pregnant women are also more prone to developing a urinary-tract infection.

Figure 19.1   Anatomy of Female Kidneys and Urinary Tract

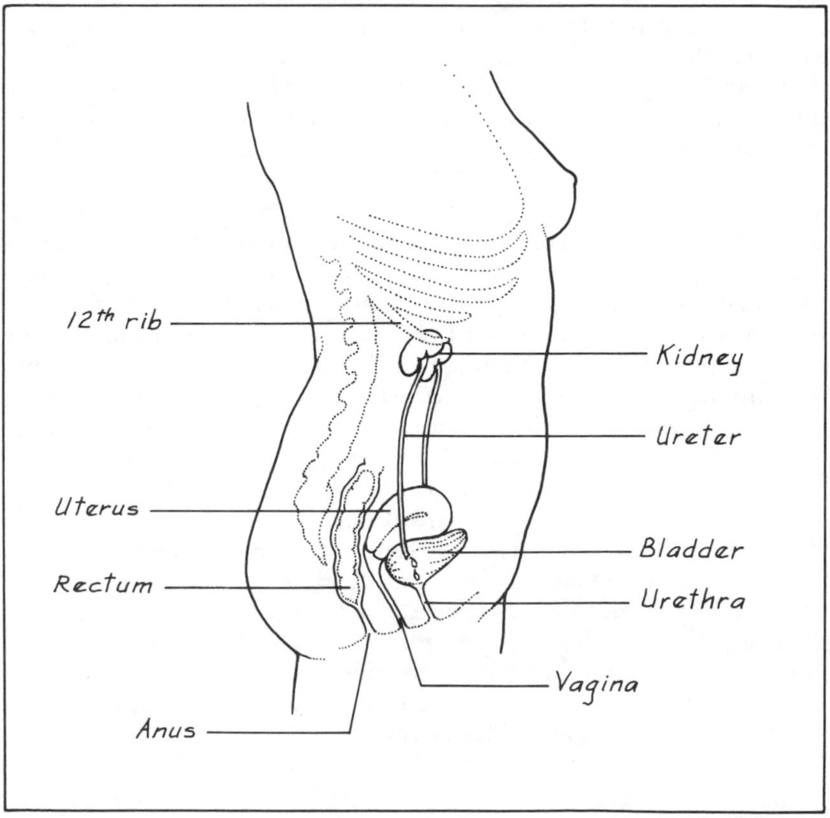

You may become even more susceptible to urinary-tract infections in the middle and later years. This is because the lower estrogen levels associated with menopause cause the lining of the urinary tract (*urothelium*) to thin out in much the same way as a lack of estrogen affects the lining of the vaginal walls. (The urinary tract and vagina arise from the same tissues in the growing embryo, so you can see why these tissues respond to low estrogen levels in a similar way.) Normally, the mucus-producing glands in the lower portion of the urethra (the *periurethral glands*) trap bacteria and secrete bacteria-fighting immune cells. These safeguards help prevent the infection from ascending to the bladder. However, the menopause-related changes in the urethral lining weaken the built-in biological protection you have.

Low estrogen levels may also cause a decline in an important "mechanical barrier" to the spread of bacteria. Along the length of the urethra are muscle fibers that help control the flow of urine from the bladder. The muscles are thickest midway up the urethra, where they create a "pressure zone" that helps contain bacteria in the lower part of the urethra. When estrogen levels fall after menopause, blood flow to the area decreases and muscle tone may weaken, causing urethral pressure to decline and allowing bacteria to migrate more easily to the bladder.

Finally, prolapse of the bladder, or *cystocele,* is more common among older women. This may make it more difficult for you to empty your bladder completely, and the residual pool of urine in the bladder may form a breeding ground for bacteria.

Symptoms include a frequent need to urinate (throughout the day *and* night) or a strong urge even when there's no need; lower-abdominal pressure; pain upon urination; and possibly blood in the urine. Infections may also stimulate urge incontinence, in which you leak a small amount of urine before you have a chance to get to the bathroom.

You should take bladder infections seriously, particularly since untreated infections can lead to permanent kidney damage. *Never* try to self-treat a urinary-tract infection with cranberry juice or other home remedies. If you have symptoms of an infection, see your physician, who will perform a few diagnostic tests to confirm your suspicions. A simple urinalysis, in which chemically treated paper is dipped into a sample of your urine, can detect white and red blood cells, possible signs of infection. Because the type of bacteria causing the infection could influence the type of drugs used to treat it, your physician may also want to perform a urine culture, in which a sample of your urine is sent to a laboratory and the bacteria in it are grown in a special culture medium.

If you have a urinary-tract infection, your doctor will prescribe antibiotics to kill the bacteria causing your symptoms. The most commonly prescribed antibiotics are Ampicillin, Macrodantin, and Septra, depending on the results of your urine culture. Since antibiotics may cause a secondary vaginal yeast infection (*monilia*), your doctor may also recommend that you use a vaginal antiyeast cream or suppository (Monistat, Femstat, or Terazol) for the full ten days that you are taking antibiotics. You should also drink plenty of fluids while you are being treated to help flush out the bladder. (This will not dilute the antibiotic concentrations in your blood, by the way.)

If you are in a lot of pain, your doctor may prescribe the analgesic Pyridium. (The drug changes the color of urine to red or orange, which may stain

There are several measures you can take to reduce your chances of developing a urinary-tract infection.

• **Drink plenty of fluids.** Ideally, you should drink a glass of water every two to three hours to flush out the bladder.

• **Urinate "when nature calls" and empty your bladder completely.** Holding your urine for long periods of time may encourage infection. If you have a cystocele (prolapse of the bladder), you can help empty the bladder by inserting a finger into your vagina and pushing up on the front of the vaginal wall as you urinate.

• **Practice safe sex.** You should urinate just before and right after having intercourse to help wash any wayward bacteria out of the urethra. During intercourse, avoid undue pressure on the front of the vaginal wall, which could irritate the urethra and cause a bout of honeymoon cystitis. If your partner enters you from behind, take care not to sweep bacteria from the rectum up to the urethra. If you are prone to developing honeymoon cystitis, you may want to consider taking a preventive dose of antibiotics after intercourse (for instance, Macrodantin or Septra). If you use a diaphragm, don't leave it in place any longer than necessary. (If you experience chronic urinary-tract infections while using a diaphragm, you should consider switching to another form of birth control. See Chapter 9.)

• **After urination or a bowel movement *always* wipe from front to back.** Regularly washing the area with a bidet or "peri" bottle (a small plastic squirt bottle filled with water that's usually recommended for cleaning the perineum in the weeks after childbirth) may further reduce the risk of infection.

• **Change tampons and menstrual pads often to discourage the growth of bacteria.**

• **Ask your physician to test the pH (acid-base balance) of your vagina.** If your physician finds that your vaginal pH is above 4.5, this usually means that the urethral pH is elevated, as well. In that case, you may want to consider using a local vaginal estrogen cream.

• **Take your symptoms seriously.** If you develop symptoms of a urinary-tract infection, report them to your doctor. *Don't* try to treat the symptoms yourself.

your underclothing, so wear a panty shield while you are taking it.) This drug is usually not needed for more than two or three days. If pain persists beyond a few days after you've begun treatment, call your doctor, who may want to reexamine you.

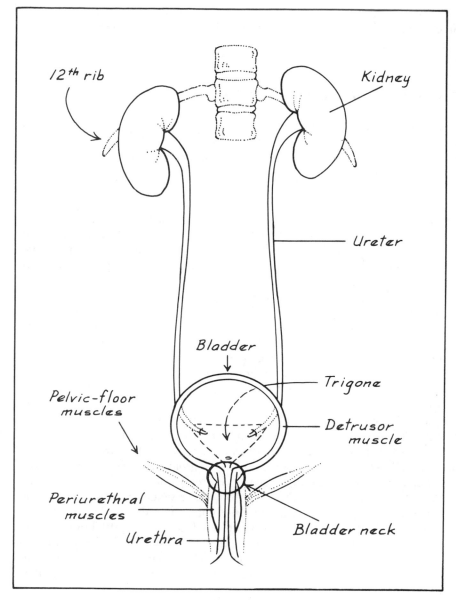

Figure 19.2 Anatomy of the Bladder

Most antibiotics work better in an alkaline environment, which is why your physician may recommend that you drink cranberry juice; the juice helps alkalinize the urine, which may increase the biological effectiveness of the antibiotic. Sodium bicarbonate, found in the antacid Citrocarbonate, may work even better than cranberry juice. While you are being treated, take one to two teaspoonfuls of Citrocarbonate mixed in a glass of cold water three times a day.

You should have a repeat urine culture performed ten days and again three months after completing the antibiotics to ensure that the infection has cleared up. Many recurrent infections are incompletely treated—often because of a failure to take the full course of antibiotics.

The Urethral Syndrome and Trigonitis

This syndrome is very common among postmenopausal women and often misdiagnosed as recurrent urinary-tract infections. The symptoms, frequency of urination, urgency, and lower-abdominal pressure, are similar to those for bladder infections, with one exception: you may experience little or no pain upon urination.

We're still not sure what causes the urethral syndrome; indeed, there may be more than one cause. One hallmark of the condition is an inflammation of the upper urethra and trigone (a triangular area at the base of the bladder; see Figure 19.2). The mucous lining of the urethra becomes thickened, raised, and covered with inflamed cells that have sloughed off. Eventually, small noncancerous polyps and cysts may develop. The urethra appears pale, with red streaks running through it.

One theory holds that the inflammation is caused by a blockage of the periurethral glands in the lower urethra and a subsequent lack of natural lubrication. (You could think of this as being equivalent to an engine running without any oil.) Low estrogen levels may also contribute to the irritation. The lining of the urethra contains estrogen receptors and, as we mentioned earlier, it may become pale and thin after menopause, sometimes causing inflammation. (Note: Even women taking oral postmenopausal estrogens can develop these symptoms.)

Some women have a buildup of connective tissue that causes scarring around the urethra, which may narrow the urethra and cause symptoms. Spasms in the muscles that help control the flow of urine from the urethra (*urethral spasms*) may be responsible for symptoms in some women, as well.

Sometimes, an infection caused by bacteria not picked up by a normal urine culture mimics the urethral syndrome. The sexually transmitted disease *chlamydia* is one such culprit. Because this bacteria "hides out" inside the cells it infects (see page 278) it may go undetected unless special laboratory tests are performed to diagnose chlamydia. Other organisms, such as mycoplasma, trichomonas, monilia (yeast), and human papilloma virus (a sexually transmitted disease that causes genital warts) have also been found to mimic the urethral syndrome.

Frequent intercourse may cause inflammation of the urethra without infection, a condition known as *honeymoon cystitis*. This is believed to be caused by mechanical trauma (the penis rubbing over the urethra).

Bubble baths, excessive vaginal douches, perineal sprays, and even tampon use have also been associated with the urethral syndrome. Spinal injuries or nerve damage have been implicated, as well.

Making a Diagnosis

Your physician will first perform a urinalysis and a urine culture to check for signs of a urinary-tract infection. Your doctor may perform urethral cultures to rule out gonorrhea and chlamydia. A cotton swab is inserted in the urethra and a sample of cells sent to a laboratory to be grown in a culture dish.

Your doctor will also perform a physical exam to screen for any physical abnormalities that may be causing symptoms, such as prolapse of the bladder (*cystocele*), rectum (*rectocele*), uterus, or intestines (*enterocele*). The physical examination will include a neurological exam to rule out any nerve damage involving the lower urinary tract. This may involve tapping your knee and ankle with a reflex hammer to check your reflexes, gently scraping the bottom of your foot to see whether your toes curl (a normal reflex), and testing the perineum (the area between the clitoris and rectum) for certain reflexes.

Your physician will perform a pressure test by inserting a finger into your vagina and pressing forward on the vaginal wall (where the urethra is located) to see whether your symptoms can be reduplicated. (You can perform this test yourself at home, as well.)

Your doctor may recommend that you undergo a *uroflowmetry* to determine the average amount of urinary flow and the time it takes to urinate. This test is usually performed by sitting on a specially designed chair and urinating into a bowl attached to a pressure-sensing device. Your physician could even ask you to urinate into a container that measures the amount of urine voided while having you use a stopwatch to track the amount of time it takes to empty your bladder.

Your physician will then perform a *urethroscopy* to look inside the urethra. The test is performed while you are lying on an examining table with your feet in the stirrups. Using a small insulin syringe (without the needle), your doctor will first insert a local anesthetic jelly into the urethra. The urethroscope, a thin, lighted tube, will then be carefully inserted into the urethra to check for visible signs of inflammation, polyps, or other abnormalities of the urethral lining and trigone. The test takes from five to ten minutes. The amount of discomfort you experience depends on the amount of inflammation present.

Treating Urethral Syndrome

Just as there are many possible causes of urethral syndrome, there are numerous ways to treat it. Your doctor will treat the most probable cause(s), depending on the results of your diagnostic work-up.

• **Antibiotics:** If your doctor suspects or finds evidence of an infection such as *chlamydia,* he or she may first prescribe antibiotics (Tetracycline, Doxycycline, or Erythromycin) for two weeks.

• **Vaginal estrogen creams:** If your symptoms persist even after taking antibiotics, or if a urethroscopic examination shows you have urethral syndrome stemming from low estrogen levels, a vaginal estrogen cream may be prescribed. (Vaginal estrogen creams placed in the vagina are well absorbed by the urethral tissues.) Generally speaking, you insert one-half applicatorful of cream into your vagina every other night for the first two weeks, followed by the same dosage twice a week for three to six months. You can also massage a small amount of cream into the vagina with your finger every night.

• **Urethral dilations:** In addition, urethral dilations may be recommended. This procedure, which can be performed in your doctor's office, is believed to work in several different ways: The dilators massage and open up inflamed or infected urethral glands, helping to increase lubrication. Dilations also massage the mucous membranes of the urethra, stretch the underlying tissues, and relieve stenosis (narrowing of the urethra), helping to improve the flow of urine.

The procedure itself takes less than ten minutes. During the procedure, you lie on an examining table with your feet in the stirrups. Our method involves inserting a small amount of estrogen cream into the urethra to act as a lubricant and also to get better local absorption of estrogen. The physician will then slowly insert and remove a series of metal dilators into the urethra, starting with the smallest in diameter and progressing to increasingly larger diameters until either the largest in diameter is inserted or you experience discomfort. After the procedure, more estrogen cream and possibly cortisone is inserted into the urethra. The procedure is performed once a week for three consecutive weeks. To help prevent a secondary infection, your doctor may recommend that you take an antibiotic (for instance, Macrodantin) every day for a month while you undergo urethral dilations.

Dilations often produce a dramatic cure for women who for years have suffered from "chronic" cystitis. Symptoms are often relieved in a matter of weeks. Theresa Strickland, a sixty-five-year-old patient at our clinic, had a history of urinary frequency, going to the bathroom every one to two hours and two to three times at night. After being diagnosed with trigonitis and urethral syndrome, she was treated with three courses of urethral dilations, together with a vaginal estrogen cream. Because her pelvic-floor muscles were weak, she began a daily routine of pelvic-floor exercises (see page 427). As a result of her treatment, Theresa now has perfectly normal bladder function and sleeps through the night.

If symptoms recur after your treatment is over, your physician may recommend that you use vaginal estrogen creams for up to one year. You may need repeat dilations, as well.

The Painful Bladder

Some women experience abdominal pain as the bladder fills, a need to urinate frequently, and relief of pain after urinating, with no signs of infection—a condition known as painful bladder syndrome or *interstitial cystitis*. The condition is associated with inflammation of the bladder wall and the development of ulcers in the lining of the bladder, which leads to decreased bladder capacity and hypersensitivity of the bladder.

No one knows yet what causes interstitial cystitis. Infection, chronic use of antibiotics, and autoimmune diseases affecting the body's connective tissue have all been implicated. Today, researchers are focusing on a possible defect in the protective outer layer of the bladder lining, which may allow some substances in urine to penetrate and inflame the bladder wall.

To make a diagnosis, your doctor will first perform a urinalysis, urine culture, a physical examination, and additional diagnostic and urologic tests to rule out other medical conditions that could cause these symptoms. A definitive diagnosis can be made only with a procedure called *cystoscopy*, in which a device called a *cystoscope* is inserted into the urethra to look at the inside of the bladder. The procedure, which involves filling the bladder with fluid to reveal the disease's characteristic strawberrylike red dots (ulcers) in the bladder lining, is usually done in the doctor's office using a local anesthetic jelly or, occasionally, in the hospital under general anesthesia. Your doctor may also perform a bladder biopsy at the same time to rule out cancer of the bladder.

There's no cure for interstitial cystitis, and treatment is geared toward alleviating or at least reducing symptoms. A variety of drug treatments have been used, including antihistamines, anticoagulants (heparin), antispasmotics, and antidepressants. These drugs are believed to improve symptoms by reducing inflammation of the bladder. Immunosuppressive drugs have also been used. However, most of these drug therapies have met with limited success.

By far the most successful treatment is a procedure in which the bladder is filled with a drug called *dimethyl sulfoxide* (DMSO). This drug has antiinflammatory effects, breaks down the connective tissue collagen, and blocks pain sensations in the nerve endings within the bladder wall. The treatment is usually done in the doctor's office. A catheter is inserted into the urethra and the bladder is filled with DMSO. After a few minutes, the solution is either drained from the bladder through the catheter or emptied by voiding into the toilet.

About 70 percent of women who are treated with DMSO experience satisfactory relief of their symptoms. The therapeutic effects of the treatment last an average of six weeks, and some women may experience relief from their symptoms for up to ten months after a single treatment. However, a minority of women may need to undergo DMSO treatments as often as once a month to control their symptoms.

Urinary Incontinence

Urinary incontinence, involuntary leakage of urine, is a very common problem, but many women are too embarrassed to talk about it. Too often, shame, guilt, anxiety, fear, embarrassment, loss of self-esteem, and depression associated with incontinence only add to the problem.

Adult diapers and pads *are only a temporary solution*. To get help for your problem, it is essential that you know how your bladder works and that you are properly evaluated by your doctor or a specialist in urinary incontinence.

How Your Bladder Works

Your bladder, located in the lower abdomen just below and in front of the uterus, is normally under voluntary control; the bladder fills with and holds urine until you decide it is time to void. This sounds simple enough, but bladder control is actually a complex interaction of numerous anatomical, neurological, and even psychological factors.

• **The bladder and urethra:** A number of muscles within and adjacent to the bladder and urethra play a role in bladder control. These include:
  The detrusor muscle: This is actually not one muscle but a network of

muscles that lie within the bladder wall and that contract and relax to allow for storage and elimination of urine. When the detrusor muscle contracts, the bladder neck opens, expelling urine from the bladder into the upper part of the urethra. Relaxation of the detrusor muscle allows the bladder to fill again.

The periurethral and urethral muscles: The urethra is made up of both circular bands of muscles and muscles that run lengthwise from the lower portion of the urethra to the lower edge of the detrusor muscle. As we mentioned earlier, a thick band of muscles around the middle of the urethra creates a "pressure zone" that helps keep urine in the bladder. Continence is maintained as long as the pressure in the urethra exceeds that of the bladder.

When the detrusor muscle contracts, the urethral and periurethral muscles relax, lowering pressure in the urethra and allowing urine to flow out of the body.

The pelvic-floor and perineal muscles: This sling of muscles, extending from the inside of the pubic bone to the anus and woven around the vagina, urethra, and rectum (see Figure 19.3), indirectly helps control the contractions

Figure 19.3   The Pelvic Floor Muscles

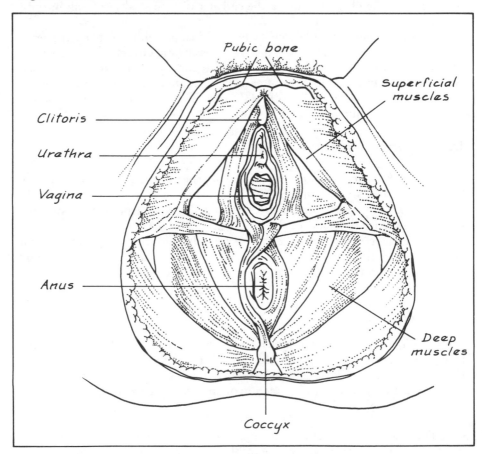

of the detrusor muscle and the urethral pressure, too. When you go to the bathroom, take note of how you relax the pelvic-floor muscles to urinate and tighten them to stop the urine stream.

• **The brain and central nervous system:** Several different areas of the brain are involved in bladder control. One part of the brain senses when the bladder is full. Another brain center can inhibit the activity of the detrusor muscle. It does so via special nerve fibers that stimulate *beta-adrenergic receptors* in the detrusor muscle, causing it to relax. Another part of the brain governs the contraction of the urethra. The brain communicates with the urethra through the same special type of nerve fibers, which stimulate *alpha-adrenergic receptors* in the bladder neck and urethra, causing them to contract and retain urine until voiding is appropriate. Activation or suppression of these receptors serves as the basis for the use of certain drugs, which can help control over- or underactivity of the bladder.

The brain stem (at the base of the brain) acts like a switchboard operator to coordinate the nerve impulses between various control centers of the brain and the bladder and urethra. Nerves leading from the spinal cord to the bladder and urethral sphincter help coordinate the contraction of the detrusor and the relaxation of the urethral muscles, which causes you to release urine.

As your bladder fills with urine, pressure gradually builds up. At a certain point, these sensations are relayed to the spinal cord and the brain, and you become aware of the need to empty your bladder. The spinal cord may signal the urethra to relax as the bladder contracts, but this reflex may be overridden by the brain, which signals the urethra to remain closed until you can get to a bathroom.

As pressure builds, you deliberately tighten the pelvic-floor muscles to help suppress contraction of the bladder's detrusor muscle. If you wait too long, pain may set in and you may even have to squeeze your legs together or hold your hands against your labia to keep urine from escaping.

Once you are in an acceptable place, you must deliberately decide to release the urine, which is a process in itself. Your brain signals the pelvic-floor muscles to relax. As a result, the bladder detrusor muscle contracts and rises, causing the urethral muscles to relax. The upper urethra funnels as it opens and, together with a decrease in urethral pressure, leads to the release of urine. How quickly this happens depends on how distracted you are, how anxious you feel, and how long you have been postponing release. Sexual arousal may sometimes stimulate or delay the release of urine.

When pressure on the bladder is relieved and no more urine comes out, the brain signals the pelvic-floor muscles to contract (even if there may be residual urine in the bladder). Contraction of the pelvic-floor muscles closes the lower urethra, squeezing any remaining urine back up into the bladder. As a result, the detrusor muscle relaxes and the bladder returns to its original position, ready to fill with urine again.

Bladder control requires a balanced contribution from all components of the system; a breakdown of even one part of the system can lead to incontinence or, more rarely, urine retention.

417

Types of Incontinence

Incontinence is classified as either *transient* or *established*. Transient incontinence is usually caused by an underlying condition that manifests itself as a problem with bladder function. Once the underlying cause has been removed, continence is restored. Bacterial infections of the urinary tract, the urethral syndrome, or an acute bladder inflammation from bladder stones can all cause temporary or transient incontinence. A number of medications may also trigger transient incontinence by increasing urine production, decreasing your ability to get to the bathroom on time, or interfering with the normal process of urination. These include diuretics, calcium channel blockers, sedatives, hypnotics, muscle relaxants, anticholinergics (drugs that suppress parts of the autonomic, or involuntary, nervous system) and other drugs that affect the autonomic nervous system.

Acute illnesses that confine you to bed, or environmental barriers to the bathroom (such as a narrow door if you use a wheelchair or walker), may also lead to incontinence by making it difficult for you to get to the bathroom in time—if at all. Even such common metabolic problems as *hyperglycemia* (high blood sugar), *hypercalcemia* (high blood-calcium levels), or *hypokalemia* (abnormally low blood-potassium levels) can cause transient incontinence by increasing urine flow.

Once the reversible causes of incontinence are ruled out, all other kinds of incontinence are classified as established incontinence. Established incontinence usually is caused by a physiological problem with the bladder, the urethra, or the brain centers or nerves that help govern bladder control. There are several different types:

•   **Urge incontinence:** With this type of incontinence, you may be overwhelmed by a sudden urge to urinate, followed by a significant leakage of urine a few seconds to a few minutes later. Frequency of urination and nighttime urination are other common symptoms of urge incontinence. Leakage can occur while you are lying down, sitting, or standing, but many patients with urge incontinence experience leakage only when standing.

The most common cause of urge incontinence is *trigonitis*, an inflammation of the triangular area of muscles at the base of the bladder (see Figure 19.2). Urge incontinence may also be caused by overactivity or instability of the detrusor muscle. Most times, the cause of detrusor instability cannot be determined. Spontaneous bladder contractions may occur as a result of damage to the central nervous system caused by a stroke, Alzheimer's disease, a brain tumor, or Parkinson's disease, or interference with the nerves leading from the spinal cord to the bladder (caused by multiple sclerosis, for example, which is common among women). Bladder infection, radiation therapy, bladder stones, and certain cancers may irritate the bladder, leading to increased contractions.

A common feature of urge incontinence is weakness of the bladder-neck support and premature or inappropriate opening of the upper urethra, a phenomenon called *funneling*. This stimulates bladder contractions and involuntary loss of urine.

418

- **Overflow incontinence:** This type of incontinence is characterized by frequent leakage of small amounts of urine or the inability to empty your bladder completely.

Overflow incontinence may be caused by either an obstruction of the urethra, an underactive detrusor muscle, or both. Obstruction may occur as a result of a cystocele, impacted feces, urethral stricture (narrowing), or a pelvic tumor. Chronic obstruction may, in turn, weaken the contractions of the detrusor muscle.

Less frequently, a lax detrusor muscle may be caused by such neurological problems as a herniated disk, nerve damage caused by diabetes, a vitamin B_{12} deficiency, alcohol abuse, or traumatic or surgical damage to the pelvic nerves. Anticholinergic medications (muscle-relaxant drugs) may also be culprits.

- **Genuine stress incontinence:** Stress incontinence is involuntary leakage of urine that occurs only during the stress of a sudden increase in abdominal pressure, such as when you cough, sneeze, lift things, or climb stairs. You may notice a loss of small to moderate amounts of urine—particularly when you cough, laugh, or sneeze—during the day and little or no leakage at night.

Stress incontinence is caused by reduced urethral pressure and is usually associated with weakened or damaged supporting ligaments around the bladder neck. Normally, these ligaments help supply an equal amount of pressure on all sides of the urethra. However, if the ligaments weaken, the urethra may shift from its normal position. As a result, there may be a loss of pressure on one side of the urethra, leading to urine leakage. Weak pelvic-floor muscles also contribute to the problem. Contributing factors include:

Genetics: Some women may be born with a genetic predisposition to stress incontinence. Heredity determines the type of muscle you have (the percentage of slow- and fast-twitch muscle fibers you have may affect your muscle strength and endurance; this probably applies to the pelvic-floor muscles, as well). Your genes also help determine your pelvic anatomy; some women have a deep rectovaginal pouch, which may be associated with displacement of the urethra.

Childbirth: Experiencing a long labor (particularly the second stage of labor when the baby is pushed out), a traumatic forceps delivery, or giving birth to large babies may weaken the urethra or stretch its supporting ligaments, causing the urethra to shift from its normal position and increasing the risk of developing stress incontinence. On the other hand, a very quick, easy delivery may suggest weak muscle support of the pelvic organs, including the urethra.

Menopause: The drop in estrogen levels associated with menopause may decrease the strength and tone of the muscles needed to maintain urethral pressure. Low estrogen levels may also decrease collagen in connective tissues and ligaments that help support the urethra and reduce blood flow, which may be responsible for up to one-third of urethral pressure.

Obesity: Excess weight may increase abdominal pressure, predisposing you to stress incontinence.

Cigarette smoking: Cigarette smokers are more likely to suffer from all types of incontinence—and genuine stress incontinence in particular—than nonsmokers. Moreover, women who smoke develop stress incontinence at a younger age than nonsmokers, possibly because they cough more often and more violently than nonsmokers.

• **Mixed incontinence:** Often women have not one type of incontinence but a combination. For instance, some 25 percent of women with symptoms of stress incontinence also have some detrusor-muscle instability. This is why a thorough medical evaluation and individualized treatment is a must.

• **True (continuous) incontinence:** Women who suffer from true incontinence are wet all the time. The cause is usually a *fistula,* a permanent opening between the bladder or ureter and the vagina. The fistula is typically caused by some kind of trauma to the tissues—for instance, prolonged labor associated with childbirth, surgery, or pelvic radiotherapy. This type of incontinence is rare, however.

What Type of Incontinence Do I Have?

Answering these basic questions can be the first step toward getting help.

1. **When you cough, sneeze, or laugh,** do you experience instant leakage of a few drops of urine (a sign of stress incontinence) or a delayed flow (suggestive of detrusor instability)?

2. **Do you experience a sudden urge to urinate** followed a few seconds later by leakage? This may be a sign of urge incontinence.

3. **Do you frequently get out of bed** in the middle of the night to go to the bathroom (a sign of urge incontinence)?

4. **Do you frequently leak urine** with and without coughing (a sign of detrusor instability)?

5. **When you void into the toilet, is the urine stream slow?** This may be a sign of a urethral obstruction or a cystocele. If you experience a small dribble of urine after you've stopped voiding, you may have a cystocele or diverticulum (small pouch) of the urethra, which may cause urine to pool and leak out after you have stopped urinating.

How Can I Test Myself for Incontinence?

There are a few simple self-tests you can perform in the privacy of your home that may help you better describe your symptoms to your physician and, in this way, aid in a diagnosis. Each of the tests described here should be performed when your bladder is full, so before each test, drink plenty of fluids (two to three eight-ounce glasses of water) to fill your bladder.

420

1. Using a postal or food scale that measures grams, weigh a dry menstrual pad and put it on. For the next hour, walk around, rock on your heels, cough ten times, wash your hands. Now weigh the pad again. (If the pad becomes completely saturated before the hour is over, remove the wet pad and replace it with a clean one. At the end of the testing time, weigh the two pads together.) This test helps determine how much urine you are leaking.

If the pad weight increases by	Urine loss is
less than 1 gram	essentially dry
2 to 10 grams	slight to moderate
10 to 50 grams	severe
more than 50 grams	very severe

Any increase in pad weight of more than one gram should be investigated further by your physician.*

2. With a full bladder, stand with your legs apart on a bathroom mat or in the bathtub. Cough and note the loss of urine that occurs when you cough. If you are leaking drops of urine, this is probably pure stress incontinence. If leakage is delayed and followed by a flow of urine, this is detrusor instability or mixed incontinence.

3. While voiding into the toilet, note the strength of the urine stream and whether you can stop it. If the urine stream is slow, you may have an obstruction of the urethra or a cystocele that is blocking the flow of urine. If you have difficulty stopping the stream of urine, this may be an indication that your pelvic-floor muscles are weak or that you have a problem with the bladder's detrusor muscle.

4. After emptying your bladder, place your finger into your vagina and bear down with the muscles you would normally use to have a bowel movement. If the front of the vaginal wall comes down as you strain, this could be a sign that you have a cystocele. If pressing on the front wall of the vagina reproduces symptoms of urgency, frequency, abdominal pain, or leakage, you may have trigonitis in addition to incontinence.

Your doctor may also ask you to keep an incontinence chart for a period of twenty-four to forty-eight hours (see page 426). In it, you will log the time of day you urinate and the estimated or measured amount of urine voided. You should also record the amount of fluids you drink during this time (particularly caffeine-containing beverages and alcohol) and any sensation you experience (such as a strong urge) preceding or during urination or the leakage of urine. This chart can help differentiate between urge and stress incontinence.

*Note: Table adapted with permission from D. R. Ostergard, ed., *Gynecologic Urology and Urodynamics: Theory and Practice*, 2nd ed. (Baltimore: Williams & Wilkins, 1985), 245–246.

Making a Diagnosis

• **Medical history:** Your physician will begin by taking a thorough medical history. Be prepared to discuss current and past medical illnesses, any medications you may be taking (*make a list*), and past experiences with infections, abdominal or vaginal surgery, radiation treatments, childbirth, and kidney stones. You should also be able to describe when your problem started, as well as the frequency, pattern, and amount of leakage you are experiencing (see How Can I Test Myself for Incontinence? on page 420). Be sure to discuss *all* your symptoms with your doctor, including pain upon urination, excessive urination at night, blood in the urine, hesitancy, straining, vaginal discharge, constipation, or fecal incontinence.

• **Laboratory tests:** You will undergo various blood and urine tests as part of the work-up, including urinalysis and urine culture to rule out possible bacterial infections, kidney-function tests, and sometimes a glucose-tolerance test.

• **Physical examination:** The next step is a physical examination. This will consist of a few quick checks for any damage to the central nervous system (see page 412). Your doctor will perform a pelvic and rectal exam to check for pelvic masses or prolapse of the bladder, urethra, or rectum. He or she will check your vaginal pH (see page 40) for signs of atrophic vaginitis. Then the doctor will insert a finger into your vagina and press on the upper wall of the vagina (where the urethra is located) to see whether your symptoms can be duplicated.

A test with a cotton swab (Q-Tip) may also be performed to screen for genuine stress incontinence. During this test, you will lie on the examining table with your feet in the stirrups as your physician inserts an anesthetic-saturated cotton swab into the urethra. You will then be asked to strain the muscles you use to have a bowel movement. A major upward change in the angle of the cotton swab as you bear down may be a sign of stress incontinence.

To get a general idea of the strength of your pelvic-floor muscles, your doctor may also insert a finger into your vagina and rectum and ask you to "pinch" or squeeze the muscle.

• **Urodynamic tests:** Your doctor may be able to make a presumptive diagnosis based on a careful history, laboratory tests, and a physical examination alone. However, if surgical correction of the problem is a possibility or if other therapies don't work, you should undergo a complete urodynamic examination. This may include one or more of the following tests:

Urethroscopy/cystoscopy: One of the first tests you may undergo is a urethroscopy/cystocopy, in which a thin, lighted tube (a urethroscope) is gently inserted into the urethra, allowing your physician to view the inside of the urethra and the bladder. The urethroscope continually pumps a small amount of carbon dioxide into the urethra during the examination to give your doctor a better view of these organs. Your doctor will look for any physical abnormalities in the urethra and bladder that may cause loss of bladder control, including estrogen-related changes in the urethra (see "The Urethral Syndrome and Trigonitis" on page 410).

During the exam, you will be asked to bear down or cough when your bladder is nearly full and also to contract your pelvic-floor muscles. This allows your doctor to check the tone of the urethra and whether the bladder neck is working as it should.

Uroflowmetry: Essentially, this test measures the amount of urine expelled through the urethra and the amount of time it takes to empty your bladder. Uroflowmetry is used to diagnose a urethral obstruction and/or narrowing of the urethra, as well as an underactive bladder. It can also be used to monitor the progress of treatment.

For this test, you will be asked to sit on a specially designed chair when your bladder is full and urinate into a bowl attached to a pressure-sensing device.

If your bladder capacity is reduced or if your bladder is not full enough (less than 200 milliliters), an accurate test cannot be performed. In this case, uroflowmetry is repeated after filling your bladder with water.

After the uroflowmetry test, your doctor will want to determine the amount of residual urine remaining in your bladder. This involves inserting a catheter into your urethra and measuring the amount of urine that comes out.

Cystometry: This test, conducted while you are standing, measures the amount of pressure in the bladder and can help determine whether you have a problem with the detrusor muscle and urge incontinence. During the test, a thin catheter containing a pressure-sensing device will be inserted into the urethra and will be used to fill the bladder with either gas or water. After your bladder is full, you will be asked to cough and/or rock on your heels.

Normally, pressure remains fairly constant as the bladder fills, rising only slightly as the bladder reaches capacity, and rising briefly, then returning to baseline when you cough or rock on your heels. A constant rise in pressure as the bladder fills or an increase in bladder pressure a few moments after you cough or sneeze indicates a problem with the detrusor muscle.

Uroprofilometry (urethra-pressure profile): This test measures the amount of pressure in the urethra and bladder and may be used to help diagnose stress incontinence. The test involves inserting a pressure-sensing catheter into the urethra and filling the bladder with water while you are lying down. Normally, pressure in the urethra should exceed pressure in the bladder. If this is not the case, then you have stress incontinence.

Pelvic-floor muscle strength: As we mentioned earlier, your pelvic-floor muscles play a key role in bladder control. This is why it is important to know how strong your pelvic-floor muscles are. Objective methods used to measure the strength of the pelvic-floor muscles are now available, but most are cumbersome and expensive. Researchers at the University of Florida are developing a more cost-effective measuring technique, which may be more widely available in the next several years. The test involves using a water-filled balloon attached to a pressure-sensing device that records on graph paper the amount of pressure applied to the balloon. As you lie on an examining table with your feet in the stirrups, the balloon is inserted into your vagina, where it records the pressure of the vagina at rest. You are then instructed to tighten the pelvic-floor muscles as hard as you can ten times for twelve seconds each time. This kind of testing will also allow you and your physician to monitor your progress as you strengthen these muscles with pelvic-floor exercises (see page 427).

423

Treating Urinary Incontinence

Treatment of urinary incontinence depends on the type of incontinence you have. Because of the side effects associated with drug therapies and the possible risks associated with surgery, you may want to try some of the nondrug approaches to managing your incontinence first.

Urge Incontinence

Bladder training: Such training is thought to help inhibit involuntary bladder contractions that cause urge incontinence. Bladder training involves gradually increasing the interval between voiding by a half an hour at a time until you can eventually go at least three hours between urinations. (For details, see A Guide to Bladder Training on the opposite page.) This type of behavioral therapy has been shown to improve urge incontinence anywhere from 40 to 100 percent.

Pelvic-floor exercises: These exercises can help suppress the urge to urinate by inhibiting contractions of the bladder's detrusor muscle. The exercises (for instructions, see Pelvic-Floor Exercises on page 427) should be performed whenever you feel a strong urge to empty your bladder. When the urge strikes, sit down, take a few deep breaths, and quickly contract the pelvic-floor muscles several times. Doing so helps the urge pass so you have more time to get to the bathroom. The exercises also send a signal to the brain that it's not time to void yet.

Biofeedback: This technique, which you can learn with the help of your doctor, can help you to regain control over your bladder by inhibiting contractions of the bladder's detrusor muscle.

Dietary measures: One of the first things you should do is eliminate caffeine from your diet. Caffeine acts as a diuretic, which may overload the bladder with urine, thus triggering incontinence. Caffeine also directly stimulates the bladder itself, causing bladder contractions. (For tips on cutting caffeine out of your diet, as well as a list of caffeine-containing foods, beverages, and drugs, see page 92.)

If nighttime leakage is a problem, you may want to restrict the amount of fluids you drink after 5:00 P.M.

Drug therapies: If nondrug therapies don't work, drugs that help inhibit bladder contractions may be used to treat urge incontinence. The most commonly prescribed medications are anticholinergic drugs, such as ProBanthine and Methantheline, and antispasmodic medications, such as *oxybutynin chloride* (Ditropan), *dicyclomine hydrochloride* (Bentyl), and *flavoxate* (Urispas).

Anticholinergic drugs have numerous side effects, including dry mouth, impaired vision, constipation, tachycardia (rapid heart rate), postural hypotension, and increased eye (intraocular) pressure. For this reason, these drugs should be used with caution if you have heart disease, glaucoma, or osteoporosis.

Other, less frequently prescribed medications include calcium channel blockers (Terodiline and Flunarizine), beta-adrenergic agonists (Bricanyl), and tricyclic antidepressants.

Surgery: Surgery is not often used to treat urge incontinence unless you experience funneling of the bladder neck along with detrusor instability. We developed a simple two-stitch operation, called the *Notelovitz hammock*, to help repair the problem (see pages 428–430).

You should first keep a record of the number of times you urinate within a twenty-four- or forty-eight-hour time period (see the incontinence chart on page 426). To start bladder training, you should schedule a trip to the bathroom every thirty or sixty minutes, depending on how frequently you urinate before the training begins. At the scheduled time, empty your bladder as completely as you can regardless of whether you feel you need to urinate. If you feel an urge to void before the next assigned time, you should suppress the urge for as long as possible by using relaxation exercises (see page 132), pelvic-floor exercises, or by distracting yourself with other activities. If you can't control the urge and feel that you may soon leak urine, you should go ahead and heed nature's call.

Throughout the bladder-training period, you should keep a daily log. If you see a decrease in the number of incontinent episodes and tolerate the initial voiding schedule well, you should progressively try to increase the interval between voiding by thirty minutes each week. Your goal is to reach a three- to four-hour interval between voidings.

Overflow Incontinence

Treatment of overflow incontinence depends on the cause. If urethral strictures are the culprits, urethral dilations (see page 413) may be used to open up the urethra. Dilations should be used along with a vaginal estrogen cream, which improves blood flow to the area, and antibiotics, which help prevent infection during the course of the treatment.

If a cystocele is responsible for overflow incontinence, surgery is required to restore the normal anatomy of the bladder and permit appropriate bladder emptying. The surgery involves tightening the muscle, connective tissues, and ligaments surrounding the bladder.

If overflow incontinence is caused by an underactive detrusor muscle rather than an obstruction, management will be geared toward reducing residual urine in the bladder and preventing infection. The drug *bethanechol chloride* (Urecholine) may be prescribed to stimulate bladder contractions. However, this drug is not consistently successful when taken orally. (An injectable form of the drug is available but must be administered by your doctor.) Because the drug may cause abdominal cramping at night, you should not take it after 6:00 P.M.

Your physician may also recommend that you try self-catheterization after voiding in the morning and again before you go to bed at night to ensure that your bladder has been completely emptied and to measure the amount of residual urine in the bladder. (Your doctor or nurse can teach you how to insert the catheter by yourself.) You may periodically need to wear a catheter for ten to fourteen days to decompress the bladder. This treatment sometimes restores bladder function. If it doesn't help, you may be instructed to press on your abdomen with your hand or fist as you urinate to ensure that your bladder empties completely.

Bladder Training Record

Instructions: Each time you void or find yourself wet, fill in the following information.

Date	Time	Continent (C) or Incontinent (I)	Urge? (Y/N)	Amount 1. Small 2. Moderate 3. Large	Associated Activity

Stress Incontinence

Surgery is usually required to correct stress incontinence, but before you undergo surgery you should first take these steps to ensure a better outcome:

•   If you have trigonitis (an inflammation of the base of the bladder), a chronic cough, a weight problem, or another condition that may aggravate stress incontinence, these should be treated first.

•   Vaginal estrogen creams should be used for a month or two before surgery, as well. Estrogen improves blood flow and urethral-closure pressure. There's some evidence that estrogen creams combined with alpha-adrenergic agonists work even better than estrogen alone at increasing urethral pressure.

•   Pelvic-floor exercises are essential because they may also improve urethral-closure pressure. (For instructions on how to perform pelvic-floor exercises, see Pelvic-Floor Exercises opposite.)

There is solid evidence that weak pelvic-floor muscles (also known as the *circumvaginal muscle*) contribute to stress urinary incontinence and possibly other types of incontinence.

Remember, the pelvic-floor muscle is the main support of the pelvic organs (see Figure 19.3). Like any other muscle in the body, it needs to be regularly conditioned to maintain its strength and tone. In short, you either use it or lose it.

To locate the circumvaginal muscle, sit on the toilet, spread your legs apart, and begin urinating. See if you can stop and start the flow of urine without moving your legs. If you can stop and start the stream, you are using the circumvaginal muscle. If you don't succeed the first time, keep trying until you have identified it.

Pelvic-floor exercises can be performed anytime, anywhere, in a seated or standing position. First contract the circumvaginal muscle and hold it for as long as you can, working your way up to eight to ten seconds. Then relax the muscle and repeat the exercise. Start with a set of fifteen contractions a day, adding ten more contractions per session each week until you can complete thirty-five to forty contractions per day.

A good way to remember to do your pelvic-floor exercises is to exercise in the morning when you wake up, during certain daily activities, or before going to bed at night. In a week or two, you should begin to notice improved control. If you do not notice improvement after several weeks, consult your physician for further evaluation.

Another option for women wishing to increase the strength of their pelvic-floor muscles is to use pelvic muscle training weights. A set of weights contains five vaginal cones that resemble tampons (including a string to remove them), ranging from 20 to 70 grams in weight. During a typical training program, you place the smallest weight in the vagina and wear it for ten to fifteen minutes two times a day. You must use your circumvaginal muscle to hold the weight in the vagina; otherwise, it will fall out. You begin by wearing the weight while you are seated, then graduate to a standing position. When you can hold the weight in place even as you cough or laugh, you are ready to progress to the next-size weight.

The pelvic-floor weights, called Femina Pelvic Muscle Training Weights, are manufactured by the Dacomed Corporation in Minneapolis, Minnesota. A set of five weights costs ninety-nine dollars. If you are interested in ordering a set, ask your physician or call Dacomed's toll-free number: (800)328-1103.

If you have genuine stress incontinence, the goal of surgery is to restore the normal anatomy of the urethra and its supports, either by lengthening the urethra, restoring the angle of the bladder neck, or increasing urethral pressure. (If bladder-neck funneling is a problem, this, too, will be surgically corrected.)

In the past, vaginal surgery was used to correct stress urinary incontinence, but this type of surgery is successful only about 60 percent of the time. If the vaginal approach failed, abdominal surgery, with a more than 80 percent success rate, was the next step.

Today, most surgery to correct stress urinary incontinence is performed abdominally, largely because most of the main supporting ligaments involved are best supported to tissues above the pelvic-floor muscles. However, vaginal surgery may still be appropriate for some women.

Numerous surgical methods are used to correct urinary stress incontinence. These include the following:

• *The Marshall-Marchetti-Kranz (MMK) Method* (also known as bladder lifting, elevating, or suspending, or the bladder tack): During this operation, the surgeon places a series of stitches down the length of the urethra on either side, then attaches the supporting ligaments to the back of the pubic bone.

• *The Burch Method:* The surgeon places a series of stitches on either side of the juncture between the urethra and the bladder neck. Then the supporting ligaments of the urethra and bladder neck are attached to another major ligament on the side wall of the pelvis.

• *The Notelovitz Hammock:* One stitch is placed on either side of the bladder neck, then tied across the middle, creating a "hammock" of supporting tissues around the urethra. The hammock of tissues is then stitched to the back of the pubic bone.

• *The Stamey Procedure:* This operation is performed through the vagina and may be appropriate for women who also need another type of vaginal surgery, such as vaginal hysterectomy or repair of a cystocele, rectocele, or enterocele. The surgeon makes an incision in the vaginal wall, then sutures together some of the surrounding ligaments to create a supportive "sling" around the urethra. The surgeon then makes a small abdominal incision just above the pubic hairline to lift and secure the urethra and its supporting ligaments back to their normal position. After the vaginal and abdominal incisions have been closed, other vaginal procedures may be performed.

• *The Sling Procedure:* This operation is usually reserved for patients in whom the MMK method has failed. Artificial material or muscle tissue from the thigh or abdominal wall is used to create a supportive sling around the urethra. The sling is then suspended from the abdominal wall.

In addition, there are other surgical considerations that you should be aware of. They include:

• If you have a large cystocele, you will need to have it repaired along with the surgery for stress urinary incontinence. (See Chapter 13.)

• If you have a rectocele or enterocele along with stress urinary incontinence, you should consider having these corrected, as well.

• Your doctor may recommend that you undergo a hysterectomy (surgical removal of the uterus) at the same time, even if your uterus is normal. Having a hysterectomy increases the success rate of surgery for stress urinary incontinence by 10 to 15 percent.

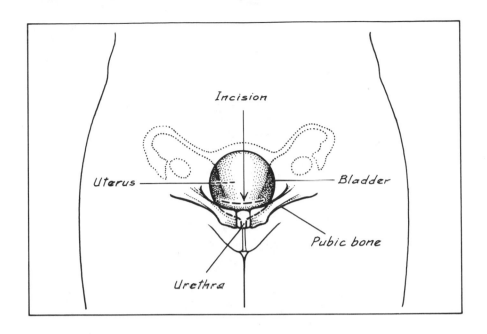

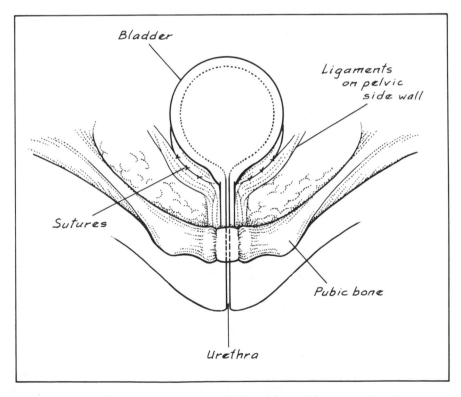

Figure 19.4   Surgery for Stress Urinary Incontinence: The Burch Method

429

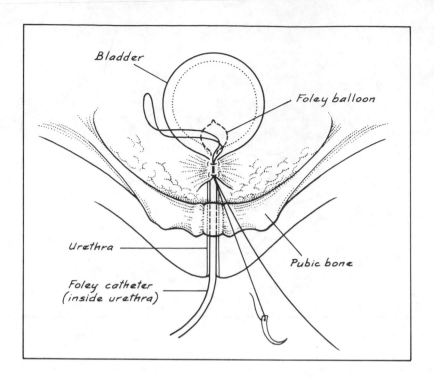

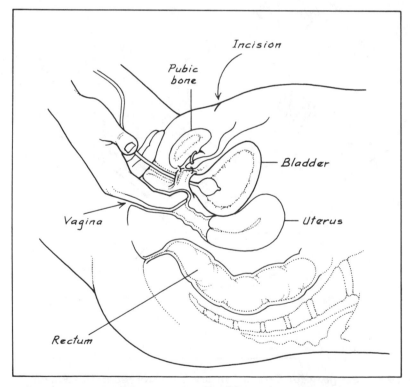

**Figure 19.5   Surgery for Stress Urinary Incontinence:
The Notelovitz Hammock**

430

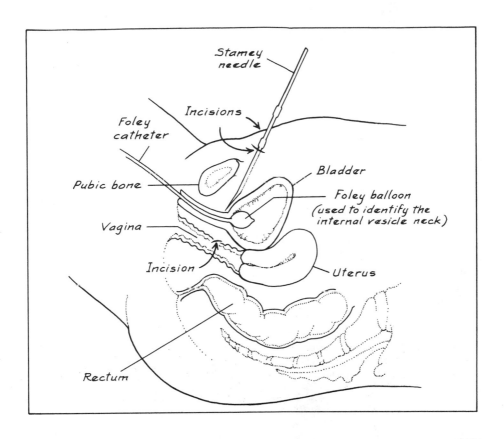

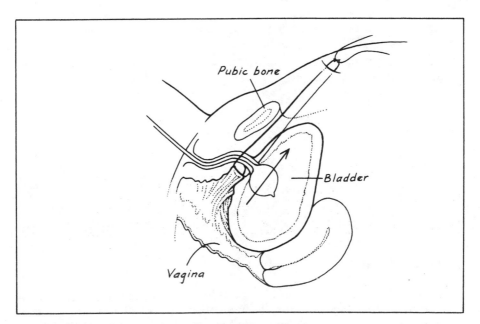

Figure 19.6   Surgery for Urinary Stress Incontinence: The Stamey Procedure

431

• If you are postmenopausal and have previously had a hysterectomy in which you retained your ovaries, it would be prudent to have your ovaries removed while you are undergoing surgery to correct stress urinary incontinence. This decreases your chances of developing hard-to-detect ovarian cancer.

• As we mentioned earlier, if you have a weight problem, you *must* lose weight *before* the operation; otherwise, the treatment has a greater chance of failing.

After the operation, you will need to let the urethra and bladder-neck area rest so that it can heal properly. For this reason, your physician may have a catheter inserted into your bladder through the abdominal wall. The catheter will remain in place until your bladder and urethra begin functioning normally again (an average of four to five days, but occasionally up to two weeks). The catheter will also be able to measure the amount of residual urine in the bladder once you begin voiding on your own. Be aware, too, that you may have to adjust the way you sit on the toilet to accommodate the new position of the urethra (and bladder).

Generally speaking, you will be able to drive two to three weeks after the operation and return to work four to six weeks after surgery. You should refrain from having sex until six weeks after surgery.

....
Preventing Stress Urinary Incontinence
....

Advice for Menopausal Women with No Symptoms
There are some steps you can take to help *prevent* stress urinary incontinence.

• Have your physician test the strength of the pelvic-floor muscles prior to menopause and afterward. If sophisticated testing equipment isn't available for an objective measurement, your physician can simply insert a finger into your vagina and rectum and have you squeeze the muscle.

• If you are not using vaginal estrogen creams, ask your physician to test the pH of your vagina during your annual examination. If the pH is above 4.5, use a vaginal estrogen cream (half an applicatorful once or twice a week) as a preventive measure. Remember, estrogen improves blood flow to the area and may help maintain urethral pressure.

• Don't wait for your pelvic-floor muscle to break down. Exercise your right to remain continent by performing the pelvic-floor exercises on page 427 daily until they increase and maintain the strength of the circumvaginal muscle.

A Final Word

Any kind of chronic bladder problems can have a tremendous impact on your life, both physically and emotionally. Whatever you do, don't wait to get help. You should undergo a complete physical, neurologic, and urologic examination to determine the cause of your problem. (When incontinence surgery fails, it may be because the wrong procedure was used to correct a problem.) Support groups are available for women to share their emotional concerns, as well (see Resources and Support below).

Resources and Support

The Simon Foundation for Continence, Box 835, Wilmette, IL 60091. Phone: (800) 23-SIMON. This nonprofit organization provides educational materials for men and women who suffer from urinary and fecal incontinence. The foundation has a wealth of information on incontinence, including books, videotapes, a quarterly newsletter, and a topic-specific reprint series. The organization also offers the "I WILL MANAGE" educational/support group for incontinence sufferers in local communities nationwide. Write or call for a free information packet.

Help for Incontinent People (HIP), P.O. Box 544, Union, South Carolina 29379. Phone: (803) 579-7900; (800) BLADDER (252 3337). Help for Incontinent People (HIP) is a nonprofit organization dedicated to improving the quality of life for people with incontinence. HIP is a leading source of education, advocacy, and support to health professionals and the general public about the causes, prevention, diagnosis, treatment, and management alternatives for incontinence. The organization publishes a quarterly newsletter (The HIP Report), a *Resource Guide of Continence Products and Services,* audio/visual programs, books, and educational pamphlets. HIP also provides referrals to physicians and support groups in your area. Call or write for additional information.

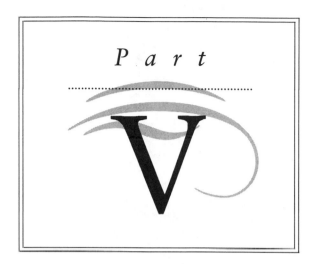

Part

V

*A Practical Primer
on Hormone
Therapy*

Chapter 20

Weighing Hormone Therapy's Benefits and Risks

You may have already heard numerous conflicting reports about the benefits and risks of hormone therapy. Many women who visit our clinic are (not surprisingly) confused and concerned. Is hormone therapy safe? Does it cause heart attacks? What about the risk of cancer? Doesn't hormone therapy cause blood clots?

In fact, hormone therapy is an excellent way to relieve many of the discomforts of menopause, such as hot flashes and vaginal dryness. It's one of the most effective ways of slowing (or stopping) the loss of bone mass after menopause. There's mounting evidence that taking estrogen after menopause *prolongs* the apparent built-in protection women have against heart disease. Indeed, the benefits of hormone therapy are so attractive that some experts believe *all* postmenopausal women should take estrogen.

However, as with any drug, there are risks. Before you (and your doctor) decide whether hormone therapy is right for you, you should carefully weigh the benefits and risks.

Replacing Hormones or Adding Them?

First, let's clear up some confusion about the term most often used to describe postmenopausal hormones: *hormone-replacement therapy*. This term is somewhat misleading because it suggests that hormones that *should* be there are being replaced. Technically, however, hormones are not being replaced; they're being *added*. Remember, after menopause, the principal type of estrogen produced by your body changes. Postmenopausal women produce more *estrone* than *estradiol,* the predominant estrogen in premenopausal women. So if hormones were being *replaced*, you would actually receive more estrone than estradiol. However, most postmenopausal hormone therapy is intended to increase the blood levels of *estradiol,* the more potent of the two hormones.

The hormone progesterone is not normally produced at all in postmeno-pausal women. When progesterone is given to menopausal women (mainly for women with an intact uterus, and primarily to protect the endometrium, which we'll discuss later), synthetic types are prescribed.

While it may seem we're overly concerned with semantics, the issue runs far deeper than words. In a sense, the term hormone-replacement therapy has become symbolic of a mind-set that has led to the medicalization of menopause. *Hormone-replacement therapy* suggests that menopause is an illness that should be treated by replacing missing hormones, in the same way that diabetes is treated by replacing insulin. This has led to the belief—by some experts, at least—that *all* menopausal women should take hormones.

However, it's perfectly *normal* for postmenopausal women to have lower levels of estrogen. Most otherwise-healthy menopausal women don't experience any serious complications relating to the drop in estrogen after menopause. Indeed, the majority of menopausal women do perfectly well without hormone therapy *provided they enter the menopause in optimal health and maintain good health throughout their postmenopausal years.*

For these reasons, we suggest you use the term *hormone-additive therapy* (HAT) or *estrogen-additive therapy* (EAT). Essentially, when you are prescribed postmenopausal hormones, you are being treated with drugs. There's nothing wrong with this so long as the benefits of the drug outweigh the risks.

The question is, Who should be treated, and how? Basically, four groups of women should consider treatment:

• women with symptoms of menopause, such as hot flashes and/or vaginal dryness, or estrogen-related psychological symptoms, such as depression, irritability, confusion, mood swings, insomnia, and early-morning awakenings

• women who experience an early menopause (either a "surgical" or natural menopause before age forty)

• women at risk of developing osteoporosis

• women who need to protect themselves against cardiovascular disease

Of course, if you don't fall into one of these categories but wish to take hormone-additive therapy, there's no reason not to (unless you are a woman for whom hormones are contraindicated). Neither is there hard evidence that by taking hormones, you'll be healthier or better off or will live longer than women who don't take hormones but adopt a healthy lifestyle in their middle and later years. With a thorough clinical evaluation and currently available technology, we can determine whether you're one of the women who would benefit from hormone therapy.

What Hormone Therapy Can Do for You

Menopausal Symptoms

Postmenopausal hormone therapy is one of the most effective ways we have of relieving hot flashes, vaginal dryness, and other bothersome symptoms of menopause.

•   **Hot flashes:** While the exact mechanism isn't known, estrogen is believed to influence the body's temperature-regulating system somehow (see page 242), reducing the number and intensity of hot flashes, and often relieving them altogether.

•   **Vaginal dryness and related symptoms:** Vaginal dryness or a discharge, itching, and a burning sensation are common symptoms related to the drop in estrogen after menopause. Estrogen increases blood flow to the vagina and thickens the vaginal epithelium (mucous lining of the vaginal walls). Estrogen also improves the pH (acid-base balance) of the vagina and relieves vaginal dryness, a common cause of pain during intercourse among postmenopausal women.

•   **Urethra and bladder:** The urinary tract develops from the same tissues as the vagina in the growing embryo, and these "estrogen-sensitive" tissues also undergo changes as a result of declining estrogen levels after menopause. The most common symptoms are urgency, frequency of urination, low abdominal pain, and tenderness without any signs of bacterial infection, a condition known as *urethral syndrome*. Estrogen helps thicken the lining of the urethra and increases blood flow to the area, therefore improving—and often curing—these symptoms. Estrogen also improves smooth muscle tone, which may result in better bladder control.

•   **Psychological changes:** Some mood changes common around the time of menopause, such as irritability, depression, insomnia, impaired memory, early-morning awakenings, and crying jags, respond well to estrogen therapy. This may be partly because estrogen improves sleep, and many of these symptoms are also signs of chronic sleep disturbances. Estrogen appears to have a "mental tonic effect" as well, enhancing the mood of women who aren't suffering from clinical depression or other emotional problems that aren't related to estrogen. (Note: Estrogen therapy *won't* cure depression.)

Are your menopausal symptoms serious enough to warrant taking hormone-additive therapy? Fill out the Menopausal Symptoms Questionnaire on page 239. You should also undergo a thorough pre- or postmenopausal checkup (see Chapter 3) to rule out other possible causes of these symptoms.

Osteoporosis

While a number of factors contribute to the development of osteoporosis, low estrogen levels after a natural menopause (or the removal of your ovaries) accelerate the rate of bone loss. As it turns out, estrogen therapy is one of the most effective means of slowing or even stopping the loss of bone mass after menopause. Estrogen therapy is associated with an average 50 percent reduction in hip fractures and a *90 percent decrease in spinal deformities* (such as loss of height and dowager's hump) among surgically menopausal women who take estrogen for ten years.

Estrogen is believed to help slow bone loss in several ways:

•   Estrogen somehow preserves bone mineral, which in turn is associated with a decrease in fractures among women who take it. The hormone is believed to increase the activity of the bone-building cells, the osteoblasts, and possibly inhibit the activity of the bone-dissolving cells, the osteoclasts.

•   Estrogen increases your body's ability to absorb calcium from the intestines.

•   Estrogen may stimulate the release of the bone-sparing hormone *calcitonin* from the thyroid gland and other tissues.

•   Estrogen stimulates the manufacture of certain "binding proteins" from the liver, which protect against calcium losses from overactivity of the adrenal and thyroid glands.

•   Estrogen increases collagen in other parts of the body (notably the skin), and it is suspected that it does the same for bone. (Collagen in bone forms the bone matrix to which calcium and phosphorous crystals adhere, giving bone its rigidity. See Bone Basics beginning on page 339.)

Estrogen may have an indirect effect, as well: By improving your sense of well-being, it may increase your level of activity. More active women are stronger and more stable, which, in turn, decreases their chances of falling.

Estrogen may work even better when combined with other drugs and/or preventive measures, such as progestogen, fluoride, and exercise (see Chapter 17).

How can you tell whether you should take hormone-additive therapy to prevent osteoporosis? The simplest, most effective way to make a decision is to have your bone density tested (see Chapter 3, page 37, and Chapter 17, page 346, for details).

Cardiovascular Disease

Perhaps one of the biggest myths about postmenopausal hormone therapy is that it will raise your risk of heart disease or stroke. Mounting evidence now suggests that postmenopausal hormones actually *protect against cardiovascular disease*. In population studies, postmenopausal women who take oral estrogen for ten years or longer have *50 percent less coronary heart disease than women who don't*. In effect, hormone therapy appears to extend the natural protection from heart disease that women enjoy in their premenopausal years.

Estrogen users appear to be protected against stroke, as well: Researchers report a 50 percent reduction in death rates due to stroke in estrogen users compared with nonusers.

How can estrogen protect against heart disease? Keep in mind that most of the research linking oral contraceptives and cardiovascular complications was done on the older birth-control pills, which contained much higher doses of estrogen and progestogen than are now given to menopausal women. Also, the estrogen in birth-control pills is a synthetic form of the hormone, which has an entirely different chemical makeup from the conjugated and other "natural" estrogens typically prescribed for women during the menopausal years. Birth-control pills contain higher levels and a different kind of progestogen, as well.

Hormone-additive therapy is thought to protect in several different ways.

- Estrogen lowers damaging LDL cholesterol by an average of 8 percent and raises protective HDL cholesterol by an average of 15 percent compared with untreated women.

- Estrogen doesn't cause your blood pressure to rise; in fact, the hormone may *lower* blood pressure.

- Estrogen doesn't appear to raise your risk of developing a blood clot. While oral estrogen does raise the levels of several coagulation proteins, these are not biologically active until they're exposed to an injured blood vessel. Plus, "normal" levels for these coagulation proteins vary widely, and it's impossible to use them to predict whether you're at a greater risk of developing a blood clot. On the other hand, natural estrogen *doesn't* significantly decrease antithrombin III, a potent anticoagulant that is a good marker for predicting whether a blood clot will develop.

In fact, *there is no study showing a cause-and-effect relationship between taking estrogen-additive therapy and the development of blood clots.* Estrogen's poor reputation comes from studies on the use of older, high-dose oral contraceptives among older women who smoked. *Smoking is the demon.*

- Long-term use of estrogen does not affect your body's ability to use blood sugars (carbohydrate metabolism). Indeed, estrogen *decreases* fasting blood-sugar levels, possibly because it prevents the breakdown of insulin. What's more, estrogen does not increase blood-insulin levels. Even diabetic women can safely use estrogen.

- Estrogen improves blood flow and appears somehow to protect the innermost lining of the blood-vessel wall from the development of artery-narrowing plaques.

- Estrogen may also protect women against the apparent artery-clogging effects of a type of LDL cholesterol called "small-molecule LDL cholesterol." Moreover, the hormone protects against spasm of the coronary arteries, which can trigger a heart attack.

When considering whether to take hormone-additive therapy to help protect against cardiovascular disease, you and your physician should consider:

1. Whether you have a family history of premature heart disease (that is, if your father or a brother has suffered *angina* (chest pain), a heart attack, or sudden death before age fifty-five or your mother or a sister has developed heart disease before age sixty).

2. Whether your parents, brothers, or sisters have had elevated blood-cholesterol levels.

3. Whether a parent or sibling has had high blood pressure or diabetes.

4. Whether your own blood pressure and blood cholesterol levels are elevated (total cholesterol above 240 mg/dl, LDL cholesterol above 140 mg/dl, triglycerides above 250 mg/dl, or HDL cholesterol below 35 mg/dl).

5. Whether you've experienced an early menopause (before age forty).

What About Progestogen?

Progestogens are prescribed to prevent overstimulation of the uterine lining by estrogen. Hence they help protect against the development of endometrial cancer among women who still have an intact uterus. (Women who have had a hysterectomy don't need to take progestogen, even if their ovaries remain intact. See Who Needs Progestogen? below.) The practice not only prevents endometrial cancer but also has a protective effect. *Indeed, women who take a progestogen for at least ten days per month have less endometrial cancer than women who take no hormones whatsoever.* (We'll talk more about hormone therapy and endometrial cancer in The Risks of Hormone Therapy on page 443.)

When the practice of prescribing a progestogen along with estrogen became more routine, it raised numerous questions about what impact, if any, progestogen would have on the therapeutic effects of estrogen, particularly estrogen's improvement of menopausal symptoms, maintenance of bone mass, and protection from cardiovascular disease. After all, most of the studies on the beneficial effects of postmenopausal hormones involved estrogen alone. The research on progestogen is continuing, but it appears that in many ways added progestogen offers some benefits of its own.

Menopausal Symptoms

Researchers began to realize that progestogen could help relieve hot flashes when a progestogen called *depomedroxyprogesterone acetate* (Depo-Provera) was used to treat women with endometrial cancer. Hot flashes were suppressed in 90 percent of the women receiving monthly injections of Depo-Provera.

Progestogen may suppress hot flashes in a totally different way from estrogen—that is, it appears to raise your body's temperature-regulating set point so hot flashes become less noticeable. Progestogen may suppress hot flashes in other ways, as well.

As for menopause-related psychological symptoms, it appears that certain types of progestogen may aggravate or induce depression and other PMS-like symptoms. Often, switching to a different type of progestogen helps (see page 459).

Who Needs Progestogen?

If you have an intact uterus	Yes
If you have had a hysterectomy (uterus removed but ovaries intact)	No
If you have had a hysterectomy and oophorectomy (uterus and ovaries removed)	No
If you have had an oophorectomy (one or both ovaries removed, uterus intact)	Yes

---

Osteoporosis

Adding progestogen—either cyclically or continuously—may actually work synergistically with estrogen to protect bone. Progestogen competes with and blocks the action of bone-dissolving cortisone by occupying the receptor for cortisone in bone cells.

Cardiovascular disease

Progestogen *does* appear to dampen the effects of estrogen on blood lipids somewhat. However, when progestogen is given cyclically (see page 459) and with intermediate to high doses of estrogen, you'll still experience an *overall increase in cardioprotective factors,* such as HDL cholesterol. One study of women taking estrogen and a progestogen showed a 6 percent increase in HDL cholesterol—about half that of women receiving estrogen alone, but still a significant rise. Contrary to popular belief, low levels of progestogens have no adverse effect on blood pressure. Again, the idea that progestogen raises blood pressure was based on studies involving the older oral contraceptives, which contained large doses of progestogen.

Progestogen doesn't appear to increase the risk of developing blood clots, either. In fact, it may even prevent blood clots from forming. We found that progestogen *increases* the activity of the anticoagulant plasminogen by 16 to 20 percent. Although we don't yet know what effect these changes have in the body, it's possible that the increased plasminogen may protect against the formation of blood clots. Higher levels of plasminogen may also help protect against a newly discovered blood lipid, known as apolipoprotein (a), which is thought to take the place of plasminogen in the artery wall and short-circuit the blood vessel's natural ability to dissolve clots.

Progestogen *does* increase insulin resistance somewhat, which may be a problem for some women, particularly diabetics. Diabetic women who take combination hormones may need to be more closely monitored.

Animal studies have also suggested that progestogen may reduce blood flow. This may somewhat dampen the increase in blood flow associated with estrogen, particularly through the coronary arteries. However, more research needs to be conducted before we know for certain whether the decreased blood flow associated with progestogen leads to an increased risk of heart disease.

In the near future, new types of progestogen and different ways of administering the hormone may be safer still. Preliminary evidence suggests that a new class of synthetic progestogens, *gestodene, desogestrel,* and *norgestimate,* as well as a form of micronized oral progesterone will have little effect on HDL cholesterol in women taking estrogen. A transdermal skin patch containing both estrogen and progestogen may also reduce the negative effects of progestogen on blood lipids.

Of course, as we mentioned earlier, cardiovascular disease is a result of many different factors, so it's hard to quantify what overall effect progestogen has. Remember, though, that it is needed only if you have an intact uterus, and it is prescribed in the lowest possible dose to protect the uterine lining from overstimulation by estrogen. So far, it appears that progestogen doesn't cancel out the good that estrogen does for your menopausal symptoms, bones, and heart and may even provide some protection of its own.

The Androgen Connection

Your body continues to produce low levels of the "male" hormone testosterone as well as other androgens after menopause. Low levels of androgens after menopause have been associated with such menopause-related symptoms as depression, headaches, decreased sex drive, and even bone loss.

Prescription androgens are occasionally used to help alleviate some of these symptoms. If you continue to have symptoms on estrogen therapy alone, your practitioner may recommend that you take an androgen along with estrogen. Preliminary evidence suggests that androgens may help in the following ways:

• **An increased sense of well-being:** Several studies have found that women who take androgen along with estrogen get more than relief from such menopausal symptoms as hot flashes. In a study by Barbara Sherwin, Ph.D., at McGill University in Montreal, those who took an androgen-estrogen combination reported a heightened sense of well-being and more energy than those who took estrogen alone. Another study investigating the mood-enhancing effects of testosterone found that those who had been receiving estrogen and androgen felt more composed, elated, and energetic than those who were given estrogen alone. Our own study of the effects of aging and menopause on women buoys these findings. In our study, higher levels of free testosterone in postmenopausal women who were not taking hormones were associated with an increased feeling of well-being (see pages 5–6).

• **Improved sex drive:** While estrogen can help relieve painful intercourse as a result of changes in the vagina, several studies now show that testosterone is critical for maintaining desire and interest in sex. Women who take androgen have higher levels of sexual desire, sexual arousal, and fantasy than women who receive estrogen alone or a placebo. Androgen users also make love more often and have more orgasms than nonusers.

• **Fewer headaches:** Women who suffer from hormonal headaches (usually migraine headaches triggered by estrogen therapy; see page 468) often find relief by taking androgen along with estrogen.

• **Relief from depression:** Androgen-estrogen combinations work even better than estrogen alone in alleviating depression associated with the hormonal changes of menopause. (Androgens *do not* boost the mood of women suffering from true clinical depression, however.)

• **Increased bone mass:** Adding androgen to estrogen therapy may help prevent bone loss, possibly by enhancing the effects of estrogen. Women with vertebral crush fractures reportedly have lower testosterone levels than women without fractures. Columbia University's Robert Lindsay, M.D., showed that the more rapid bone loss in the early menopausal years is associated with low blood levels of estrogen *and* the androgen *androstenedione*. Others have found virtually no bone loss—and no new collapsed vertebrae in osteoporosis patients who received estrogen and testosterone for thirty years. In a recent study of ours, women taking estrogen alone maintained bone mass in the lumbar spine, while those who took an estrogen along with testosterone experienced a 3 percent *increase* in bone mass after twelve months, and a 4 percent increase after twenty-four months.

While some researchers worried that giving androgen to women would raise their blood-cholesterol levels, to date, most studies involving estrogen combined with a nonoral androgen have found little or no change in blood lipids. However, oral androgen may reduce protective HDL cholesterol.

On the other hand, oral androgen appears to reduce triglycerides and may help offset the *rise* in blood triglycerides often triggered by oral estrogen. In one recent study we conducted, women taking an estrogen-androgen combination experienced a 20 percent decrease in blood triglycerides. So there may actually be a role for androgen in the prevention of cardiovascular disease.

Androgens aren't without side effects, however. Your skin may become more oily, increasing the possibility of developing acne. Mild hirsutism, or hair growth (including facial hair), occurs in about 15 to 20 percent of patients. Sometimes simply lowering the dosage of androgen helps alleviate these symptoms. Giving the diuretic *spironolactone* (Aldactone, Aldactazine) often helps, too.

Androgens *don't* protect against overstimulation of the uterine lining by estrogen, either. So if your uterus is intact and you are being treated with an estrogen-androgen combination, you will most likely be prescribed a progestogen to guard against endometrial cancer.

The Risks of Hormone Therapy

Cancer: The Greatest Fear

Over the past several years, headlines that estrogen therapy increased the risk of endometrial cancer and possibly breast cancer spread a wave of fear among women taking estrogen—or those who were thinking about taking it. Let's look at the facts to help dispel some of your greatest fears:

•   **Endometrial cancer:** It's true that estrogen alone can increase the risk of endometrial cancer by about 10 to 20 percent among postmenopausal women who still have an intact uterus. (During the recent scare about a link between estrogen and endometrial cancer, many women who had had a hysterectomy and didn't need to worry stopped treatment.) However, the absolute numbers are still relatively low: from one case of endometrial cancer per thousand to twenty cases per thousand. Moreover, the type of cancer involved is rarely life-threatening. It is usually picked up at a much earlier stage than some other types of endometrial cancer, and the cure rate is almost 100 percent.

Since the first reports of an increased risk of endometrial cancer associated with the use of estrogen came out, physicians have begun prescribing progestogens along with estrogen for at least ten days per cycle. This regimen more closely resembles a woman's natural menstrual cycle and prevents overstimulation of the uterine lining by estrogen alone. As a result, the incidence of endometrial cancer among women taking combination hormone therapy *is less than that of women who take no hormones whatsoever.*

• **Breast cancer:** The risk of breast cancer is a concern mainly because of the prevalence of this illness: Remember, one in nine women will develop breast cancer in her lifetime. The fear of breast cancer was fueled by a 1989 Swedish study involving 23,244 women thirty-five years and over. While the study showed that women using a combination of estrogen and progestogen experienced overall about 10 percent more breast cancers than expected, reflecting only a slightly elevated risk of breast cancer, which would be perfectly acceptable given the benefits associated with the use of postmenopausal estrogens. The researchers also reported that, however, among the 850 women in the study who took estrogens for nine years or more, the risk increased to 70 percent above expected levels.

More recently, however, a thorough analysis of the data—a *meta analysis* (a combination of all previous epidemiological studies)—shows that the risk of developing breast cancer is not all that great (see Table 20.1). After fifteen years of estrogen-additive therapy, your risk of developing breast cancer may increase by roughly 30 percent which, in statistical terms, is *not* significant. No studies have shown an increase in deaths from breast cancer among estrogen users, and some have actually shown an increase in the cure rate of breast cancer among women taking postmenopausal hormones. It's not known whether the hormone therapy itself played a role in the higher cure rate or whether the women were screened more diligently, helping to catch their cancers in the early stages, when the cure rate is high.

Among women with a family history of breast cancer, however, those who have never taken estrogen have a twofold greater risk than those who have never taken it, which is why most women whose mothers or sisters have been diagnosed with breast cancer may be advised *not* to take estrogen.

The exact mechanisms by which estrogen may increase the risk of breast cancer are not known. Estrogen doesn't appear to be an initiator of cancer;

TABLE 20.1 *Postmenopausal Estrogen Use and Breast Cancer Risk: Results of Major Studies (circles)*

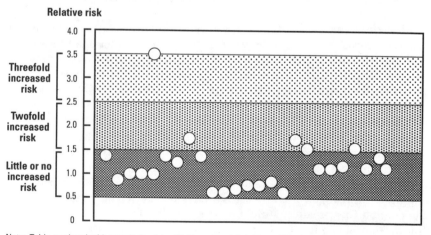

Note: Table reprinted with permission from W. Dupont and D. L. Page. "Menopausal Estrogen Replacement Therapy and Breast Cancer." *Archives of Internal Medicine*, 151 (January 1991), 67–72. Copyright © by 1991 The American Medical Association.

that is, it does not turn a normal cell into a cancerous cell. Rather, estrogen appears to be a *promoter* of cancer by stimulating cells that have already become cancerous to grow more rapidly.

More research needs to be conducted before we fully understand the role of postmenopausal hormone therapy in the development of breast cancer. At this point, the benefits to some women (particularly those at risk of developing heart disease and osteoporosis) clearly outweigh the slightly increased risk of breast cancer. Remember, ten times more women die of cardiovascular disease than of breast cancer. Keep in mind, too, that postmenopausal hormone therapy isn't the only possible breast cancer–related risk factor to consider: A high-fat diet may contribute to up to 30 percent of breast cancers (see Chapter 18), and reducing the fat in your diet certainly would be a prudent policy for lowering your risk of breast cancer. In addition, 80 to 90 percent of breast cancers are cured when caught early, which is why close surveillance of all women on hormone-additive therapy is essential. We advise weekly breast self-examination, possibly two breast examinations annually by a health-care professional, and most definitely yearly mammograms.

The data on the risk of breast cancer are not conclusive enough to change the way we prescribe postmenopausal hormones. But studies do point to the need for additional research. Until we know more, it's safe for women who would benefit most from postmenopausal hormones—those with a family history of heart disease, for example—to take them, provided they're closely monitored. Fibrocystic breast disease is not a reason to forego estrogen therapy, but it may be a reason to use an added progestogen—even if you have had a hysterectomy.

• **Other types of cancer:** If you have had melanoma (the most serious type of skin cancer), you should *not* take estrogen therapy, since melanoma may be fueled by estrogen. However, other types of cancer, including cancer of the colon and cervix and certain types of ovarian cancer, generally are not a contraindication to estrogen therapy. If you have a history of these types of cancer, ask your doctor about taking estrogen.

One published study has noted an increase in lung cancer among men being treated with estrogens for heart disease, which leads to the suspicion that cigarette smokers who also take estrogen may be at an increased risk of developing lung cancer. Although no researchers have formally investigated the issue, we do know that the lungs contain a rich supply of estrogen receptors. It's possible that estrogen may act as a "Trojan Horse," carrying the carbon residues from cigarette smoke into the lung cells and in this way helping to promote lung cancer.

Other Complications

• **Gallstones:** One or two studies have shown a slight increase in the risk of developing gallstones among women who take estrogen. It's still not clear, however, whether the estrogen actually *caused* the development of gallstones. At any rate, this complication is very rare. If you or your physician suspect you may have gallstones, you may want to undergo an ultrasound scan of your gallbladder before beginning hormone-additive therapy.

- **Liver disease:** If you have significant hepatitis or suffered residual liver damage as a result of a past bout with hepatitis, we recommend the use of a patch, pellets, or some other nonoral form of estrogen that bypasses the liver altogether.

If You Take Hormone-Additive Therapy, Will You Get Monthly Periods Again?

This is one of the more pressing questions among women who must take a combination of estrogen and progestogen to protect against endometrial cancer, particularly when the cessation of monthly bleeding is seen as one of the *benefits* of menopause. Indeed, resumption of menstruallike bleeding is the chief reason women give for *not* taking hormones prescribed to them, or for stopping hormone-additive therapy soon after they've begun taking it.

Actually, the bleeding you experience is *not* a real menstrual period in the true sense of the word, since it is the shedding of an artificially stimulated endometrium. *How much* bleeding you expect and *when* you can expect it depends on which one of three estrogen-progestogen regimens you take.

1. Twenty-five-day cyclic regimen: If you take estrogen for twenty-five days, an added progestogen for days fifteen through twenty-five, followed by five days of no medication, you can expect to experience some bleeding during the five-day interval in which you are taking no hormones.

2. Continuous cyclic regimen: If you take an estrogen every day without a break, along with an added progestogen during the first two weeks of every month, you will experience some bleeding during the middle of the month.

3. Continuous combined regimen: If you take an estrogen and progestogen every day, you may experience some irregular bleeding and light spotting for the first four months. (Sixty percent of women on this regimen won't bleed at all during the first four to six months.) After six months, few women will experience any bleeding.

For most women, the menstrual effects of combined estrogen-progestogen therapy are minimal. (A minority of women may experience heavy bleeding, menstrual cramps, and pain. See Chapter 21 for ways to alleviate these symptoms.) Keep in mind, too, that the benefits of hormone-additive therapy—prevention of fractures ten years from now or protection from cardiovascular disease—far outweigh the minor inconvenience of menstruallike bleeding.

Who Should Not Take Hormones?

The list of women who *should not* take hormones is actually quite short. If you have unexplained vaginal bleeding, breast or endometrial cancer, or have had a recent heart attack, you definitely should *not* take hormones. If you've had ovarian cancer, you should check with your physician about taking estrogen. Some types of ovarian cancer have estrogen receptors whose recurrence or spread might be stimulated by the estrogen in hormone-additive therapy.

Some women will need to be monitored more closely while taking hormone-additive therapy, including women with seizure disorders, hypertension, fibroid tumors of the uterus, high blood cholesterol, migraine headaches, previous superficial blood clots in the legs (thrombophlebitis), endometriosis, and gallbladder disease.

Do You Really Need Hormones?

Since estrogen-additive therapy (and possibly combined estrogen-progestogen therapy) can improve a woman's odds against developing heart disease and protect against osteoporosis, why not treat all women?

To begin with, diet and exercise provide ample protection against heart disease. A lifetime of exercise and good eating habits protects against osteoporosis, as well. As a protection against heart disease and osteoporosis, hormone therapy should be considered an *adjunct* to such lifestyle habits as a low-fat diet, not smoking, and participation in an exercise program.

Can you get even better results by combining exercise and estrogen-additive therapy? Yes and no. The combination of estrogen-additive therapy and exercise doesn't appear to lower blood lipids more than estrogen therapy alone. On the other hand, it really does pay to combine exercise with hormone therapy, because hormone-additive therapy does not increase cardiovascular fitness or build bone, both of which also protect against heart disease and osteoporosis. Moreover, we found that exercise and hormone therapy combined is even more effective than hormone therapy alone in lowering blood pressure. In our study, women who took estrogen alone experienced a 3.8 percent decline in blood pressure, while those who took estrogen *and* exercised registered an even greater 6 percent drop in blood pressure.

As for protecting your bones, 75 percent of women *won't* develop osteoporosis. If your bone mass is high at the time of menopause, you probably don't need to take hormone-additive therapy, *provided you take steps to retard bone loss after menopause with adequate calcium in your diet and regular exercise.*

Before you decide whether to take hormone-additive therapy, you should first learn the facts. (If you've just read this chapter, you've already done some of your homework.) Second, discuss the issue with your doctor. Make sure that he or she is well informed. Third, make up your own mind. Your doctor may recommend hormone-additive therapy, but the final decision rests with you.

Whatever you decide, be sure you are regularly monitored by your physician. If you decide not to take hormone therapy, your physician will want to ensure that an indication (such as accelerated bone loss) doesn't develop later on. (See "The Postmenopausal Checkup" beginning on page 139.) If you do decide to take hormone therapy, you should be monitored to ensure that the treatment is effective, safe, and not producing serious side effects.

If you feel you need the benefits of hormone-additive therapy and wish to start taking it, the next chapter will acquaint you with the various types of hormone preparations available to you and will give you practical pointers on taking hormone-additive therapy.

Chapter 21

....

A User's Guide to Postmenopausal Hormones

A wide array of hormonal preparations is available today—from pills to patches to pellets. You should be aware, however, that all are not equal in terms of their effectiveness or potential side effects. Nor do all women respond to the same medication in the same way. Cost and convenience also factor into the equation, particularly when you must take postmenopausal hormones for many years. To get the most benefit from hormone-additive therapy with the fewest side effects, you should first acquaint yourself with the various types of hormonal preparations available to you.

What Is Available to You?

Estrogen

Unlike birth-control pills, which contain synthetic estrogens, most estrogens prescribed for menopausal women are "natural" estrogens, which are much safer and are associated with far fewer side effects. (*Natural estrogens* is actually a bit of a misnomer, since the most widely used, *conjugated equine estrogens*, come from horses, not humans.)

Estrogen can be administered in several different ways, and the route of administration sometimes *does* make a difference (see Table 21.1).

• **Oral estrogens:** The most commonly prescribed form of estrogens are oral estrogens, which are fairly easy to swallow in terms of cost and convenience. There are several types of oral preparations: *Conjugated equine estrogens* (Premarin) are derived from the urine of pregnant mares and contain many different types of estrogen, some unique to horses. *Micronized estradiol* (Estrace); *esterified estrogens* (Estratab); and *estropipate* (Ogen) are considered "natural" estrogens because they closely mimic human estrogens. *Ethinyl estra-*

TABLE 21.1   *How Various Estrogen Preparations Affect Estrogen Levels in Your Body*

(a) Oral conjugated equine estrogens (1.25 mg)

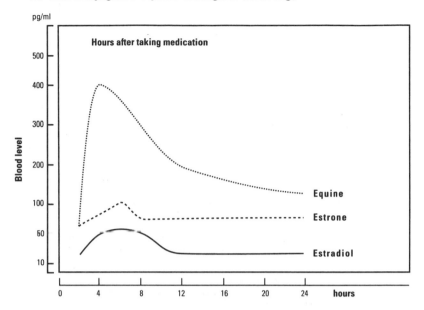

Note: Table adapted with permission from Paul G. Whittaker, "Metabolism of Oral Estrogen," *International Journal of Fertility* (Supplement, 1986): 21–28. Copyright © 1986 by U.S. International Foundation for Studies in Reproduction, Inc., Scandinavian Association for Studies in Fertility, and International Federation of Fertility Societies.

(b) Oral estradiol (2mg)

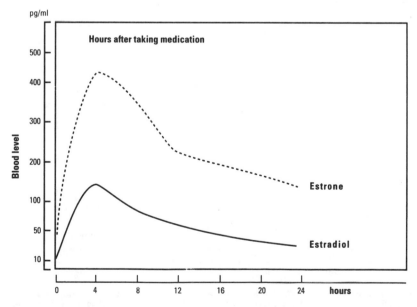

Note: Table adapted with permission from H. Kuhl, "Pharmacokinetics of Oestrogens and Progestogens," *Maturitas* 12 (1990): 171–197. Copyright © 1990 by Elsevier Scientific Publishers Ireland Ltd.

451

(c) Estradiol vaginal cream (0.2mg)

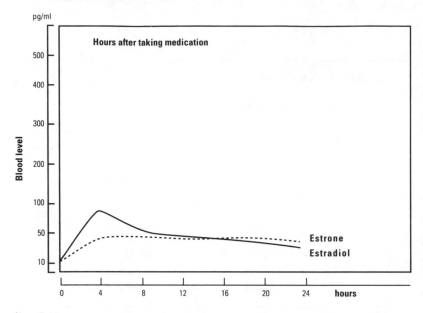

Note: Table adapted with permission from L. A. Rigg, H. Hermann, and Samuel S. C. Yen, "Absorption of Estrogens from Vaginal Creams," *The New England Journal of Medicine* 298, no. 4 (January 26, 1978): 195–97.

(d) Estraderm patch (0.5 mg/day)

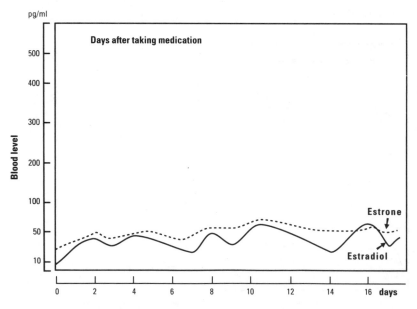

Note: Table adapted with permission from M. S. Powers, L. Schenkel, P. E. Darley, W. R. Good, J. C. Balestra, and V. A. Place, "Pharmacokinetics and pharmacodynamics of transdermal dosage forms of 17 beta-estradiol: Comparison with conventional oral estrogens used for hormone replacement," *American Journal of Obstetrics and Gynecology* 152, no. 8 (August 15, 1985): 1099–1106.

(e) Estradiol pellet (100mg)

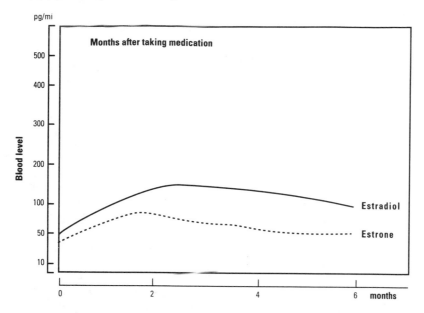

Note: Table adapted with permission from M. H. Thom, W. P. Collins, and J. W. W. Studd, "Hormonal Profiles in Postmenopausal Women after Therapy with Subcutaneous Implants," *British Journal of Obstetrics and Gynaecology* 88 (April 1981): 426–433.

diol (Estinyl) and *quinestrol* (Estrovis) are synthetic hormones whose chemical structure is markedly different from that of human estrogens.

One potential drawback to oral estrogens is that they pass through the liver before entering your bloodstream. The liver acts on the estrogen in several ways. To begin with, all estrogens (except *ethinyl estradiol,* found in oral contraceptives) are converted to *estrone,* which is less potent than *estradiol.* (Before the estrone enters your cells, your body converts estrone back into estradiol.) Second, some of the estrogen is bound by proteins produced by the liver, rendering it incapable of entering your cells. Third, some of the estrogen is metabolized, or broken down, by the liver. Because of these changes, only from 5 to 40 percent of the oral estrogen you take is "free" and therefore biologically active.

On the other hand, some oral estrogens, which have been used now for fifty years, have stood the test of time, while newer forms of estrogen, such as the patch, still need longer experience to prove their ability to prevent fractures and protect against heart disease. Most of the scientific studies showing a beneficial effect of estrogen on bone mass and protection from cardiovascular disease in the United States have involved oral estrogens. Indeed, the fact that oral estrogens do pass through the liver is one reason why they help raise levels of protective HDL cholesterol.

• **Transdermal skin patch:** This is a paper-thin, half dollar–sized, transparent oval patch with adhesive on one side. When placed on your skin (usually your lower abdomen or back; see Tips for Using the Skin Patch on page 457), the patch slowly releases a small amount of estradiol each day. The estradiol

Postmenopausal Hormonal Preparations

Brand name	Type of estrogen	Available dosages	Manufacturer
Oral estrogens			
Premarin	Conjugated equine estrogen	0.3 mg 0.625 mg 0.9 mg 1.25 mg 2.5 mg	Ayerst
Estrace	Micronized estradiol	1.0 mg 2.0 mg	Mead Johnson
Estratab	Esterified estrogens	0.3 mg 0.625 mg 1.25 mg 2.5 mg	Solvay
Ogen	Estropipate	0.625 mg 1.25 mg 2.5 mg 5.0 mg	Abbott
Estinyl	Ethinyl estradiol	0.02 mg 0.05 mg 0.5 mg	Schering
Estrovis	Quinestrol	0.1 mg	Parke-Davis
Estrogen vaginal creams			
Premarin	Conjugated equine estrogens	0.625 mg	Ayerst
Estrace	17 beta-estradiol	0.1 mg	Mead Johnson
Ogen	Estropipate	1.5 mg	Abbott
Ortho Dienestrol	Dienestrol	0.01%	Ortho
Estragard	Dienestrol	0.01%	Solvay
Diethyl-stilbestrol suppositories	Diethylstilbestrol	0.1 mg 0.5 mg	Lilly
Parenteral estrogens (injections, pellets, patches)			
Depo-Estradiol	Estradiol cypionate	1 mg	Upjohn
Delestrogen	Estradiol valerate	10 mg 20 mg 40 mg	Squibb
Estraval	Estradiol valerate	10 mg 20 mg	Solvay

Brand name	Type of estrogen	Available dosages	Manufacturer
Estrapel	Estradiol pellet	25 mg pellet	Bartor, Progynon
Estraderm	Transdermal estradiol	0.05 mg/day 0.1 mg/day	Ciba-Geigy
Progestogens			
Provera	Medroxyprogesterone acetate	10 mg	Upjohn
Curretab	Medroxyprogesterone acetate	10 mg	Solvay
Cyrin	Medroxyprogesterone acetate	10 mg	Ayerst
Amen	Medroxyprogesterone acetate	10 mg	Carnick
Aygestin	Norethindrone acetate	5 mg	Ayerst
Norlutate	Norethindrone acetate	5 mg	Parke-Davis
Norlutin	Norethindrone	5 mg	Parke-Davis
Megace	Megesterol acetate	20 mg 40 mg	Bristol-Myers
Ovrette	Norgestrel	0.075 mg	Wyeth
Micronor	Norethindrone	0.35 mg	Ortho
Nor-Q.D.	Norethindrone	0.35 mg	Syntex
	Micronized oral progesterone	100 mg	—
	Progesterone vaginal suppositories	25 mg 50 mg	—
Oral androgens			
Oreton	Methyltestosterone	5 mg	Schering
Metandren	Methyltestosterone	5 mg	Ciba
Halotestin	Fluoxymesterone	5 mg	Upjohn
Fluoxy-mesterone	Fluoxymesterone	5 mg	Solvay
Ora-Testryl	Fluoxymesterone	5 mg	Squibb
Injectable androgens			
Depo-testosterone	Testosterone cypionate	50 mg/ml	Upjohn
Depo-Testadiol Delatestryl	Testosterone enanthate	100 mg/ml	Squibb

Brand name	Type of estrogen	Available dosages	Manufacturer
Androgen pellets			
Testopel	Testosterone pellets	75 mg	Bartor
Androgen ointments			
	Testosterone propionate	2% in a petrolatum base	
Estrogen/androgen combinations			
Estratest tablets	Esterified estrogens Methyltestosterone	1.25 mg 2.5 mg	Solvay
Estratest H.S. tablets	Esterified estrogens Methyltestosterone	0.625 mg 1.25 mg	Solvay
Premarin with Methyl-testosterone	Conjugated equine estrogens Methyltestosterone	1.25 mg 10 mg	Ayerst
Premarin with Methyl-testosterone	Conjugated equine estrogens Methyltestosterone	0.625 mg 5 mg	Ayerst
Depo-Testadiol	Estradiol cypionate Testosterone cypionate	2 mg 50 mg	Upjohn

Note: Table adapted from R. D. Gambrell, *Estrogen Replacement Therapy* (Durant, OK: Essential Medical Information Systems, Inc., 1990). Adapted and reproduced with permission from the publisher.

is absorbed through the skin and directly into the bloodstream, thus bypassing the intestines and liver. With the patch and other nonoral forms of estrogen therapy (discussed below) there's less binding, less breakdown of estrogen by the liver, and—theoretically—easier access of the hormone to the cell. As a result, these types of estrogen can be more potent than oral estrogens, and lower doses should be used.

The patch must be changed twice weekly. Your physician will usually prescribe the lower strength (0.05 mg) first, increasing the dosage (to .10 mg) if your symptoms don't subside after a few months. (The patch can be divided into quarters or halves by your pharmacist for an even lower dose, but a special cutter must be used to seal in the medication after dividing it.)

One advantage of the estrogen patch is that the slow, steady release of estrogen into your bloodstream helps keep blood-estrogen levels fairly stable, thus preventing the peaks and valleys in blood-estrogen levels sometimes associated with pills (see Table 21.1). Although the patch hasn't been used long

• **To help prevent skin irritation,** rotate the areas to which you apply the patch. The best place to use the patch is on the back just above the buttock.

• **If skin irritation occurs,** move the patch to another site. Your doctor may prescribe a low-dose steroid cream to clear up persistent skin irritations.

• **If the patch falls off** in the shower or while exercising, leave it off until after you've finished, dry the skin thoroughly, then reapply the patch.

enough for researchers to perform quantifiable studies showing whether it reduces the number of bone fractures or heart attacks among its users, theoretically it should work.

The patch has a few disadvantages, as well. Some 20 percent of women using the patch will experience a skin reaction. The estrogen in the patch may be poorly or inadequately absorbed, especially in warm, humid climates. Also, the lower blood-hormone levels associated with the patch may be inadequate protection against osteoporosis and heart disease for some women. (Your doctor can monitor your blood estradiol levels to ensure that you are getting adequate protection against heart disease and osteoporosis.) Finally, some women may have trouble remembering to change the patch twice a week. It's best to establish a regular schedule (a calendar appears on the patch's packaging, making it easier to remember the schedule).

• **Vaginal creams (Estrace, Estraguard, Ogen, Ortho Dienestrol, Premarin):** Estrogen cream is ideal for women whose main complaint is vaginal dryness or urinary symptoms because the cream goes right to the heart of the problem— the estrogen-deprived vaginal (and urethral) tissues. Because the cream is applied directly to the tissues that need it most, many women think of vaginal estrogen as a "local" treatment that is "safer" than other forms of estrogen that circulate throughout the body. After all, estrogen cream affects only the vaginal and urethral tissues and doesn't circulate in the bloodstream, right? Not exactly. What most women don't realize is that estrogen cream is quickly absorbed through the vaginal walls and into the bloodstream, so, in effect, this "local" treatment (if large enough quantities are used) can have a systemic effect. This isn't a problem for most women. In fact, the vagina's ability to absorb estrogen can actually be a therapeutic advantage for some women (see vaginal use of oral tablets, on page 458). But women who wish to minimize their exposure to systemic estrogen, such as those with a family history of breast cancer, could be getting a bigger dose of estrogen than they bargained for when using estrogen creams.

When used in low doses (¼ to ½-applicatorful every other day), estrogen creams are perfectly safe, and the amount of estrogen that is absorbed from the vagina into the bloodstream is quite low (see Table 21.1). Even if you have a family history of breast cancer, you can still use vaginal creams. (We recommend that women with a family history of breast cancer use Estrace cream, since it contains only the hormone estradiol and your blood hormone levels can be easily monitored while you're using the cream.)

The biggest drawback to creams is that some women find them messy. Newer forms of vaginal estrogens, many of which may be available in the United States within the next five years, should help solve this problem. Until some of these newer preparations become available, wear a sanitary napkin or panty liner to protect your clothes while using vaginal creams.

• **Vaginal use of oral tablets:** An alternative to oral estrogen for women who can't use the skin patch involves placing half a tablet of oral Estrace into the vagina every two to three days. This treatment results in moderate blood levels of estrogen that may last for up to thirty-six hours. Since only 25 to 50 percent of the usual oral dosage is used, this method is more cost-effective than oral estrogens, too. The only disadvantages are that you must break the tablets in half yourself and, because the tablets are colored purple, they may stain your undergarments. (Wearing a panty shield or panty liner helps solve this problem.)

• **Pellets:** Estrogen-containing pellets—each about the size of a saccharine tablet—can be injected in the fat tissue just under the skin (usually in the lower abdomen or buttock) by a physician. Once injected, the pellet slowly releases its medication into the bloodstream and is absorbed by the body.

The chief advantage of this method is that one or two pellets containing 25 milligrams of estradiol each provide steady blood levels of estrogen for three to four months after you receive it. The pellets are usually prescribed for women who experienced little or no relief of their symptoms from oral estrogens or for those who experienced side effects from oral estrogens. (Testosterone pellets may be used along with the estrogen for women who experience a decreased sex drive or other problems that respond well to androgen therapy.)

The main drawback to the pellet is that it is difficult to remove if you experience any unwanted side effects. (This is rare, since most women using the pellets experience *relief* from their symptoms after finding oral estrogens ineffective.) Since it's also difficult to tell when the pellet has been spent, your blood-hormone levels will have to be monitored more closely while using this form of estrogen therapy. And, of course, you will have to see your physician and undergo a minor surgical office procedure each time your supply of estrogen runs out (about every three to four months).

• **Intramuscular injection:** Several injectable forms of estrogen are available that last up to four weeks. However, injections are associated with peaks and valleys in blood-estrogen levels and for this reason are not usually recommended. If you do receive injections, your blood-hormone levels will have to be frequently monitored and the dose of estrogen adjusted accordingly.

What Estrogens Will Be Available in the Near Future?
Several new forms of estrogen are now being investigated in the United States and may be available within the next five years.

• **Vaginal tablet (Vagifem):** An estrogen tablet with the unique ability to coat the vaginal walls is now used in Europe, and is currently under investigation in the United States. The estrogen in the tablet is not absorbed through the vaginal walls or into the bloodstream so the therapeutic effects of the drug remain localized in the vagina. For this reason, it may be safer for some women than vaginal creams, most of which *do* raise blood-estrogen levels, depending on the dosage.

• **Estradiol ring (Estring):** This thin, flexible rubber ring is worn in the vagina much like a diaphragm. It gradually releases a small amount of estrogen in the vagina. The rings can be left in place during intercourse and can be easily removed to regulate or change the drug dosage being given. (Some researchers are also experimenting with a vaginal ring containing a combination of estrogen and progesterone to help protect the endometrial lining from overstimulation by estrogen alone.) The main advantage is that the ring is not as messy as vaginal creams.

• **Gel (Oestragel):** A new estradiol-containing gel now available in Europe may make estrogen-additive therapy as simple as using a moisturizing cream or lotion every day. The gel, which is squeezed out of a tube in measured doses, may be applied to the arms, shoulders, waist, thighs, or other parts of the body (except for the breast) in much the same way as you'd apply a moisturizing cream or lotion. The gel dries rapidly (usually within two minutes), leaves no sticky residue, and has no odor. The gel provides the same steady blood-hormone levels as the patch, but the overall blood levels of estradiol are higher among gel users than patch users.

What About Generic Estrogen Preparations?
Generic drugs are usually less expensive than their name brand counterparts, and there are generic equivalents to many of the commonly prescribed estrogen preparations, particularly conjugated estrogens. You should be aware, however, that most generic conjugated estrogens contain fewer estrogens than name brands. And while generic preparations initially are absorbed more rapidly into the bloodstream, resulting in higher peak blood levels of estrogen, after about eight hours, the levels of estrogen circulating in the bloodstream for generic brands tend to be lower than those for name brands. It's still not known whether these differences affect the overall efficacy of generic drugs. Until we know more, we recommend that you request name brand drugs from your pharmacist instead of generic brands.

Progestogen

• **Oral progestogens:** Most progestogens today are given orally in one of the following three dosing regimens:

1. If you take estrogens for twenty-five days, you'll take an added progestogen for days fifteen through twenty-five, followed by five days of no medication, which is what's known as a *twenty-five-day cyclic regimen*.
2. If you take an estrogen every day without a break, you'll take an added progestogen during the first two weeks of every month, which is known as a *continuous cyclic regimen*.
3. You may also take an estrogen and a progestogen every day, in a *continuous combined regimen*.

All regimens protect equally well against endometrial cancer, but there are several chemically different types of oral progestogens, and sometimes the choice of progestogen you use does make a difference.

Medroxyprogesterone acetate (Provera, Curretab, Amen): This is the most widely used progestogen in the United States and has one of the longest track records for safety and effectiveness. For this reason, your physician may recommend that you begin hormone-additive therapy with this type of progestogen. This is particularly true if you have a past history of breast problems (such as fibrocystic breast disease). Some physicians believe this type of progestogen may inhibit benign breast disease and possibly protect against breast cancer. However, these progestogens may not be the best choice for women being treated for mood swings and other estrogen-dependent psychological symptoms, since studies have linked medroxyprogesterone acetate with an increase in moodiness and depression.

19 Nortestosterone derivatives (Aygestin, Norlutate, Norlutin, Ovrette): These progestogens are fairly potent, but if used in low-enough doses, they don't affect blood lipids and may better protect the endometrium than other progestogens.

Your physician may recommend these progestogens if you have a past history of heavy or prolonged menstrual periods (they help reduce bleeding somewhat) or if you are taking estrogen to help relieve menopause-related emotional symptoms.

Megesterol acetate (Megace): This progestogen is used primarily for the treatment of breast and endometrial cancers. However, Megace is also a good treatment for hot flashes among women with breast or endometrial cancer. The drug should be used in collaboration with an oncologist (cancer specialist) to ensure you get the proper dosage of the medication. If the cancer is estrogen- or progesterone-sensitive, you'll need to take a full chemotherapeutic dose.

Micronized oral progesterone: This formulation of natural progesterone doesn't adversely affect blood lipids and doesn't cause the mood swings associated with some synthetic hormones. While the drug has not yet received approval from the U.S. Food and Drug Administration, your physician may be able to buy it from independent pharmacists.

• **Progestasert IUD:** The progestogen-containing intrauterine device, Progestasert, may be an ideal way for postmenopausal women taking estrogen to protect themselves against endometrial cancer. The IUD, inserted into the uterus by a physician, slowly releases a small amount of progestogen. Since it is administered locally, it doesn't adversely affect blood lipids.

What Progestogens Will Be Available in the Near Future?
Most of the progestogens used today can produce side effects similar to those associated with the "male" hormone androgen, including acne, weight gain, and negative changes in blood-cholesterol levels. However, three new types of progestogens now available in Europe, *gestodene, desogestrel,* and *norgestimate,* have few androgenlike properties, so these side effects are unlikely to occur.

460

Androgens

Androgens are available in the form of oral tablets, injections, and pellets.

• **Oral:** Tablets containing 1.25 milligrams to 2.5 milligrams of methyltestosterone are taken daily and usually along with an oral estrogen from the first through the twenty-fifth day of the month (to minimize side effects).

• **Injection:** A long-acting type of testosterone may be given by injection. The dose is usually 50 to 75 milligrams of testosterone every four weeks. Because blood levels of testosterone are high right after you receive the injection, then decline over the four-week interval, you may experience a gradual decline in its therapeutic effects.

• **Implants:** Testosterone pellets may be used along with estrogen pellets (one or two estrogen pellets with one testosterone pellet). Effects usually last from three to four months.

• **Ointment:** Testosterone propionate ointment can be applied locally to the clitoris.

Estrogen-Androgen Combinations

• **Oral:** Several estrogen-androgen tablets are available in this country. Some (Estratest and Estratest H.S.) contain esterified estrogen and methyltestosterone. Combination products of conjugated estrogens are also available (Premarin with methyltestosterone), but they are not as well balanced as those containing esterified estrogen.

• **Injection:** A combination estrogen-androgen injectable, Depo-Testadiol, usually relieves symptoms for four weeks.

A Symptoms Guide to Hormone-Additive Therapy

The type and amount of estrogen and progestogen you take depends largely on your reason for taking it.

Menopausal Symptoms

• **Hot flashes:** Most types of estrogen (pill, patch, pellet, or injection) work equally well in relieving hot flashes. (Estrogen creams generally are *not* prescribed for these symptoms.) Your physician will prescribe the lowest possible dose of estrogen to control your symptoms.

It may take three to four weeks before you feel the full effects of estrogen on your symptoms. Since peak blood-estrogen levels occur from four to six hours after taking oral estrogens, you should take your medication just before bedtime. If you take your estrogen in the morning, you may continue to be bothered by early-morning awakenings and night sweats because, by this time, blood-estrogen levels have fallen (see Table 21.1). Some women may have to take oral estrogen twice a day: once in the morning and once at night. If after three months your symptoms still haven't subsided, your physician will gradually increase the dosage as needed or will change to another route of administration.

If your uterus is intact, you'll have to take progestogen, either cyclically or continuously (see page 459) along with the estrogen.

Three to five years is the average length of time that hormones are used to control hot flashes. However, in some women, symptoms persist—and treatment may be required—for many years. Some 30 percent of women over sixty need hormone-additive therapy for hot flashes. Therapy generally is tapered off over a few months, then stopped altogether.

You should note that the low dose of estrogen used to relieve hot flashes may be too low for protection against cardiovascular disease or osteoporosis. If one of your objectives is to protect your heart and/or bones, you may need to take a larger dose for a longer period of time. Check with your physician.

• **Vaginal dryness and related symptoms:** Vaginal creams are the treatment of choice for vaginal dryness and urethral and bladder-related symptoms. Systemic estrogens (oral, patch, pellets) are not as effective in relieving vaginal symptoms. In one study we conducted in conjunction with Dr. Gloria Bachmann at the University of Medicine and Dentistry of New Jersey in New Brunswick, 44 percent of women taking oral estrogens still complained of vaginal dryness.

Note: You should *not* use estrogen cream as a lubricant during intercourse; our research has shown that estrogen can be absorbed by the penis into the man's bloodstream (see page 251).

A low dose (one-fourth to one-half an applicatorful) is usually prescribed because estrogen is well absorbed from the vagina. Using your finger to massage a small amount of estrogen into the vagina helps reduce absorption of the hormone into the bloodstream. You should use estrogen creams two to three times a week for three to six months. You may need a "maintenance" dose of estrogen cream twice a week thereafter.

Even women with a history of breast cancer can probably use Estrace cream (one-fourth an applicatorful), since blood-hormone levels can be easily monitored. Creams are also recommended for some urinary symptoms (see Chapter 19). The dosage is one-half an applicatorful three times a week for three to six months.

• **Psychological symptoms:** Systemic estrogens (pills, pellets, or patches) work best. Some women may find that nonoral types of estrogen (pellets or patches) work better than pills because there's less of a binding effect on the drug by the liver, which increases the bioavailability and effectiveness of the drug. If you are sensitive to fluctuations in hormone levels, the patch and pellets also provide more stable blood-estrogen levels than oral estrogen.

Progestogens are another matter: If you need to take a progestogen, some—particularly *medroxyprogesterone acetate* (Amen, Curretab, Provera)—may aggravate or induce depression and other PMS-like psychological symptoms. If this is the case, ask your physician to prescribe *19 Nortestosterone derivatives* (Aygestin, Norlutate, Norlutin, Ovrette), which are less likely to trigger depression. Micronized oral progesterone may in fact be the best.

462

Osteoporosis

As a rule, if you have relatively normal bone mass (that is, you have lost less than 30 percent of your bone mass), you can choose the type of estrogen and its route of administration. If you have lost more than 30 percent of your bone mass, we recommend oral estrogen, especially conjugated equine estrogens, since their ability to maintain bone mass has been better documented than that of the skin patch or other forms of estrogens.

Most of the research with oral estrogen has shown that the type of estrogen used doesn't make much difference as long as the dose is adequate. Here are the minimum doses for the most widely prescribed oral estrogen preparations:

Premarin	0.625 to 0.9 mg/day
Estrace	1–2 mg/day
Ogen	1.25 mg/day
Estratab	0.625 mg to 1.25 mg/day
Estinyl	20 mcg/day

How long will you need to take hormones? It depends on how much bone mass you have to start with. If you are maintaining bone mass, you may take hormone therapy for ten to fifteen years, up to age sixty-five. If you have established osteoporosis or are at very high risk of developing osteoporosis, we recommend that you take hormones for the rest of your life, provided you have no contraindications and provided you don't experience any serious side effects during your treatment. Why so long? When you stop taking hormone therapy, you could experience a substantial decrease in bone density.

Again, if you have experienced a natural menopause and have your uterus intact, you should take a progestogen along with estrogen to protect against endometrial cancer. It may also help to add bone mass.

Cardiovascular Disease

Hormone therapy for the prevention of cardiovascular disease should be tailored to women who are, for one reason or other, at increased risk of developing heart and vascular problems.

• **If you have high blood pressure:** As we mentioned earlier, oral estrogens actually *lower* blood pressure. For the minority of women whose blood pressure rises after beginning hormone therapy or for women whose hypertension is related to the hormone *renin*, the estrogen patch should be used.

• **If you have diabetes:** If your blood triglycerides are elevated, you should use the patch, since oral estrogens have been associated with an increase in blood triglycerides. If your levels of HDL cholesterol are not too low, you could also consider using an oral estrogen-androgen combination, since the androgens appear to offset the rise in blood triglycerides associated with oral estrogens. Otherwise, oral estrogens are fine because they actually *lower* blood-sugar levels.

- **If you have a history of blood clots:** Women with previous deep venous thrombosis *can* take estrogen therapy, particularly if the blood clot was from a nonrecurring cause. (For instance, a woman who developed phlebitis after a caesarean section twenty years ago can safely use hormone-additive therapy.)

What kind of estrogen is best? If you have a remote deep venous thrombosis, the type of estrogen you take makes no difference. If you have recently developed a blood clot from a nonrecurring cause (for instance, after a hysterectomy), you should use the skin patch, which has less of an effect on coagulation factors produced by the liver.

Should you stop estrogen-additive therapy before surgery? It's probably not necessary, but some surgeons may recommend that you do so for one month prior to surgery. Immediately after surgery, you should use the skin patch.

A precautionary note: All women with a history of blood clots should be closely monitored. Your physician can test for levels of fibrinogen, anticoagulants, such as antithrombin III activity, and the overall marker of the clotting mechanism—prothrombin time. We advocate the use of a junior aspirin (60 milligrams) every third day. Aspirin helps decrease platelet adhesiveness and encourages dilation of the blood vessels. (Remember, however, you should take aspirin regularly only while under a doctor's supervision. See page 321.) You should also exercise, which increases blood flow through your body and may raise levels of certain anticoagulants. Moreover, *you should not smoke.* Cigarette smoking increases the "stickiness" of blood platelets, decreasing clotting time, increasing blood thickness, and increasing the likelihood that a blood clot will form. Plus, cigarette smoking appears to damage the lining of arteries and depresses the production of the anticoagulant prostacyclin by the blood-vessel wall, both of which may increase the risk that a blood clot will form.

- **If you have high blood cholesterol and/or a family history of cardiovascular disease:** Most of the studies showing a protective effect are based on the use of conjugated oral estrogens (Premarin). We found that *estropipate* (Ogen) was also highly effective in reducing blood cholesterol, especially among women with elevated cholesterol (above 260 mg/dl). After twelve months, total cholesterol of the women taking Ogen in our study fell 3.4 percent, LDL cholesterol dropped 8.3 percent, and HDL cholesterol rose 9.7 percent. If you have high cholesterol and decreased HDL cholesterol, you can take oral Premarin, Ogen, Estratab, or other equivalents.

If your triglycerides are elevated, however, the patch may be a better choice, as oral estrogens may raise triglycerides. (If you have elevated triglycerides *and* fairly high levels of HDL cholesterol, your physician may recommend an estrogen-androgen combination. Oral androgens have been found to lower triglycerides.)

As for progestogen, very low doses of *19 Nortestosterone* or *micronized oral progesterone* are preferable because they have been shown to have the least effect on blood lipids. You should take the minimum dose needed to protect against endometrial cancer. You should also take a *cyclic* rather than a *continuous* regimen of progestogen, since this further limits the amount of time you are exposed to progestogen.

464

Note: The transdermal estrogen patch also alters blood lipids—but usually only after four to six months of treatment. The main positive effect of the patch is to lower levels of LDL cholesterol rather than increase those of protective HDL cholesterol. So if your HDL levels are low, in our opinion you should use oral estrogen.

• **If you have established coronary heart disease:** It's not known whether hormone therapy will be useful in women with established coronary heart disease, but hormone-additive therapy may be useful as an adjunct to other treatments, such as angioplasty. And since estrogen works so well at raising HDL cholesterol and lowering LDL cholesterol, it should be used for the treatment of patients with high blood cholesterol (*hypercholesterolemia*). Of course, if you have high cholesterol levels, you should also eat a low-fat diet and exercise regularly. You may also need to take specific cholesterol-lowering drugs.

How Do I Know Whether Hormones Are Working— and Are Safe for Me?

Hormone therapy is monitored for three reasons: efficacy, safety, and side effects.

Effectiveness

Remember, estrogen works only for as long as you take it. When you stop, bone loss may resume, cholesterol levels may rise, and some women may experience hot flashes and other menopausal symptoms once again. (Hot flashes usually abate if hormone-additive therapy is gradually tapered off.)

How will you know whether hormone therapy is working? It depends on the reason for its use:

• **Menopausal symptoms:** You'll know whether hormone therapy is working to relieve hot flashes and other symptoms of menopause simply by the way you feel. If your symptoms persist, you may need a larger dose of estrogen, or you may want to try a different route of administration. Additional, more objective tests, such as vaginal pH and the maturation index of cells in the vaginal walls (see page 249) can be used to monitor the effectiveness of estrogen creams in treating atrophic vaginitis.

• **Osteoporosis:** Having your bone density tested using dual-energy X-ray absorptiometry (DEXA) (see page 346) is an ideal way to monitor how well hormone therapy is working. A simple urine test that monitors the ratio of calcium to creatinine (a by-product of metabolism) can also be used to monitor the effectiveness of your treatment, as well. A blood test that measures levels of alkaline phosphatase (see page 350) and can tell whether new bone formation has been stimulated may also be helpful.

• **Heart disease:** Levels of total cholesterol, HDL cholesterol, LDL cholesterol, triglycerides, and the ratio of HDL to total cholesterol can be used as a gauge of whether hormone therapy is conferring protection against heart disease.

• **Biological efficacy:** Every woman responds a little differently to hormone therapy. If you don't seem to be responding to treatment, a blood test can be used to detect the levels of estrogen (estradiol and estrone) circulating in your bloodstream and to determine whether your body is absorbing the drugs. Blood-estrogen levels don't always tell the whole story, however. Sometimes, estrogen circulating in the bloodstream can be "bound" by proteins and is not biologically available. We call this the "estrogen-binding syndrome." Therefore, in addition to blood-hormone tests, your physician may also measure levels of FSH (follicle-stimulating hormone) to determine the biological efficacy of the hormones you're taking. High levels of FSH indicate that while estrogen may be absorbed, most of the estrogen is not available in a form your body can use. Often, switching the route of administration (from pills to patch, or to vaginal use of pills, for instance) will help improve the biological activity of the drug.

Safety

As we mentioned earlier, the addition of progestogen to estrogen therapy provides ample protection against endometrial cancer. Nevertheless, it's a good idea for women to be monitored for possible signs of endometrial and breast cancers. The following guidelines should be of help:

• **Endometrial sampling:** This test involves removing a small sample of endometrial tissue from the uterus and examining it under a microscope to check for any abnormalities, such as *hyperplasia* (overgrowth of cells). The test is generally recommended annually for women taking hormone-additive therapy to ensure that the endometrial lining isn't being overstimulated by estrogens, and *any time* a woman taking hormonal-additive therapy experiences an abnormal bleeding pattern.

Some physicians recommend a baseline evaluation of the endometrium before starting hormone-additive therapy. Others (ourselves included) prefer to wait until after you've taken hormones for three months. This allows you time to adjust to the medication and gives your physician a chance to determine what effect the drug regimen has on your endometrium. (For more on this test, see page 393.)

• **Ultrasound:** If your cervical canal is tightly narrowed (*stenosed*) or if you are extremely sensitive to pain, your physician may instead use ultrasound to measure the thickness of your uterine lining. This is a painless procedure that takes about ten minutes (see page 393).

An endometrial thickness of less than 5 millimeters is considered normal. If your uterine lining is more than 5 millimeters thick, additional tests, such as hysteroscopy or dilatation and curettage (D&C), may be required (see Chapter 18).

• **Regular breast examinations:** We recommend weekly breast self-examinations (for instance, "always on Sundays") to get you into the habit of performing these lifesaving examinations (see page 48 for directions on how to perform BSE) and also to give you more experience in performing the test, which ultimately makes it more accurate. You may also want to consider having two breast examinations a year by a health-care professional. And you should *definitely* undergo yearly mammograms.

Minor Side Effects

Most minor side effects of hormone therapy are rare. When they do occur, bothersome side effects can often be ameliorated by changing the form of estrogen or progestogen you use or altering the dosing schedule.

•   **Discomforts associated with menstruallike bleeding:** For most women taking combined estrogen-progestogen therapy, the menstrual effects are minimal. However, a minority of women may experience heavy bleeding, menstrual cramps, and pain. These discomforts can usually be relieved by taking an anti-inflammatory, prostaglandin-inhibiting pain reliever, such as aspirin, ibuprofen (Advil, Nuprin, Medipren, or the prescription brand Motrin), naproxen (Anaprox), or *mefenamic acid* (Ponstel). These drugs may decrease heavy bleeding by 50 percent, as well.

If you do experience fairly heavy bleeding and use tampons, be aware that some superabsorbency tampons have been associated with an increased risk of toxic-shock syndrome (TSS)—the greater the absorbency, the greater the risk (see page 234). To reduce your risk, use the least-absorbent tampon for your needs and change your tampon regularly (every four hours). You should see your physician immediately if while using tampons you suddenly develop a high fever, vomiting, diarrhea, and muscle pain, especially if these symptoms are accompanied by a sunburnlike rash.

•   **Weight gain:** Some women may gain weight after beginning hormone therapy; but our research and that of others has shown that the average weight gain is only about five pounds—*if you gain any weight at all*. If you do gain weight after beginning hormone therapy, try readjusting your metabolic balance by eating less food and exercising more. If the weight you gain is mostly fluid, your physician may recommend that you take a diuretic.

•   **Gastrointestinal problems:** Nausea and stomach upset may occur with some types of oral estrogens. This can be relieved by taking your pill with a little bit of food. If that doesn't help, you can change the type of oral estrogen you take or switch to one of the nonoral types. (Note: Taking hormones with food increases their absorption.)

•   **Breast tenderness:** If you notice increased breast tenderness after beginning hormone-additive therapy, you may find relief by changing the way in which you take the hormone (switching to a Monday through Friday regimen rather than taking the drug seven days a week, for instance). Decreasing the dosage to the bare minimum required to treat your condition helps, too. Your physician may recommend that you try a diuretic, an estrogen-androgen combination, or tamoxifen (Nolvadex), a drug used in the treatment of breast cancer, which sometimes helps to reduce breast tenderness. Cutting back on caffeine often improves symptoms (see page 92). Some women find relief by taking a vitamin E supplement (400 IU) twice daily.

•   **Sensitivity to estrogens:** Although rare, some women are extremely sensitive to estrogen, developing such unusual symptoms as hyperactivity or even severe abdominal pain. If your doctor suspects you have a sensitivity to estrogen, he or she might recommend that you try a different type of estrogen or a different route of administration. If these changes fail to solve the problem, you may be advised to stop taking estrogen altogether.

•   **Hormonal headaches:** Estrogen and progestogen may trigger headaches and migraines among some women, particularly those with a history of migraines (see page 235). Reducing the dose of estrogen often relieves the headaches. In one study of eighty-seven women who experienced migraine headaches while receiving estrogen, 58 percent experienced a reduction in symptoms after the dosage of estrogen was reduced. Taking estrogen continuously helps, too, since many women have estrogen-withdrawal headaches (see page 248). Taking a nonoral type of androgen along with estrogen often alleviates headaches, as well.

When deciding which method of hormone-additive therapy is best for you, you will of course want to choose the most effective method for your particular needs. But you should also consider which method would be most convenient for you. Too often, women stop taking hormone therapy because the method they're using becomes burdensome in one way or another. If one form of hormone therapy becomes problematic for you, try another. (But give each method a chance to work—try one method for at least three months before switching to another.) Together, you and your physician should be able to find a perfect fit.

Epilogue

....

Menopause is not a disease; rather, it is a perfectly natural transition. Most women will pass through this important biological milestone without much trouble at all. Nevertheless, the drop in estrogen associated with menopause may increase your risk of developing two serious and potentially life-threatening illnesses: heart disease and osteoporosis. Moreover, your menopause occurs at a time in your life when your risk of developing various other chronic and serious ailments, such as arthritis, diabetes, and cancer, naturally rises with age. In effect, the middle years bring a completely new set of health needs for women. You can make a smoother transition through the menopausal years and increase your chances of staying healthy and active in your later years by understanding the changes your body is going through and preparing well in advance for them, in much the same way that you may have prepared for pregnancy during your childbearing years.

You should begin by finding a physician who understands your changing health needs and with whom you feel comfortable. After you have found a physician, be sure to see your doctor at least once a year for regular medical checkups, possibly more often if you have any special health concerns or medical problems. You should have an annual examination by your doctor even if you are not experiencing any symptoms, since many of the early warning signs of potentially serious problems are silent. Your doctor has a wide array of screening and diagnostic tests to spot any signs of trouble early, when medical intervention is most effective.

Your lifestyle habits, including your diet, your level of physical activity, the way you cope with emotional stress, and your use of alcohol, tobacco, and drugs, take on increasing importance in your middle years. In fact, making a few key changes in the way you live your life—reducing your intake of fat, exercising regularly, finding positive ways of managing stress, limiting your use of alcohol, using over-the-counter and prescription medications with care, and quitting smoking—can dramatically increase your odds of living longer and, perhaps more important, living better throughout your middle and later years.

Contrary to popular belief, you won't necessarily have to take hormones after menopause. Numerous women do just fine without postmenopausal hormone therapy *provided they enter the menopausal transition years in optimal health and maintain good health throughout the middle years.* If you do experience severe hot flashes and other menopausal symptoms, or if you are at a greater risk of developing heart disease or osteoporosis, hormone therapy is one of the most effective means available of treating these problems. But again, it's only one of many treatment options available to you. Before making a decision about hormone therapy or any other drug therapy, for that matter, you should find out as much as you can about each medication's benefits and risks.

Your middle and later years have the potential to be some of the best years of your life. You can make the most of these years by taking good care of yourself—beginning right now!

Appendix

··

Standard Height and Weight Tables

You may have breathed a sigh of relief (and moved a button over a notch or two on your waistband) when, in 1990, the U.S. Department of Agriculture (USDA) released its new Suggested Weights for Adults. After all, the new guidelines suggest that you can weigh a little more than previously accepted weight standards—particularly in your middle and later years—and still expect good health and a long life.

Americans generally weigh more now than when the first height and weight tables were issued by the Metropolitan Life Insurance Company in 1959. Those tables, derived from the pooled data of twenty-six insurance companies in the United States and Canada, reflected the weights at which mortality is lowest—or longevity highest—and were intended to promote "sound concepts of weight control." In 1983, the Metropolitan Life Insurance Company issued revised tables with higher weights after a new population study found that today's adults "can weigh more than their 1959 counterparts and still anticipate favorable longevity." The higher weight of the average American is reflected in the new USDA tables, as well. Indeed, many critics claim the USDA guidelines describe what *is*, not what should be, and that the new recommendations give an already-overweight population permission to get fatter.

Keep in mind that the suggested weights—even those in the Metropolitan tables— are just that: a suggestion. The weights in these tables are averages derived from studies of large populations, without regard for individual differences. Therefore, you may find that you look fine and feel great at a weight that's higher than those in the weight tables. Or you may feel fat at the weight the tables say is right for you. For these reasons, you should work with your physician to determine your ideal weight—the weight that is right for you. This means knowing your percentage of body fat as well as your weight.

	Metropolitan Life, 1959 Ideal weight ranges for women by frame size			Metropolitan Life, 1983 Ideal weight ranges for women by frame size			USDA, 1990 Suggested Weights for Adults*	
Height†	Small	Medium	Large	Small	Medium	Large	19–34 years old	≥35 years old
5'0"	98–106	103–115	111–127	103–115	112–126	122–137	97–128	108–138
5'1"	101–109	106–118	114–130	105–118	115–129	125–140	101–132	111–143
5'2"	104–112	109–122	117–134	108–121	118–132	128–144	104–137	115–148
5'3"	107–115	112–126	121–138	111–124	121–135	131–148	107–141	119–152
5'4"	110–119	116–131	125–142	114–127	124–138	134–152	111–146	122–157
5'5"	114–123	120–135	129–146	117–130	127–141	137–156	114–150	126–162
5'6"	118–127	124–139	133–150	120–133	130–144	140–160	118–155	130–167
5'7"	122–131	128–143	137–154	123–136	133–147	143–164	121–160	134–172
5'8"	126–136	132–147	141–159	126–139	136–150	146–167	125–164	138–178
5'9"	130–140	136–151	145–164	129–142	139–153	149–170	129–169	142–183
5'10"	134–144	140–155	149–169	132–145	142–156	152–173	132–174	146–188

Note: Metropolitan Life tables (1959 and 1983) reprinted with permission from the Metropolitan Life Insurance Company.

* The USDA table makes no distinction between suggested weights for men and women, noting only that "the higher weights in the ranges generally apply to men, who tend to have more muscle and bone; the lower weights more often apply to women, who have less muscle and bone."

† All height figures are without shoes; all weight figures are without clothing.

Determining Your Skeletal Frame Size

Measure your elbow breadth using the instructions on pages 27–28. Compare your measurement with those in the tables here. These tables list the elbow measurements for women of medium frame at various heights. Measurements lower than those listed indicate that you have a small frame while higher measurements indicate a large frame.

Height (in 1-inch heels)	Elbow Breadth (inches)
4'10"–4'11"	2¼"–2½"
5'0"–5'3"	2¼"–2½"
5'4"–5'7"	2⅜"–2⅝"
5'8"–5'11"	2⅜"–2⅝"
6'0"	2½"–2¾"

Note: Instructions for determining body frame by elbow breadth on pages 27–28 and tables here are reprinted with permission from the Metropolitan Life Insurance Company.

Determining Your Body-Mass Index

Find your present weight in the left-hand column and read across to the column with your height. If your height or weight doesn't appear on this chart, you can calculate your body-mass index using the following equation:

$$(702.95 \times \text{Weight}) \div (\text{Height} \times \text{Height})$$
$$\text{(in pounds)}. \qquad \text{(in inches)}$$

For example, if you are 4 feet 11 inches (59 inches) tall and weigh 110 pounds, your body-mass index would be

$$(702.95 \times 110) \div (59 \times 59) = 22.21$$

A body-mass index of 27.3 means you are moderately overweight; one of 32.3 indicates severe obesity.

Height: (in)

Weight: (lb)	58	59	60	61	62	63	64	65	66	67	68	69	70	71	72	73	74
110	23.0	22.2	21.5	20.8	20.1	19.5	18.9	18.3	17.8	17.2	16.7	16.2	15.8	15.3	14.9	14.5	14.1
115	24.0	23.2	22.5	21.7	21.0	20.4	19.7	19.1	18.6	18.0	17.5	17.0	16.5	16.0	15.6	15.2	14.8
120	25.1	24.2	23.4	22.7	21.9	21.3	20.6	20.0	19.4	18.8	18.2	17.7	17.2	16.7	16.3	15.8	15.4
125	26.1	25.2	23.4	23.6	22.9	22.1	21.5	20.8	20.2	19.6	19.0	18.5	17.9	17.4	17.0	16.5	16.0
130	27.2	26.3	25.4	24.6	23.8	23.0	22.3	21.6	21.0	20.4	19.8	19.2	18.7	18.1	17.6	17.2	16.7
135	28.2	27.3	26.4	25.5	24.7	23.9	23.2	22.5	21.8	21.1	20.5	19.9	19.4	18.8	18.3	17.8	17.3
140	29.3	28.3	27.3	26.5	25.6	24.8	24.0	23.3	22.6	21.9	21.3	20.7	20.1	19.5	19.0	18.5	18.0
145	30.3	29.3	28.3	27.4	26.5	25.7	24.9	24.1	23.4	22.7	22.0	21.4	20.8	20.2	19.7	19.1	18.6
150	31.4	30.3	29.3	28.3	27.4	26.6	25.7	25.0	24.2	23.5	22.8	22.2	21.5	20.9	20.3	19.8	19.3
155	32.4	31.3	30.3	29.3	28.4	27.5	26.6	25.8	25.0	24.3	23.6	22.9	22.2	21.6	21.0	20.4	19.9
160	33.4	32.3	31.2	30.2	29.3	28.3	27.5	26.6	25.8	25.1	24.3	23.6	23.0	22.3	21.7	21.1	20.5
165	34.5	33.3	32.2	31.2	30.2	29.2	28.3	27.5	26.6	25.8	25.1	24.4	23.7	23.0	22.4	21.8	21.2
170	35.5	34.3	33.2	32.1	31.1	30.1	29.2	28.3	27.4	26.6	25.8	25.1	24.4	23.7	23.1	22.4	21.8
175	36.6	35.3	34.2	33.1	32.0	31.0	30.0	29.1	28.2	27.4	26.6	25.8	25.1	24.4	23.7	23.1	22.5
180	37.6	36.4	35.2	34.0	32.9	31.9	30.9	30.0	29.1	28.2	27.4	26.6	25.8	25.1	24.4	23.7	23.1
185	38.7	37.4	36.1	35.0	33.8	32.8	31.8	30.8	29.9	29.0	28.1	27.3	26.5	25.8	25.1	24.4	23.8
190	39.7	38.4	37.1	35.9	34.8	33.7	32.6	31.6	30.7	29.8	28.9	28.1	27.3	26.5	25.8	25.1	24.4
195	40.8	39.4	38.1	36.8	35.7	34.5	33.5	32.4	31.5	30.5	29.6	28.8	28.0	27.2	26.4	25.7	25.0
200	41.8	40.4	39.1	37.8	36.6	35.4	34.3	33.3	32.3	31.3	30.4	29.5	28.7	27.9	27.1	26.4	25.7
205	42.8	41.4	40.0	38.7	37.5	36.3	35.2	34.1	33.1	32.1	31.2	30.3	29.4	28.6	27.8	27.0	26.3
210	43.9	42.4	41.0	39.7	38.4	37.2	36.0	34.9	33.9	32.9	31.9	31.0	30.1	29.3	28.5	27.7	27.0
215	44.9	43.4	42.0	40.6	39.3	38.1	36.9	35.8	34.7	33.7	32.7	31.8	30.8	30.0	29.2	28.4	27.6
220	46.0	44.4	43.0	41.6	40.2	39.0	37.8	36.6	35.5	34.5	33.5	32.5	31.6	30.7	29.8	29.0	28.2
225	47.0	45.4	43.9	42.5	41.2	39.9	38.6	37.4	36.3	35.2	34.2	33.2	32.3	31.4	30.5	29.7	28.9
230	48.1	46.5	44.9	43.5	42.1	40.7	39.5	38.3	37.1	36.0	35.0	34.0	33.0	32.1	31.2	30.3	29.5
235	49.1	47.5	45.9	44.4	43.0	41.6	40.3	39.1	37.9	36.8	35.7	34.7	33.7	32.8	31.9	31.0	30.2
240	50.2	48.5	46.9	45.3	43.9	42.5	41.2	39.9	38.7	37.6	36.5	35.4	34.4	33.5	32.6	31.7	30.8
245	51.2	49.5	47.8	46.3	44.8	43.4	42.1	40.8	39.5	38.4	37.3	36.2	35.2	34.2	33.2	32.3	31.5
250	52.3	50.5	48.8	47.2	45.7	44.3	42.9	41.6	40.4	39.2	38.0	36.9	35.9	34.9	33.9	33.0	32.1

Body Mass Index	Classification
27.3 to 32.2	Moderate obesity
32.3 and over	Severe obesity

Body Composition Standards for Women

TABLE A.1 *Average Percentage of Body Fat Among Women in the Middle Years*

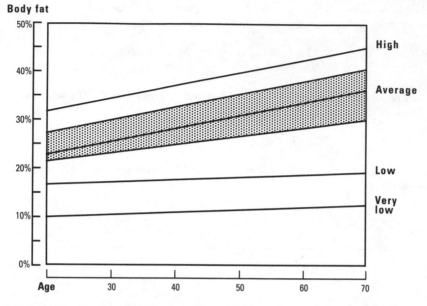

Note: Body composition standards for women reprinted with permission from Michael L. Pollock, Ph.D. Copyright © 1989 by Michael L. Pollock, Ph.D.

Bone Density and Fracture Risk in Women

Bone-density measurements taken from the spine and hip (actually, the upper thighbone) can help predict your risk of developing osteoporosis. If your percentage of bone mass falls below 80 percent of the average woman's peak bone mass in the spine or below 70 percent in the hip, you are considered at risk; the lower your bone mass, the greater your risk.

TABLE A.2 *Average Bone Density in Women and Subsequent Risk of Fractures**

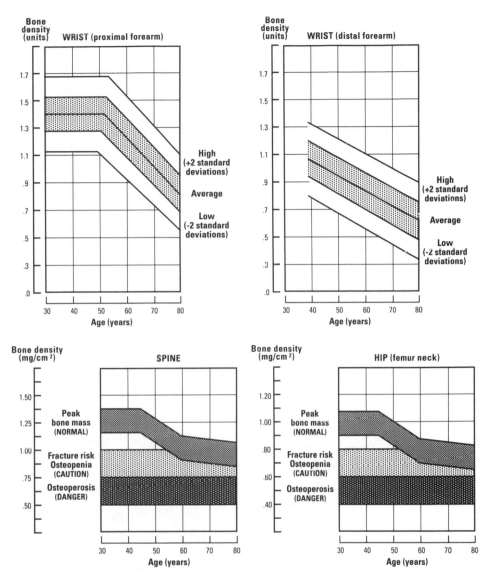

*These values are based on studies of white women. Normal values for blacks are about 6 percent higher than for whites. Those for Asians are about 7 percent lower.

Note: Tables for bone density measurement of the wrist copyright © 1993 Morris Notelovitz, M.D., Ph.D. Tables for bone density measurements of the hip and spine reprinted with permission of Richard B. Mazess, Ph.D., Professor Emeritus, University of Wisconsin Bone Mineral Laboratory.

Fitness Norms for Women in Midlife

Maximal Oxygen Uptake (VO$_2$ Max) (ml/kg min)

Norm	Age			
	30–39	40–49	50–59	60–69
Excellent	37 or less	35 or less	30 or less	25 or less
Above Average	34–37	32–34	27–29	24–25
Average	31–33	26–31	25–27	22–23
Below Average	29–31	24–25	22–25	20–22
Poor	29 or greater	23 or greater	21 or greater	19 or greater

Note: Fitness norms for maximal oxygen uptake reprinted from *Y's Ways to Physical Fitness*, 3rd ed. (Champaign, IL: Human Kinetics Publishers, 1989), with permission of the YMCA of the USA, 101 N. Wacker Drive, Chicago, IL 60606.

Resting Heart Rate (beats per minute)

Norm	Age				
	26–35	36–45	46–55	56–65	Over 65
Excellent	54–59	54–59	54–60	54–59	54–59
Good	60–64	62–64	61–65	61–64	60–64
Above Average	66–68	66–69	66–69	67–69	66–68
Average	69–71	70–72	70–73	71–73	70–72
Below Average	72–76	74–78	74–77	75–77	73–76
Poor	78–82	79–82	78–84	79–81	79–84
Very Poor	84–94	84–92	85–96	85–96	88–96

Note: Fitness norms for resting heart rate reprinted from *Y's Ways to Physical Fitness*, 3rd ed. (Champaign, IL: Human Kinetics Publishers, 1989), with permission of the YMCA of the USA, 101 N. Wacker Drive, Chicago, IL 60606.

Body Composition (percent body fat)

Norm	Age				
	26–35	36–45	46–55	56–65	Over 65
Excellent	14–16	16–19	17–21	18–22	16–20
Good	18–20	20–23	23–25	24–26	22–26
Above Average	21–23	24–26	26–28	27–29	27–29
Average	24–25	27–29	29–31	30–32	30–32
Below Average	27–29	30–32	32–34	33–35	32–34
Poor	31–33	33–36	35–38	36–38	35–37
Very Poor	36–49	38–48	39–50	39–49	38–41

Note: Fitness norms for body composition reprinted from *Y's Ways to Physical Fitness*, 3rd ed. (Champaign, IL: Human Kinetics Publishers, 1989), with permission of the YMCA of the USA, 101 N. Wacker Drive, Chicago, IL 60606.

Sit and Reach Test (inches)

	Age				
Norm	26–35	36–45	46–55	56–65	Over 65
Excellent	23–26	22–25	21–24	20–23	20–22
Good	20–22	19–21	18–20	18–19	18–19
Above Average	19–20	17–19	17–18	16–17	16–17
Average	18	16–17	15–16	15	14–15
Below Average	16–17	14–15	14–15	13–14	12–13
Poor	14–15	11–13	11–13	10–12	9–11
Very Poor	8–13	6–10	4–10	3–9	2–8

Note: Fitness norms for the sit and reach test reprinted from *Y's Ways to Physical Fitness*, 3rd ed. (Champaign, IL: Human Kinetics Publishers, 1989), with permission of the YMCA of the USA, 101 N. Wacker Drive, Chicago, IL 60606.

Sit-Ups (number of repetitions)

	Age				
Norm	26–35	36–45	46–55	56–65	Over 65
Excellent	40–54	34–50	28–42	25–38	24–36
Good	33–37	27–30	22–25	18–21	18–22
Above Average	29–32	24–26	18–21	13–17	14–16
Average	25–28	20–22	14–17	10–12	11–13
Below Average	21–24	16–18	10–13	7–9	6–10
Poor	16–20	10–14	6–9	4–6	2–4
Very Poor	1–12	1–6	0–4	0–2	0–1

Note: Fitness norms for sit-ups reprinted from *Y's Ways to Physical Fitness*, 3rd ed. (Champaign, IL: Human Kinetics Publishers, 1989), with permission of the YMCA of the USA, 101 N. Wacker Drive, Chicago, IL 60606.

Push-Ups (number of repetitions)

	Age			
Norm	30–39	40–49	50–59	60–69
Excellent	27 or more	24 or more	21 or more	17 or more
Above Average	20–26	15–23	11–20	12–16
Average	13–19	11–14	7–10	5–11
Below Average	8–12	5–10	2–6	1–4
Poor	7 or less	4 or less	1 or less	1 or less

Note: Fitness norms for push-ups reprinted from the *Canadian Standardized Test of Fitness-Operations Manual*, 3rd ed. (1986), with permission from the Canadian Association of Sports Sciences in cooperation with Fitness Canada, Fitness and Amateur Sport, Goverment of Canada.

477

TABLE A.3 *Fitness Norms for Women in Midlife: Walking Field Test*

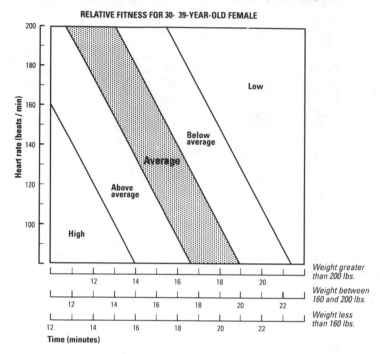

RELATIVE FITNESS FOR 30- 39-YEAR-OLD FEMALE

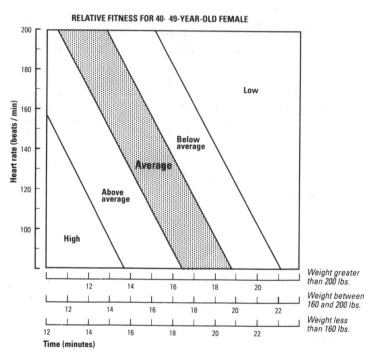

RELATIVE FITNESS FOR 40- 49-YEAR-OLD FEMALE

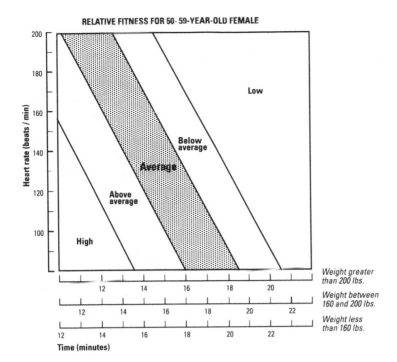

RELATIVE FITNESS FOR 50- 59-YEAR-OLD FEMALE

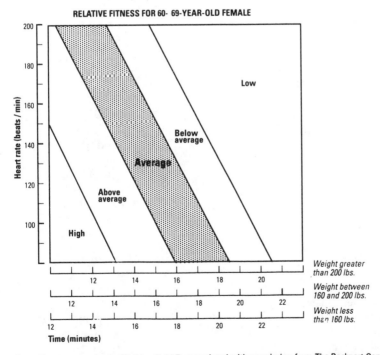

RELATIVE FITNESS FOR 60- 69-YEAR-OLD FEMALE

Note: Fitness norms for the Walking Field Test reprinted with permission from The Rockport Company, Inc. Copyright © 1992 by The Rockport Company, Inc. All rights reserved.

479

Calories Burned Per Minute During Common Exercise and Activities

Use the chart here as a guide for estimating the number of calories you use during exercise and to help determine the number of calories you should consume each day (page 57). Remember to count only those activities that you engage in for at least twenty minutes on a regular basis. Keep in mind, too, that the numbers in this chart are *estimates*. The number of calories you burn depends not only on the type of activity you engage in but also on its duration and the intensity with which it is carried out. So individual variation in the number of calories expended on a particular activity can be quite large. The figures here are based on a person weighing 154 pounds. You'll burn fewer calories if you weigh less than this and more calories if you weigh more.

To estimate the number of calories you burn for a particular activity, multiply the number of calories in the chart here by the number of minutes you engage in the activity. Use the smaller number if your level of activity is mild to moderate; use the larger number if your level of activity is more strenuous.

Activity	Calories per minute
Archery	3.7–5
Backpacking	6–13.5
Badminton	5–11
Basketball	
Nongame	3.7–11
Game	8.5–15
Bicycling	
Recreational	3.7–10
Bowling	2.5–5
Canoeing (rowing and kayaking)	3.7–10
Calisthenics	3.7–10
Dancing	
Social and square	3.7–8.5
Aerobic	7.5–11
Golf	
Using power cart	2.5–3.7
Walking, carrying bag, or pulling cart	5–8.5
Handball	10–15
Hiking (cross-country)	3.7–8.5
Horseback Riding	3.7–10
Jogging/Running (flat surface)	
5.5 mph (11 min./mile)	10.1
6.0 mph (10 min./mile)	12.0
7.0 mph (8:35 min./mile)	14.0
8.0 mph (7:30 min./mile)	15.6
9.0 mph (6:40 min./mile)	17.5
10 mph (6 min./mile)	19.6
11 mph (5:30 min./mile)	21.7
12 mph (5 min./mile)	24.5

Activity	Calories per minute
Mountain Climbing	6–12
Paddleball/Racquetball	10–15
Rope Skipping	10–14
Sailing	2.5–6
Scuba Diving	6–12
Shuffleboard	2.5–3.7
Skating (ice or roller)	6–10
Skiing (snow)	
Downhill	6–10
Cross-country	7.5–15
Snowshoeing	8.5–17
Squash	10–15
Soccer	6–15
Softball	3.7–7.5
Stair Climbing	5–10
Swimming	5–10
Table Tennis	3.7–6
Tennis	5–11
Volleyball	3.7–7.5
Walking (flat surface)	
2.0 mph (30 min./mile)	2.5
2.5 mph (24 min./mile)	3.0
3.0 mph (20 min./mile)	3.7
3.5 mph (17 min./mile)	4.2
3.75 mph (16 min./mile)	4.9
4.0 mph (15 min./mile)	5.5
4.5 mph (13 min./mile)	7.0
5.0 mph (12 min./mile)	8.3
Weight Training (resistance)	10

Note: Table reprinted with permission from Michael L. Pollock and Jack H. Wilmore, *Exercise in Health and Disease: Evaluation and Prescription for Prevention and Rehabilitation* (Philadelphia: W. B. Saunders Company, 1990).

Basal Body Temperature Chart

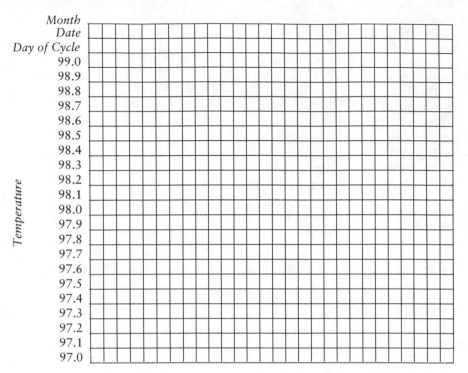

Month
Date
Day of Cycle

Temperature

99.0
98.9
98.8
98.7
98.6
98.5
98.4
98.3
98.2
98.1
98.0
97.9
97.8
97.7
97.6
97.5
97.4
97.3
97.2
97.1
97.0

To predict your time of ovulation using a basal body temperature chart:

1. Start taking your temperature on the first day of your menstrual cycle (the day your period begins), marking the month and date on the chart here. Mark the dates of your period with an *x* (see the sample chart on page 203).

2. Shake the thermometer down to 96 degrees Fahrenheit (or 35 degrees Celsius) before you go to bed at night (or just before taking your temperature in the morning).

3. Take your temperature (either orally or rectally, whichever you prefer; just be sure to use the same method every time) *before getting out of bed in the morning.* Leave the thermometer in place for a minimum of three minutes. The longer you leave it in place, the more reliable the reading will be.

4. Record and plot your temperature on the chart here. Your temperature will increase about 0.4 to 0.8 degrees Fahrenheit *after* you have ovulated and will remain at this higher level until a day or two prior to your next menstrual period.

5. Your most fertile period begins six days before you are expected to ovulate (using charts from previous cycles) and continues until your basal body temperature remains elevated for at least five days.

482

Hot Flash Diary

In the daily log here, record the number of hot flashes you experience per hour and any triggers you may notice. (You may want to make copies of the hot flash diary before filling it out, or make your own daily logbook so you can track your hot flashes for two weeks.)

	Hot flash	Trigger
12:00 A.M.		
1		
2		
3		
4		
5		
6		
7		
8		
9		
10		
11		
12:00 P.M.		
1		
2		
3		
4		
5		
6		
7		
8		
9		
10		
11		

Note: Hot Flash Diary adapted with permission from Ann M. Voda, R.N., Ph.D., *Menopause: Me and You: A Personal Handbook for Women*. Copyright © 1984 by Ann M. Voda, R.N., Ph.D., College of Nursing, University of Utah, Salt Lake City. All rights reserved.

Figure A.1   Body Charts for Skin Self-Exam and Hot Flash Diary

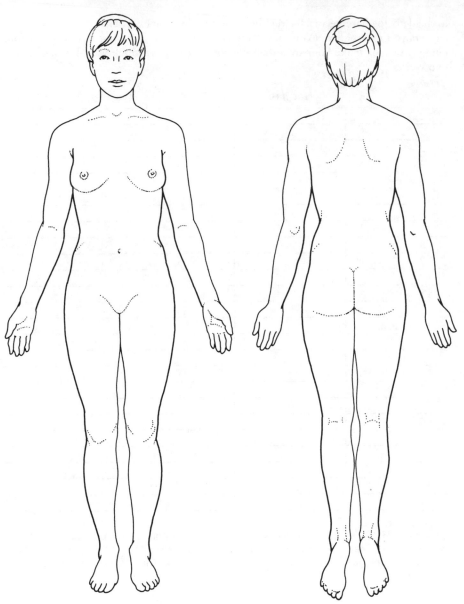

Recommended Dietary Allowances for Women, Revised 1989

	Age (years) or condition		
	25–50	51+	Pregnant/Lactating
Fat-soluble vitamins:			
Vitamin A (IU)	4,000	4,000	5,000
Vitamin D (IU)	200	200	400
Vitamin E (mg α-TE)*	8	8	10
Vitamin K (mcg)	65	65	65
Water-soluble vitamins:			
Vitamin C (mg)	60	60	70
Thiamin (mg)	1.1	1.0	1.5
Riboflavin (mg)	1.3	1.2	1.6
Niacin (mg NE)	15	13	17
Vitamin B_6 (mg)	1.6	1.6	2.2
Folate (mcg)	180	180	400
Vitamin B_{12} (mcg)	2.0	2.0	2.2
Minerals:			
Calcium (mg)	800	800	1,200
Phosphorus (mg)	800	800	1,200
Magnesium (mg)	280	280	320
Iron (mg)	15	10	30
Zinc (mg)	12	12	15
Iodine (mcg)	150	150	175
Selenium (mcg)	55	55	65

* Although International Units are no longer used as a measure of Vitamin E, many food and supplement labels still list Vitamin E in International Units. The recommended dietary allowance of Vitamin E expressed in International Units is 12 IU for adult women and 15 IU for pregnant and lactating women.

Food item	Amount	Calories	Carbohydrates (g)	Total fat (g)	Saturated fat (g)	Unsaturated fat (g)	Cholesterol (mg)	Sodium (mg)
			Breads, Cereals, Crackers					
Breads								
bagel	1	163	30.9	1.4	NA	NA	NA	198
corn bread	1 piece	178	27.5	5.8	1.7	NA	NA	263
cracked-wheat	1 slice	66	12.5	0.9	NA	NA	NA	108
mixed-grain	1 slice	64	11.7	0.9	NA	NA	NA	103
pita pocket	1 pocket	106	20.6	0.6	NA	NA	NA	215
raisin	1 slice	70	13.2	1.0	NA	NA	NA	94
roman-meal	1 slice	70	13.0	1.0	NA	NA	NA	140
rye	1 slice	66	12.0	0.9	NA	NA	NA	174
pumpernickel	1 slice	82	15.4	0.8	NA	NA	NA	173
white	1 slice	64	11.7	0.9	NA	NA	NA	123
whole-wheat	1 slice	61	11.4	1.1	NA	NA	NA	159
Breakfast cereals								
cornflakes	1 cup	110	25.0	1.0	NA	NA	NA	310
granola	¼ cup	127	20.7	4.1	3.0	0.4	0	76
oatmeal, cooked								
instant	¾ cup	104	18.1	1.7	NA	NA	0	286
quick	¾ cup	108	18.9	1.8	0.3	0.7	0	280
raisin bran	½ cup	86	22.0	0.4	0.0	0.1	0	178
shredded wheat	1 oz.	102	22.6	0.6	NA	NA	NA	3
wheat flakes	1 cup	99	22.6	0.5	0.1	0.2	NA	270
Muffins								
blueberry	1 muffin	126	19.5	4.3	NA	NA	NA	200
bran	1 muffin	112	16.7	5.1	NA	NA	NA	168
corn	1 muffin	130	20.0	4.2	1.2	NA	NA	192
English	1 muffin	135	26.2	1.1	NA	NA	0	364
Pancakes (4-inch size)								
frozen batter	3	210	42.2	1.6	NA	NA	NA	857
from mix	3	180	38.2	1.0	NA	NA	NA	710
frozen	3	246	46.6	3.7	NA	NA	NA	777
Waffles								
from mix	1 7-inch	206	27.2	8.0	2.7	NA	NA	515
frozen	2 waffles	190	28.4	6.4	NA	NA	NA	470

Food item	Amount	Calories	Carbohydrates (g)	Total fat (g)	Saturated fat (g)	Unsaturated fat (g)	Cholesterol (mg)	Sodium (mg)
Breads, Cereals, Crackers *(cont.)*								
Pasta (cooked)								
macaroni	1 cup	159	33.7	0.7	NA	NA	0	1
spaghetti	1 cup	159	33.7	0.7	NA	NA	0	1
Crackers								
cheese	5 pieces	81	7.8	4.9	NA	NA	NA	180
graham	2 squares	60	10.8	1.5	NA	NA	NA	66
ground-wheat	5 crackers	70	9.0	3.0	NA	NA	NA	135
Ritz	4 crackers	70	9.0	4.0	NA	NA	NA	120
rye	2 wafers	45	9.9	0.2	NA	NA	NA	115
saltines	2 crackers	26	4.4	0.6	NA	NA	NA	80
Triscuit	3 crackers	60	10.0	2.0	NA	NA	NA	90
Milk, Eggs, and Other Dairy Products								
Milk								
whole (3.3%)	8 oz.	150	11.4	8.2	5.1	0.3	33	120
low-fat (2%)	8 oz.	121	11.7	4.7	2.9	0.2	18	122
low-fat (1%)	8 oz.	102	11.7	2.6	1.6	0.1	10	123
skim	8 oz.	86	11.9	0.4	0.3	0.0	4	126
buttermilk	8 oz.	99	11.7	2.2	1.3	0.0	9	257
Creams								
sour cream	1 tbsp.	26	0.5	2.5	1.6	0.0	5	6
half and half	1 tbsp.	20	0.6	1.7	1.1	0.0	6	6
whipping cream								
heavy, fluid	1 tbsp.	52	0.4	5.6	3.5	0.2	21	6
pressurized	1 tbsp.	8	0.4	0.7	0.4	0.0	2	4
whipped topping								
frozen	1 tbsp.	13	0.9	1.0	0.9	0.0	0	1
nondairy creamers								
liquid	½ oz.	20	1.7	1.5	1.3	0.0	0	12
powdered	1 tsp.	11	1.1	0.7	0.7	0.0	0	4
Yogurt								
whole	8 oz.	139	10.6	7.4	4.8	0.2	29	105
low-fat	8 oz.	144	16.0	3.5	2.3	0.1	14	159
nonfat	8 oz.	127	17.4	0.4	0.3	0.0	4	174
frozen low-fat	4 oz.	100	22.0	1.0	NA	NA	2	60

Food item	Amount	Calories	Carbohydrates (g)	Total fat (g)	Saturated fat (g)	Unsaturated fat (g)	Cholesterol (mg)	Sodium (mg)
Milk, Eggs, and Other Dairy Products (*cont.*)								
Eggs								
whole	1 large	75	0.6	5.0	1.6	2.6	213	63
yolk	1 large	59	0.3	5.1	1.6	2.6	213	7
white	1 large	17	0.3	0	NA	NA	0	55
Egg substitutes								
frozen	¼ cup	96	1.9	6.7	1.2	3.7	1	120
liquid	1.5 oz.	40	0.3	1.6	0.3	0.8	0	33
powdered	.35 oz.	44	2.2	1.3	0.4	0.2	57	79
Cheeses								
American	1 oz.	106	0.5	8.9	5.6	0.3	27	406
cheddar	1 oz.	114	0.4	9.4	6.0	0.3	30	176
cottage cheese								
creamed	1 cup	217	5.6	9.5	6.0	0.3	31	850
1% low-fat	1 cup	164	6.2	2.3	1.5	0.0	10	918
2% low-fat	1 cup	203	8.2	4.4	2.8	0.1	19	918
cream cheese	2 tbsp.	99	0.8	9.9	6.2	0.4	31	84
Monterey Jack	1 oz.	106	0.2	8.6	NA	NA	NA	152
mozzarella								
whole-milk	1 oz.	80	0.6	6.1	3.7	0.2	22	106
part-skim	1 oz.	72	0.8	4.5	2.9	0.1	16	132
ricotta								
whole-milk	½ cup	216	3.8	16.1	10.3	0.5	63	104
part-skim	½ cup	171	6.4	9.8	6.1	0.3	38	155
Swiss cheese	1 oz.	107	1.0	7.8	5.0	0.3	26	74
Ice cream								
vanilla								
10% milk fat	½ cup	134	15.8	7.5	4.4	0.2	29	58
16% milk fat	½ cup	174	16.0	11.8	7.3	0.4	44	54
ice milk	½ cup	92	14.5	2.8	1.7	0.2	9	52
sherbet	½ cup	135	29.3	1.9	1.2	0.0	7	44
sorbet	½ cup	110	28.0	0.1	NA	NA	NA	9
Meat and Poultry								
Chicken								
dark meat w/skin								
fried	3.5 oz.	285	4.1	16.9	4.6	3.9	92	89
roasted	3.5 oz.	253	0.0	15.8	4.4	3.5	91	87
stewed	3.5 oz.	233	0.0	14.7	4.1	3.2	82	70

Food item	Amount	Calories	Carbohydrates (g)	Total fat (g)	Saturated fat (g)	Unsaturated fat (g)	Cholesterol (mg)	Sodium (mg)
Meat and Poultry (*cont.*)								
dark meat w/o skin								
fried	3.5 oz.	239	2.6	11.6	3.1	2.8	96	97
roasted	3.5 oz.	205	0.0	9.7	2.7	2.3	93	93
stewed	3.5 oz.	192	0.0	9.0	2.5	2.1	88	74
white meat w/skin								
fried	3.5 oz.	246	1.8	12.1	3.3	2.7	87	77
roasted	3.5 oz.	222	0.0	10.9	3.1	2.3	84	75
stewed	3.5 oz.	201	0.0	10.0	2.8	2.1	74	63
white meat w/o skin								
fried	3.5 oz.	192	0.4	5.5	1.5	1.3	90	81
roasted	3.5 oz.	173	0.0	4.5	1.3	1.0	85	77
stewed	3.5 oz.	159	0.0	4.0	1.1	0.9	77	65
Turkey (roasted)								
dark meat								
w/skin	3.5 oz.	221	0.0	11.5	3.5	3.1	89	76
w/o skin	3.5 oz.	187	0.0	7.2	2.4	2.2	85	79
light meat								
w/skin	3.5 oz.	197	0.0	8.3	2.3	2.0	76	63
w/o skin	3.5 oz.	157	0.0	3.2	1.0	0.9	69	64
ground turkey	3.5 oz.	225	0.0	14.0	4.5	3.2	92	74
Beef								
brisket, braised								
with fat	3.5 oz.	391	0.0	32.4	13.2	1.2	93	61
fat removed	3.5 oz.	241	0.0	12.8	4.6	0.4	93	72
chuck arm pot roast, braised								
with fat	3.5 oz.	350	0.0	26.0	10.7	1.0	99	60
fat trimmed	3.5 oz.	231	0.0	10.0	3.8	0.4	101	66
chuck blade roast, braised								
with fat	3.5 oz.	383	0.0	30.4	12.7	1.1	103	63
fat trimmed	3.5 oz.	270	0.0	15.3	6.2	0.5	106	71
flank steak, broiled								
with fat	3.5 oz.	254	0.0	16.3	7.0	0.5	71	82
fat trimmed	3.5 oz.	243	0.0	15.0	6.4	0.5	70	83
ground beef, panfried								
extra lean	3.5 oz.	255	0.0	16.4	6.5	0.6	81	70

Food item	Amount	Calories	Carbohydrates (g)	Total fat (g)	Saturated fat (g)	Unsaturated fat (g)	Cholesterol (mg)	Sodium (mg)
Meat and Poultry (*cont.*)								
ground beef *(cont.)*								
lean	3.5 oz.	275	0.0	19.1	7.5	0.7	84	77
regular	3.5 oz.	306	0.0	22.6	8.9	0.8	89	84
eye of round, roasted								
with fat	3.5 oz.	243	0.0	14.2	5.8	0.5	73	59
fat trimmed	3.5 oz.	183	0.0	6.5	2.5	0.2	69	62
sirloin steak, broiled								
with fat	3.5 oz.	280	0.0	18.0	7.5	0.7	90	63
fat trimmed	3.5 oz.	208	0.0	8.7	3.6	0.4	89	66
Pork								
bacon								
broiled/fried	3 pieces	109	0.1	9.4	3.3	1.1	16	303
center loin, with fat								
broiled	3.5 oz.	316	0.0	22.1	8.0	2.5	97	70
panfried	3.5 oz.	375	0.0	30.5	11.0	3.5	103	72
roasted	3.5 oz.	305	0.0	21.8	7.9	2.5	91	64
center loin, fat trimmed								
broiled	3.5 oz.	231	0.0	10.5	3.6	1.3	98	78
panfried	3.5 oz.	266	0.0	15.9	5.5	2.0	107	85
roasted	3.5 oz.	240	0.0	13.1	4.5	1.6	91	69
ham, cured (canned)								
lean	3.5 oz.	120	0.0	4.6	1.5	0.4	38	1255
regular	3.5 oz.	190	0.0	13.0	4.3	1.5	39	1240
sausage links	1 link	48	0.1	4.1	1.4	0.5	11	168
sausage patties	1 patty	100	0.3	8.4	2.9	1.0	22	349
Veal								
chuck (braised/ roasted/stewed)	3 oz.	200	0.0	10.9	5.2	NA	NA	41
loin (broiled)	3 oz.	199	0.0	11.4	5.5	NA	NA	55
rib roast	3 oz.	229	0.0	14.4	6.9	NA	NA	57
Organ meats								
chicken liver	3.5 oz.	157	0.9	5.5	1.8	0.9	631	51
beef liver	3.5 oz.	161	3.4	4.9	1.9	1.1	389	70
beef tongue	3.5 oz.	283	0.3	20.7	8.9	0.8	107	60

Nutritional Values of Selected Foods

Food item	Amount	Calories	Carbohydrates (g)	Total fat (g)	Saturated fat (g)	Unsaturated fat (g)	Cholesterol (mg)	Sodium (mg)
			Meat and Poultry (*cont.*)					
Luncheon meats								
bologna								
beef	1 slice	72	0.2	6.6	2.8	0.3	13	226
turkey	1 slice	60	0.6	4.5	1.4	1.1	20	222
chicken roll	2 slices	90	1.4	4.2	1.2	0.9	28	331
corned beef	1 oz.	43	0.0	1.7	0.7	0.1	13	270
frankfurters								
beef	1 frank	180	1.0	16.3	6.9	0.8	35	585
beef and pork	1 frank	144	1.2	13.1	4.8	1.2	22	504
chicken	1 frank	116	3.1	8.8	2.5	1.8	45	617
turkey	1 frank	100	0.6	8.1	2.7	2.1	39	472
ham								
lean (5% fat)	1 slice	37	0.3	1.4	0.5	0.1	13	405
regular (11% fat)	1 slice	52	0.9	3.0	1.0	0.3	13	373
pastrami	1 oz.	99	0.9	8.3	3.0	0.3	26	348
turkey breast	1 slice	23	0.0	0.3	0.1	0.1	9	301
			Fish and Shellfish					
Fish (baked)								
bass	4 oz.	287	3.0	19.4	NA	NA	NA	68
cod	3 oz.	89	0.0	0.7	0.1	0.2	47	66
fish filets (frozen, batter-dipped)	3 oz.	180	15.0	10.0	NA	NA	NA	230
flounder	3.5 oz.	202	0.0	8.2	NA	NA	NA	237
grouper	3 oz.	100	0.0	1.1	0.3	0.3	40	45
haddock	3 oz.	95	0.0	0.8	0.1	0.3	63	74
halibut	3 oz.	119	0.0	2.5	0.4	0.8	35	59
mackerel	3 oz.	223	0.0	15.1	3.6	3.7	64	71
ocean perch	3 oz.	103	0.0	1.8	0.3	0.5	46	82
salmon, pink (canned)	3 oz.	118	0.0	5.1	1.3	1.7	NA	471
sardines in oil	2	50	0.0	2.8	0.4	1.2	34	121
snapper	3 oz.	109	0.0	1.5	0.3	0.5	40	48
sole, filet	1	80	0.6	0.8	NA	NA	NA	162
trout	3 oz.	129	0.0	3.7	0.7	1.3	62	29
tuna fish								
in oil	3 oz.	169	0.0	7.0	1.3	2.5	15	301
water-packed	3 oz.	111	0.0	0.4	0.1	0.1	15	303

Nutritional Values of Selected Foods

Food item	Amount	Calories	Carbohydrates (g)	Total fat (g)	Saturated fat (g)	Unsaturated fat (g)	Cholesterol (mg)	Sodium (mg)
			Fish and Shellfish (*cont.*)					
Shellfish								
clams	3 oz.	126	4.4	1.7	0.2	0.5	57	95
crab	3 oz.	87	0.0	1.5	NA	NA	NA	237
crab cakes	1 cake	93	0.3	4.5	0.9	1.4	90	198
lobster	3 oz.	83	1.1	0.5	0.1	0.1	61	323
mussels	3 oz.	147	6.3	3.8	0.7	1.0	48	313
oysters	3 oz.	117	6.7	4.2	1.1	1.3	96	190
scallops, fried	2 large	67	3.1	3.4	0.8	0.9	19	144
shrimp								
steamed	3 oz.	84	0.0	0.9	0.2	0.4	166	190
fried	3 oz.	206	9.8	10.4	1.8	4.3	150	292
			Fruits and Vegetables					
Fruits								
apples	1 medium	81	21.1	0.1	0.1	0.1	0	1
apricots	3 medium	51	11.8	0.4	0.0	0.1	0	1
bananas	1 medium	105	26.7	0.6	0.2	0.1	0	1
blueberries	1 cup	82	20.5	0.6	NA	NA	0	9
cantaloupe	1 cup	57	13.4	0.4	NA	NA	0	14
cherries	10 medium	49	11.3	0.7	0.1	0.2	0	0
dates (dried)	10	228	61.0	0.4	NA	NA	0	2
fruit cocktail								
in syrup	½ cup	93	24.2	0.1	0.0	0.0	0	7
in juice	½ cup	56	14.7	0.0	0.0	0.0	0	4
grapefruit								
pink	½ medium	37	9.5	0.1	0.0	0.0	0	0
white	½ medium	39	9.9	0.1	0.0	0.0	0	0
grapes	1 cup	58	15.8	0.3	0.1	0.1	0	2
oranges	1 medium	59	14.4	0.4	0.0	0.1	0	0
peaches								
raw	1 medium	37	9.7	0.1	0.0	0.0	0	0
canned, in syrup	1 cup	190	51.0	0.3	0.0	0.1	0	16
canned, in juice	1 cup	109	28.7	0.1	0.0	0.0	0	11
pears								
raw	1 medium	98	25.1	0.7	0.0	0.2	0	1
canned, in syrup	1 cup	188	48.9	0.3	0.0	0.1	0	13
canned, in juice	1 cup	123	32.1	0.2	0.0	0.0	0	10
pineapple								
raw	1 cup	77	19.2	0.7	0.0	0.2	0	1

Nutritional Values of Selected Foods

Food item	Amount	Calories	Carbohydrates (g)	Total fat (g)	Saturated fat (g)	Unsaturated fat (g)	Cholesterol (mg)	Sodium (mg)
Fruits and Vegetables *(cont.)*								
pineapple *(cont.)*								
canned, in syrup	1 cup	199	51.5	0.3	0.0	0.1	0	3
canned, in juice	1 cup	150	39.2	0.2	0.0	0.1	0	4
plums	1 medium	36	8.6	0.4	0.0	0.1	0	0
prunes								
canned, in syrup	5	90	23.9	0.2	0.0	0.0	0	2
dried	5	100	26.3	0.2	0.0	0.0	0	1
raisins	⅔ cup	300	79.1	0.5	0.2	0.1	0	12
strawberries								
raw	1 cup	45	10.5	0.6	0.0	0.3	0	2
frozen,								
sweetened	1 cup	245	66.1	0.3	0.0	0.2	0	8
frozen,								
unsweetened	1 cup	52	13.6	0.2	0.0	0.1	0	3
watermelon	1 cup	50	11.5	0.7	NA	NA	0	33
Vegetables								
asparagus								
fresh, boiled	½ cup	22	4.0	0.3	0.1	0.1	0	4
canned	½ cup	24	3.0	0.8	0.2	0.3	0	NA
avocado, raw								
California	1 medium	306	12.0	30.0	4.5	3.5	0	21
Florida	1 medium	339	27.1	27.0	5.3	4.5	0	14
baked beans								
vegetarian	1 cup	235	52.1	1.1	0.3	0.5	0	1008
w/pork	1 cup	247	49.1	2.6	1.0	0.3	17	1113
beets								
fresh, boiled	½ cup	26	5.7	0.0	0.0	0.0	0	42
canned	½ cup	27	6.1	0.1	0.0	0.0	0	NA
pickled	½ cup	75	18.6	0.1	0.0	0.0	0	301
broccoli								
raw, chopped	½ cup	12	2.3	0.2	0.0	0.1	0	12
boiled	½ cup	23	4.3	0.2	0.0	0.1	0	8
frozen	½ cup	25	4.9	0.1	0.0	0.1	0	22
brussels sprouts								
fresh, boiled	½ cup	30	6.8	0.4	0.1	0.2	0	17
frozen	½ cup	33	6.5	0.3	0.1	0.2	0	18
cabbage								
green	½ cup	8	1.9	0.1	0.0	0.0	0	6
red	½ cup	10	2.1	0.1	0.0	0.0	0	4
coleslaw	½ cup	42	7.5	1.6	0.2	0.8	5	14

Nutritional Values of Selected Foods

Food item	Amount	Calories	Carbohydrates (g)	Total fat (g)	Saturated fat (g)	Unsaturated fat (g)	Cholesterol (mg)	Sodium (mg)
Fruits and Vegetables (*cont.*)								
carrots								
raw	1 medium	31	7.3	0.1	0.0	0.1	0	25
canned	½ cup	17	4.0	0.1	0.0	0.1	0	176
frozen	½ cup	26	6.0	0.1	0.0	0.0	0	43
cauliflower								
raw	½ cup	12	2.5	0.1	0.0	0.0	0	7
boiled	½ cup	15	2.9	0.1	0.0	0.1	0	4
frozen	½ cup	17	3.4	0.2	0.0	0.1	0	16
celery	1 stalk	6	1.5	0.1	0.0	0.0	0	35
chick-peas								
boiled	1 cup	269	45.0	4.3	0.4	1.9	0	11
canned	1 cup	285	54.3	2.7	0.3	1.2	0	413
corn								
fresh, boiled	½ cup	89	20.6	1.1	0.2	0.5	0	14
canned	½ cup	66	15.2	0.8	0.1	0.4	0	NA
cream style	½ cup	93	23.2	0.5	0.1	0.3	0	365
frozen	½ cup	67	16.8	0.1	0.0	0.0	0	4
cucumber, raw	½ cup	7	1.5	0.1	0.0	0.0	0	2
green beans								
fresh, boiled	½ cup	22	4.9	0.2	0.0	0.1	0	2
canned	½ cup	13	3.1	0.1	0.0	0.0	0	170
frozen	½ cup	18	4.2	0.1	0.0	0.0	0	9
kidney beans								
boiled	1 cup	225	40.4	0.9	0.1	0.5	0	4
canned	1 cup	208	38.1	0.8	0.1	0.4	0	889
lentils, boiled	1 cup	231	39.9	0.7	0.1	0.3	0	4
lettuce								
romaine	½ cup	4	0.7	0.1	0.0	0.0	0	2
iceberg	½ cup	3	0.4	0.0	0.0	0.0	0	2
lima beans								
fresh, boiled	1 cup	217	39.3	0.7	0.2	0.3	0	4
canned	1 cup	191	35.9	0.4	0.1	0.2	0	809
mixed vegetables								
canned	½ cup	39	7.6	0.2	0.0	0.1	0	122
frozen	½ cup	54	11.9	0.1	0.0	0.1	0	32

* Excerpts from Jean A. T. Pennington and Helen Nichols Church, *Food Values of Portions Commonly Used*, 14th ed. (New York: HarperCollins, 1980, 1985). Copyright © Jean A. T. Pennington, Ph.D., and Helen Nichols Church, B.S. Reprinted by permission of HarperCollins Publishers.

Index

Progesterone (*cont.*)
   hormone therapy with, 438,
      459–460, 462, 464
   hot flashes and, 243
   menstrual cycle and, 9
   PMS treatment and, 217, 229
   pre- and postmenopausal levels of,
      10–11
   weight and, 289
   See also Hormones; Progestogen
Progestogen
   benefits vs. risks of, 442–443
   bone density and, 357
   cardiovascular disease and, 324–325
   challenge, 41
   endometrial cancer and, 392, 395
   headaches and, 249
   hormone therapy with, 459–460,
      462, 464
   hot flashes and, 243, 245
   injections (Depo Provera), 193, 442
   See also Hormones; Progesterone
Progestogen-only birth control pills,
   191
Progestsert IUD, 460
Prolactin, PMS and, 217, 219. *See also*
   Hormones
Prolapsed organs, 335–336, 409
   checkup for, 40–41
   hysterectomy for, 259–261
   treatment for, 266–267
Proliferative phase, menstrual cycle, 9
Prostacyclin, 320
Prostaglandin inhibitors, 230, 236
Prostaglandins
   menstrual migraines and, 235
   PMS and, 219
   See also Hormones
Prostate surgery, 275
Protein, 71–73, 76
Protein-sparing modified fast (PSMF),
   294–295
Proto-oncogenes, 369
Psychological disorders, PMS and, 219,
   224. *See also* Emotional
   health
Psychotropic drugs, 230
Psychotherapy
   finding a counselor for, 137
   stress reduction and, 133
   See also Emotional health; Stress
Psyllium seed (Metamucil), 315, 319
Pulse, taking your, 109
Push-ups, 111
Pyridinoline (PYR), 350

Pyridium, 409–410
Pyridoxine, 84

Quantitative computerized tomography
   (CT scan), 348–349
Quinestrol, 453

Radiation therapy, 387
Radical hysterectomy, 257
Radiographic densitometry, 37, 347
Radon, cancer and, 372
Recommended dietary allowances
   (RDAs), 485
Reconstructive surgery, 381, 387–389
Rectum
   cancer of, 389–391
   checkup of, 41
   prolapse of, 266
Red blood cell count, stroke and,
   333–334
Relaxation response, 132–133. *See
   also* Stress
Replens, 251
Reproductive system, 7–8
   postmenopausal checkup of, 39–41
   See also Contraception; Fertility and
      pregnancy; Hysterectomy and
      surgical menopause;
      Menopause facts; Menstrual
      problems; Sexuality
Resolve, 215
Resources and support
   alcohol, tobacco, and drugs,
      154–155
   cancer, 405–406
   cardiovascular disease, 337
   cosmetic concerns, 177
   diet, 95
   exercise, 125
   hysterectomy, 268
   menopause and aging, 17
   menopause facts, 255
   osteoporosis, 367
   stress management, 138
   urinary tract problems, 433
   weight control, 300
Resting heart rate, measuring, 109
Retin-A, 160
Rheumatoid arthritis, 84
Riggs, Dr. Lawrence, 363
Roller-ball electrocoagulation, 235,
   267
Rosenman, Dr. Ray H., 330
RU-486, 198
Rubinow, Dr. David, 217